Multiple Sclerosis

CURRENT CLINICAL NEUROLOGY

Daniel Tarsy, MD, SERIES EDITOR

Multiple Sclerosis

*Etiology, Diagnosis,
and New Treatment Strategies*

Edited by

Michael J. Olek, DO

*Department of Neurology, Multiple Sclerosis Center,
University of California, Irvine, CA*

Foreword by

Howard L. Weiner, MD

*Department of Neurology, Multiple Sclerosis Center,
Brigham and Women's Hospital
and Massachusetts General Hospital,
Harvard Medical School, Boston, CA*

HUMANA PRESS ✳ TOTOWA, NEW JERSEY

Due diligence has been taken by the publishers, editors, and authors of this book to assure the accuracy of the information published and to describe generally accepted practices. The contributors herein have carefully checked to ensure that the drug selections and dosages set forth in this text are accurate and in accord with the standards accepted at the time of publication. Notwithstanding, as new research, changes in government regulations, and knowledge from clinical experience relating to drug therapy and drug reactions constantly occurs, the reader is advised to check the product information provided by the manufacturer of each drug for any change in dosages or for additional warnings and contraindications. This is of utmost importance when the recommended drug herein is a new or infrequently used drug. It is the responsibility of the treating physician to determine dosages and treatment strategies for individual patients. Further it is the responsibility of the health care provider to ascertain the Food and Drug Administration status of each drug or device used in their clinical practice. The publisher, editors, and authors are not responsible for errors or omissions or for any consequences from the application of the information presented in this book and make no warranty, express or implied, with respect to the contents in this publication.

This publication is printed on acid-free paper. ∞
ANSI Z39.48-1984 (American Standards Institute) Permanence of Paper for Printed Library Materials.

Cover illustration: Human Multiple Sclerosis Brain Section (1000X magnification)B-Cells infiltrating through a small blood vessel into a multiple sclerosis lesion [Immunocytochemical Staining]

Cover design by Patricia F. Cleary.

Production Editor: Wendy S. Kopf.

For additional copies, pricing for bulk purchases, and/or information about other Humana titles, contact Humana at the above address or at any of the following numbers: Tel.: 973-256-1699; Fax: 973-256-8314; E-mail: humana@humanapr.com, or visit our Website: http://humanapress.com

Photocopy Authorization Policy:

Authorization to photocopy items for internal or personal use, or the internal or personal use of specific clients, is granted by Humana Press Inc., provided that the base fee of US $25.00 per copy is paid directly to the Copyright Clearance Center at 222 Rosewood Drive, Danvers, MA 01923. For those organizations that have been granted a photocopy license from the CCC, a separate system of payment has been arranged and is acceptable to Humana Press Inc. The fee code for users of the Transactional Reporting Service is: [1-58829-033-6/05 $25.00].

Printed in the United States of America. 10 9 8 7 6 5 4 3 2 1
e-ISBN: 1-59259-855-2
Library of Congress Cataloging in Publication Data

Multiple sclerosis : etiology, diagnosis, and new treatment strategies /
edited by Michael J. Olek.
        p. ; cm. -- (Current clinical neurology)
  Includes bibliographical references and index.
  ISBN 1-58829-033-6 (alk. paper)
  1. Multiple sclerosis.
  [DNLM: 1. Multiple Sclerosis--therapy. 2. Multiple Sclerosis--diagnosis.
3. Multiple Sclerosis--etiology. WL 360 M95639 2005] I. Olek, Michael J.
II. Series.
  RC377.M8475 2005
  616.8'34--dc22

                                                                    2004020727

Dedication

To my parents, Loretta and Francis, whose selfless love and paramount guidance have conferred upon me a life graced with wisdom, respect, and compassion.

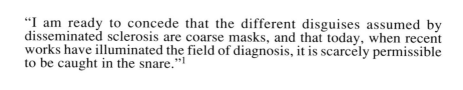

"I am ready to concede that the different disguises assumed by disseminated sclerosis are coarse masks, and that today, when recent works have illuminated the field of diagnosis, it is scarcely permissible to be caught in the snare."[1]

[1]Lectures on the Diseases of the Nervous System Delivered at La Salpetriere, JM Charcot, translated by George Sigerson, London: The New Sydenhan Society, MDCCCLXXVII, Volume LXXII, p. 185.

Series Editor's Introduction

The diagnosis and treatment of multiple sclerosis (MS) used to be very simple. Diagnosis was based on the presence of multiple lesions scattered in space and time with some support from lumbar puncture. Specific treatments were nonexistent. Corticosteroids were the only available treatment and, in desperation, were sometimes even administered intrathecally without much evidence for efficacy. The belief that multiple sclerosis is caused by a combination of host genetic susceptibility and environmental triggers is a very old one but remains the leading hypothesis. The explosion of new information concerning pathology, pathophysiology, clinical classification, imaging, and treatment during the past decade or so is truly impressive and is beginning to provide hope that this disease will come under better control in the near future. Yet, at the present time, we still remain at a waystation in its understanding and management. We may understand the enemy a little bit better, but are still very limited in our therapeutic options.

Multiple Sclerosis: Etiology, Diagnosis, and New Treatment Strategies provides a comprehensive and state of the art overview of MS. The chapters emphasize current criteria for diagnosis and subtype classification and incorporate the rapidly developing body of pathologic information, much of which can now be accessed during life with a dazzling array of new and emerging magnetic resonance imaging (MRI) techniques. As discussed by several of the authors in this volume, clinical and MRI criteria have become intertwined in the very influential McDonald criteria, which allow for earlier diagnosis. This appears to be extremely important since emerging data suggest that early treatment with disease-modifying drugs during the more acute inflammatory phase may impact progression of the disease. Despite modest gains in the treatment of early and relapsing MS, chronic progressive MS remains a major therapeutic challenge. The discovery of axonal pathology, imaging techniques able to identify and quantify brain atrophy, and greater awareness of the cumulative effects of MS on cognitive function receive much deserved attention in this volume.

Before these new developments, it was recognized that the identifiable clinical manifestations of MS were only the tip of the iceberg. One has to feel that the discoveries made in the past decade also represent only the tip of the iceberg. As described by Drs. Dangond and Olek in the last two chapters of this book, we are at the threshold of new discoveries and knowledge which should finally control this common and dreaded disease.

Daniel Tarsy, MD
Beth Israel Deaconess Medical Center
Harvard Medical School
Boston, MA

Foreword

The understanding of pathology and treatment in multiple sclerosis (MS) has progressed exponentially since the 1990s as a result of increased basic and clinical research. To date, five medications are now approved by the Food and Drug Administration and available for use in patients with MS. In addition to the elucidation of the basic mechanisms involved in the pathogenesis of the immune system, the approval of these medications can be attributed to the diligence of the pharmaceutical companies.

The advent and evolution of magnetic resonance imaging (MRI) has revolutionized the diagnosis and treatment of MS. Not only has image quality improved with the advent of higher Tesla magnets and fast fluid-attenuated inversion recovery techniques, but expanded areas of utilization such as three- and four-dimensional techniques, magnetic resonance spectroscopy, functional MRI, atrophy measures, and magnetization transfer ratio imaging have also arisen. Formal guidelines for the use of MRI in MS have been recently published and incorporated into clinical trials. In addition, MRI is now included in the current McDonald criteria, which allows for earlier diagnosis of MS which will result in earlier treatment, ultimately benefiting patient care.

New treatment strategies are being developed based on a detailed understanding of the immune process as well as pathological findings showing specific patterns of disease in terms of myelin destruction and axonal loss. The current knowledge of the immune system is presented in terms of the relevance to clinical application. From broad immunosuppression to specific antibody therapies, we have been able to broaden our clinical trial capability and consider combination therapy based on the mechanisms of actions of various medications on the immune system. In addition, new therapies on the horizon, such as bone marrow transplant and myelin repair, are presented.

Also included are state-of-the-art presentations on neuropsychological aspects and pregnancy-related issues facing patients with MS. Inclusion of these issues in designing clinical trials is crucial in the development of treatments that will cover all aspects of this long-term degenerating neurological disease.

Multiple Sclerosis: Etiology, Diagnosis, and New Treatment Strategies addresses all the current immunological, imaging techniques, neuropsychological, and pregnancy issues and shows their relationship to the development of new and improved therapies to combat this devastating neurological disorder.

Howard L. Weiner, MD
Multiple Sclerosis Center
Department of Neurology
Brigham and Women's Hospital
and Massachusetts General Hospital
Harvard Medical School
Boston, MA

Preface

Multiple Sclerosis: Etiology, Diagnosis, and New Treatment Strategies synthesizes current concepts about the evaluation, treatment, and future directions in multiple sclerosis (MS). In addition to discussing the current medications for treating relapsing-remitting MS (Avonex, Betaseron, Copaxone), this book focuses on recently approved medications (Novantrone and Rebif), new indications for medications (CHAMPS Trial), and medications in development (Oral Interferon Tau, Oral Copaxone, Oral Cellcept). Immunosuppressive therapy for progressive disease as well as symptomatic therapy is also discussed.

The evaluation of MS has been greatly enhanced by magnetic resonance imaging (MRI) and newer imaging techniques, such as magnetic resonance spectroscopy, functional MRI, and three-dimensional MRI, which was pioneered at Harvard University. These modalities have also aided in clinical trials leading to the first Food and Drug Administration approved medication to treat MS. The role of MRI is reviewed in Chapter 3.

The role of immunological research in MS is paramount. Special attention is given to the immunological mechanisms involved in the autoimmune process and in developing treatment strategies based on these concepts. We present the current thinking and latest discoveries in immunology as it relates to MS. Groundbreaking B-cell research has been pioneered at the University of California, Irvine. The basic understanding of the autoimmune mechanism and its application to specific immunotherapies is explored in Chapters 5 and 6. Immune markers are crucial for understanding and following the disease and are covered in detail.

Multiple Sclerosis: Etiology, Diagnosis, and New Treatment Strategies provides insight into the future of MS treatment. The mechanism and application of myelin repair is presented in detail in Chapter 11. Future therapies such as bone marrow transplant, combination therapy, and specific immunomodulatory treatment are discussed in Chapter 12. These therapies are based largely on basic immunologic research.

This book should prove valuable to general neurologists and primary care physicians who treat many patients with MS. We hope they find it useful.

Michael J. Olek, DO
Multiple Sclerosis Center
Department of Neurology
University of California
Irvine, CA

xi

Contents

Contributors

ROHIT BAKSHI, MD • Center for Neurological Imaging, Partners Multiple Sclerosis Center; Departments of Neurology and Radiology, Brigham and Women's Hospital, Harvard Medical School, Boston, MA

CHRISTINA CAON, MSN, RN • Multiple Sclerosis Center, Wayne State University School of Medicine, Department of Neurology, Detroit, MI

DARCY COX, PsyD • Department of Neurology, University of California, San Francisco, CA

FERNANDO DANGOND, MD • Department of Neurology, Brigham and Women's Hospital and Harvard Medical School, Boston, MA

MICHAEL DEMETRIOU, MD, PhD • Department of Microbiology and Molecular Genetics, School of Medicine, University of California, Irvine, CA

PIERRE DUQUETTE, MD • Department of Neurology, Hospital Notré-Dame, University of Montreal, Montreal, Quebéc, Canada

LAURA JULIAN, PhD • Department of Medicine, University of California, San Francisco, CA

OMAR A. KHAN, MD • Department of Neurology, Wayne State University School of Medicine, Detroit, MI

MICHAEL J. OLEK, DO • Multiple Sclerosis Center, Department of Neurology, University of California, Irvine, CA

YUFEN QIN, MD • Department of Neurology, University of California, Irvine, CA

DEREK R. SMITH, MD • Multiple Sclerosis Center, Beth Israel-Deaconess Medical Center and Harvard Medical School, Department of Neurology, Boston, MA

DANIEL TARSY, MD • Department of Neurology, Beth Israel-Deaconess Medical Center and Harvard Medical School, Boston, MA

ALEX C. TSELIS, MD, PhD • Department of Neurology, Wayne State University School of Medicine, Detroit, MI

STANLEY VAN DEN NOORT, MD • Department of Neurology, University of California, Irvine, CA

NORMAN WANG, MD • Department of Neurology, University of California, Irvine, CA

HOWARD L. WEINER, MD • Multiple Sclerosis Center, Department of Neurology, Brigham and Women's Hospital and Massachusetts General Hospital, Harvard Medical School, Boston, MA

ROBERT ZIVADINOV, MD, PhD • Buffalo Neuroimaging Analysis Center, The Jacobs Neurological Institute and Baird MS Research Center, Department of Neurology, University at Buffalo, State University of New York, Buffalo, NY

Signs and Symptoms of Multiple Sclerosis

Stanley van den Noort, MD

INTRODUCTION

The signs and symptoms of multiple sclerosis (MS) range from those that command the immediate attention of patient and doctor to those that escape the attention of patient and family over the course a lifetime. For nearly a century, we have discovered some examples of MS found at autopsy that were never recognized by the family. In the modern era, we find examples of MS on magnetic resonance imaging (MRI) scans done for other reasons, such as a motor vehicle accident.

The author believes that the best classification of the symptoms begins with those that involve the mind, sensation, and movement, those that result from brainstem lesions and involve autonomic dysfunction.

HIGHER CORTICAL SYMPTOMS

We are increasingly cognizant that axonal destruction, as well as demyelination, proceeds together even early in the disease process *(1)*. The responsible lesions that affect the mind are usually subcortical and pericallosal. Individually, these lesions are almost always asymptomatic. Over time, they may collectively degrade the highest intellectual functions, with special deficits in the ability to make complex decisions using multiple variables and to remember complex networks that tie together information. The personality may change subtly. Lesions that separate and disrupt the integration of neural systems can reproduce almost any psychiatric disorder. Depression, anxiety, paranoia, obsessions, loss of inhibition, and variants of neurosis may be encountered *(2)*. The author has seen frank psychosis consistent with schizophrenia.

In the last year, the author saw a young woman for whom the first symptom of MS was visual hallucinations and a dream in which she saw herself get up, go downstairs, and kill her husband. This same dream would recur with visual effects of great clarity in full color, and the sequence and details were always the same. She also saw large animals in great detail and in full color. It is probable that these

From: *Current Clinical Neurology: Multiple Sclerosis*
Edited by: M. J. Olek © Humana Press Inc., Totowa, NJ

were examples of peduncular hallucinations caused by lesions in the posterior hypothalamus. Vivid visual hallucinations are almost always organic. Separating these phenomena from psychiatric disorders is often difficult. When they are acute, one can sometimes surmise that the sudden change in personality or behavior is so out of context that an organic process can be suspected. However, when these symptoms are subtle, it is usual to find a psychiatric illness that can delay the diagnosis of MS for years or even decades *(3,4)*.

A disproportionate percentage of patients with MS have migraine headaches. This can involve visual phenomena, hemiparesis, transient alterations of sensation and speech, and even transient global amnesia. These can complicate the diagnostic process. The author once treated a medical student who experienced a classic migraine in the physiology laboratory and then developed persistent ataxia, which was the first manifestation of his MS. Between attacks, migraineurs are photophobic, sonophobic, and unable to tolerate smells.

If one asks the average patient with MS to list his or her major problems, the patient usually lists fatigue *(5)*, impaired sleep, and impaired memory as highly significant. If one asks the average middle-aged or young adult what bothers him or her the most, it is common for this same list to be identified. This is particularly true in American lifestyles, which are often more frantic and complex than those in other societies and cultures *(6)*. The number of things that I am required to remember in the eighth decade of my life is far greater than that required of the average individual a century ago. Often these things are not really important, and if we are slightly depressed or distracted, these failures of recall are misinterpreted as signs of decreased brain function. The separation of these relatively normal or average symptoms from those that trouble the patient with MS is often difficult to achieve. Neuropsychological testing in good hands can be extremely helpful *(7)*. It is also expensive and can be misleading. The author has had several instances of patients with MS who had been extremely successful in their careers and were recognized by others or by themselves as not functioning at that same level of performance. In some cases, neuropsychological testing may be approximately normal, when, in fact, the intellect has declined from a high level to a more average level *(8)*.

In summary, some slowing of performance, some impairment of memory, and some degradation of ability to handle a checkbook or other average task are commonly encountered in MS. When recognized by the patient, this creates anxiety. When recognized by a spouse, it often becomes a rift in a marriage, and divorce is common. When recognized by an employer, it often results in dismissal, with drastic consequences for the patient. It is not rare for a person who has been regarded as depressed and ineffective for several decades to finally be diagnosed with MS. A majority of patients with MS are able to manage their work, their families, and their responsibilities without impairment for the duration of their lifespan, which is no different than that of the average person.

Other cortical disturbances, such as stuttering, may be seen. Aphasia is rare in MS. Distortions of sensation of cortical or subcortical nature on one side of the body are not uncommon. Often, these result in a slight increase in threshold for pain accompanied by an excessive response to painful stimuli above the threshold for pain. The normal individual has mechanisms to suppress perception of a shoe, a piece of clothing, or some minor disturbance of sensation that could be uncomfortable. Loss of suppressor systems leads to preoccupation with a modest discomfort in a hand or shoulder. This obsession, in turn, may result in surgical procedures, which are not usually helpful. Psychoses may occur and cause various higher cortical symptoms, but they are rare in MS.

In speech, the inability to find a word or to occasionally say a wrong word is endemic in normal individuals in our society and usually does not indicate a disease process. Rarely, patients with MS may have seizures of a focal or general nature. There is a slightly higher percentage of epilepsy in patients with MS than in the general population. There is a recent report of compulsive scratching of a body part or similar compulsions in patients with left frontal atrophy. The author had a patient with MS who was bright and was an executive. He had become obsessed with a minor lesion on his chin, which he compulsively scratches, producing an ulcer *(9)*. He had not responded to high doses of a serotonin reuptake inhibitor. It was necessary to restrict his hands at night with gloves and to bandage the area to prevent scratching. He had not previously shown features of obsessive-compulsive disorder.

There are new computerized techniques for psychometric assessment that may be used in an MS clinic setting, and these will accelerate the diagnostic process. In complex circumstances, particularly those that involve divorce settlements, changes in employment status, and the assessment of intellect in professionals, the old approach of neuropsychological testing by an individual who is familiar with the types of deficits found in patients who have MS is helpful.

The separation of symptoms resulting from MS from those symptoms related to emotional responses and psychiatric pathology in the average person without MS is frequently difficult if not impossible. A neurologist who is trained and experienced in psychiatric problems is probably best equipped to cope with these issues. Having a psychologist and a consulting psychiatrist as part of an MS clinic is highly desirable but almost never affordable. A social worker who can examine the effects of the illness on the patient's human environment and recommend practical steps to solve problems is of great value.

The current American economy and its structure are unkind to many of these patients who are quickly fired for nonperformance or inadequate performance after many years of service without adequate analysis *(10)*. The no-fault divorce procedures can produce similar unfair solutions.

SENSORY SYMPTOMS

Distortions of sensation on one side of the body are common in MS and can lead to many diagnostic errors and therapeutic misadventures. Nearly 15% or more of patients diagnosed with MS have had inappropriate surgery for their MS symptoms in the decade before diagnosis. Perhaps most common among these is podiatric surgery on toes and feet. The hand with presumed carpal tunnel syndrome or a presumed tardy ulnar palsy is another common site. Surgery on the cervical or lumbar discs mistakenly believed to cause the patient's symptoms is common. Dental procedures to deal with facial discomforts are also seen.

In disorders of sensation involving the opposite side from head to toe arise from demyelinating lesions in the cerebral hemisphere, thalamus, and adjacent areas. In other instances, the impaired sensation only involves the arm, leg, and trunk on one side. In some patients, for reasons unknown, one can have impaired perception of pin on the entire side of the body, except for the area of the scalp innervated by C2–3, which is spared. These sensation impairments often lead to distortions of normal sensation or phantom sensations, which present diagnostic challenges. The author has had patients who, when touched on the toe with a pin, will complain of a sharp pain in the shoulder on the ipsilateral side. Dysesthesias, crawling sensations, and electrical shocks are often reported by the patient. In some instances, there is a replica of a thalamic syndrome on the ipsilateral or contralateral side. It is likely that this occurs with lesions well below the thalamus.

One of the most common distortions of sensation involves proprioception. This is often more severe in the hand than in the foot, presumably because of cervical cord lesions in the dorsal root entry zone. This finding is more common in MS than in any other illness. Some patients will present with a hand that has no position sense (the useless hand of Oppenheim). With this severe deficit, motor performance is impaired as well and probably results from the inability to organize a movement in the absence of appropriate sensation. The most common example of this occurs when one goes to the dentist and receives local anesthesia that numbs the tongue and lip on one side. No motor nerves have been blocked, but for 1 or 2 hours after this procedure, one is often modestly dysarthric. Movement requires some degree of sensation to proceed normally. Patients with lesions in the dorsal columns of the spinal cord usually have proprioceptive defects on both sides. This results in the inability to stand with eyes closed (Romberg's sign) and is often associated with band-like constricting sensations about a limb or the trunk. These patients often complain of inability to take a deep breath, and truncal discomforts leading to the diagnostic pursuit of problems in the various organs commonly results in therapeutic misadventures. A central cord syndrome in which pain perception is lost while touch is preserved is rare in MS but can occur. Focal itching is common and can be a distressing symptom. Meralgia paresthetica is common and may be related to a normally subclinical meralgia paresthetica exaggerated by inability to self-regulate. Neuralgic pains of a sudden lancinating unpleasant character are usually seen in a trigeminal distribution. However, glossopharyngeal neuralgia may also be seen in MS. Shooting pains in other parts of the body are also seen. The author has several patients who have paroxysmal or steady otalgia on one side, which can be quite distressing for them. Disturbances of sensation in the tongue, cheek, and pharynx are rare. Classic trigeminal neuralgia is quite common in MS and is the most common cause of trigeminal neuralgia in patients younger than 50 years. It is often triggered by talking, chewing, tooth brushing, or touching the face as in classic tic douloureux.

Babinski described electrical sensations from head to toe on neck flexion in soldiers with gunshot wounds of the neck. Lhermitte described this phenomenon as common in patients with MS. It still may be seen in neck injuries and cervical cord damage from other causes. These paroxysms are severe and distracting. Partial sensations of a more restricted range are also seen.

Transverse myelitis on one side often causes a loss of sensation, which involves precisely half of the perineum. It may also cause loss of sensation involving both sides of the perineum. MS is a common cause of numbness of the perineum. Bilateral loss of sensation in the perineum resulting from MS is the one sensory symptom that the author treats with high-dose IV Solu-Medrol for 4 days.

Although MS is believed to be a painless disorder, neuropathic pain of great severity, which is the most difficult to manage, is common. This often represents a form of phantom pain that responds poorly to analgesics and most other measures.

Sensation is often difficult to examine and requires repeated examinations over short intervals of time. Hysteria and malingering can produce diagnostic dilemmas. It is common for patients with neurological diseases, including MS, to present impairments of sensation, which appear to be hysterical. This often represents an attempt to convince the examiner of the severity of the problem and that there is some loss of sensation. This is also often seen in the eye. Many patients will describe monocular diplopia and multiple images, leading to a hysterical diagnosis when, in fact, they are describing competing images that are often overlapping and may be compounded by astigmatism. There is no rule that patients with MS cannot have hysterical personalities.

Sensory examinations are usually best done for only a short time and, if necessary, repeated at a later time. The author once had a visual field examination at the end of a busy day and produced a chaotic visual field finding, which caused great concern. A repeat examination after a sound night's sleep produced a normal visual field. In testing cutaneous sensation, the author prefers to use a sharp corsage pin (safety pins are too dull and needles are too sharp). The pinwheels produce accommodation and may be misleading. The author also uses a 128 tuning fork to test vibratory sensation. For position sense, it is best to grasp the finger or toe by the sides and use an up-and-down technique while the patient closes his or her eyes. It often takes some time for patients to learn, assess, and report the direction of movement as opposed to whether the final position of the digit is up or down. The author also likes to test sensation of movement in the second toe, which is much more difficult for patients and much more sensitive, as a test of proprioception. The Romberg sign is also of great value and should be done with the feet bare and close together. With eyes open, the normal individual, and most patients with MS, can sustain that posture without a problem. However, when the eyes are closed, they may fall in almost any direction. If that direction is always in the arms of the examiner, it may raise other questions. The author likes to watch the tendons on the dorsum of the foot and the dance of those tendons when the eyes are closed. This was part of the description of the sign by Dr. Romberg.

MOTOR SYMPTOMS

The motor problems in MS are, again, various and complicated. The most common motor manifestation is a paraparesis or quadriparesis primarily resulting from cord lesions. This often begins with a slowing of gait, a tendency for one of the legs to give way, and, when coupled with spasticity, may produce calf discomfort after walking some distance, closely resembling claudication. If the anterior tibial muscles are weak, tripping will be the predominant presentation. When spasticity is present, extensor spasms and spontaneous ankle clonus are often present. With a severe paraparesis, there may be flexor spasms that represent a form of the triple flexion response. These are triggered by discomfort of the skin, a full bladder, or a full rectum. These cause the legs to pull up with contraction of the psoas and hamstring muscles. In early mild cases, these signs are frequently difficult to elicit, but the symptom should be taken seriously. Based on the author's experience, flexor spasms are best controlled with pramipexole, a nonergot dopamine agonist.

The extensor plantar response first described by Babinski is part of a triple flexion response, with dorsiflexion of the great toe after noxious stimulation of the lateral aspect of the sole. It is said that it was Babinski's nurse who told him that when she took off patients' shoes, their great toes went up. The author can often avoid the necessity of testing for this sign by watching the shoes being removed.

The extensor spasms of the legs are often most prominent on awakening. In the hand and foot there is a slowness of repetitive movements. In the upper limbs it is important to try and establish the motor level of the lesion by sequentially testing the strength of the arm muscles. If the lesion is above C5, one may see impairment of the shoulder shrug on that side. Tendon reflexes may be reduced or exaggerated, depending on the level of the lesion and the integrity of the tendon reflex arc. It is often found that the arm is a little spastic, but the tendon reflexes are absent because of lesions in the dorsal root entry zone that interrupt the reflex circuit. For the author, spasticity in the arm is best elicited by a rapid passive movement of the hand from pronation to supination, which will usually produce a catch and then a give. One can also demonstrate the catch and give in the biceps. With higher motor lesions, one often encounters a dystonic hemiparesis marked by extension of the arm as opposed to the more common spastic flexion of the arm. With dystonia, there is no giveway on further stretching, and the affected muscles are the antagonists of those that have spasticity. With dystonia, the fist is often flat. One can have segmental weakness of a single nerve root owing to MS, which is often misinterpreted as resulting from a disc compression of a nerve root. In MS, weakness often seems most prominent in the finger extensors and intrinsic hand muscles; in the legs, the weakest muscles are usually the iliopsoas and the peroneal muscles.

SECONDARY SYMPTOMS OF WEAKNESS

Any limb paresis causes a reduction in spontaneous movements, resulting in edema. This edema results from only a lack of movement and can only be reduced by vigorous exercise or by placing the limb in a position above the heart so water can run downhill. A sling, recliner chair, and footstool do little for this edema. Even diuretics are not smart enough to tell water to run uphill and are usually ineffective. Elastic stockings are usually useless because the patient cannot put them on. Raising the foot of the bed 3 inches on a block while the head is flat with a thin pillow works best.

CRANIAL NERVE/BRAINSTEM SYMPTOMS

The cranial nerves and brainstem present an array of complex symptoms and signs. Distortions of smell are described in MS, but they are rarely a symptom and are usually not tested. Retrochiasmatic lesions in the visual pathway can occasionally cause symptoms, but that is quite uncommon. Hemianopsia is rare in MS. A decline in vision in one eye with a central loss of vision is the classic optic neuritis (ON) that often introduces or occurs in the context of MS. It is usually unilateral. Bilateral ON occurring at the same time may be seen in Devic's syndrome (neuromyelitis optica). This is a variation of MS more common in Asian and South American people. The central loss of vision impairs reading. The loss is usually greater for red than for other colors and allows one to find a scotoma (using a red pinhead will find scotomas not recognized by a white pinhead). This can be demonstrated with simple confrontation using a corsage pin with a red top. Sometimes one will find some degree of central scotoma and visual acuity decline in the other eye. This may result from a previous ON that was not recognized by the patient. This loss of vision results in some instability of the light reflex in that it contracts to light, but the contraction is not sustained. If one is dexterous and can use the swinging light sign (Marcus-Gunn), it shows that the pupil will dilate with light when the light is moved from the eye that has contracted normally (afferent pupillary defect). The author does not have those motor skills, and if he did have them, he would not spend much time on this sign. What the author sees is a pupil that contracts to light and then dilates again quickly and may oscillate. This is called hippus and provides an objective confirmation of visual fatigue in that eye. ON is regularly attended by pain on eye movement and a degree of photophobia in the affected eye. The impairment of central vision may be minor, moving from 20/20 to 20/30 or may be near total blindness with a preserved rim of visual function at the periphery. There is often color blindness in the affected eye that is easily tested with Ishihara plates, if available. ON usually begins rather quickly over hours or a day, may get worse for a few days, then stabilize and gradually recover over weeks to months. Recovery is usually fairly good, and residual defects are usually not severe *(11)*. If the other eye is normal, then the residual incapacity is of little consequence. However, if the normal or unaffected eye is damaged by some previous illness or by amblyopia exanopsia, the functional deficit may be major. Early treatment with high-dose IV methylprednisolone or dexamethasone for 3–5 days is often helpful *(12,13)*. ON that is near the disk may be attended by papilledema with hemorrhages. Most cases of ON are retrobulbar, and the disk at first is normal. Over time, the residual atrophy can be seen as pallor of the optic disk. When patients with past ON have fever or temperature rise from exertion, the central scotoma may reappear until the body temperature declines (Uhthoff's phenomenon). ON can occur as a disease *sui generis*, which is not followed by any further attacks on the nervous system. In some cases, ON attacks may move from one eye to the other and then back and forth with increasing residual visual deficits. In some cases, the ON precedes or follows an episode of transverse myelitis, which again may be mild or severe. However, in an eventual majority of cases, ON is an early manifestation of MS attended by several or many lesions on the MRI, which are typical of MS *(14)*.

Ischemic ON can be a problem in the differential diagnosis. It usually develops more quickly and in an older age group and blindness is usually more severe; and return of vision is not to be expected. In some cases, vasculitis may respond to vigorous IV immunosuppression with steroids and/or cyclophosphamide. It is necessary to treat quickly. Leber's optic atrophy is a hereditary disorder that produces rapid loss of vision in childhood, almost always in boys. However, in women with Leber's optic atrophy, there may be white matter lesions in the brain and/or spinal cord as well. Embolic occlusion of the ophthalmic artery and thrombosis of the ophthalmic veins can produce confusion in diagnosis. Vitamin B_{12} deficiency is believed to produce ON. Methanol poisoning usually produces bilateral blindness. Tobacco/alcohol amblyopia has become much less frequent but still can occur.

The third, fourth, and sixth cranial nerves may all be affected in MS. Lesions in the brainstem may produce gaze deficits, nystagmus, oscillopsia, oculomotor dysmetria, abnormal saccadic eye movements, and a common disorder called internuclear ophthalmoplegia (INO). This results from a lesion in the brainstem that interrupts the coordination of the third and sixth cranial nerves essential to effect conjugate lateral gaze. Typically, there is failure to adduct one eye when the other eye is abducted. This is usually attended by nystagmus in the abducted eye. This is one of the most common deficits seen in MS. It is easily recognized when it is severe but somewhat more difficult to recognize in milder cases. New neurophysiologic recording techniques can demonstrate INO and other complex gaze defects in a large percentage of patients with MS. This may be key in adding a second lesion disseminated in time and space. Although unilateral INO may be seen in vascular disease, bilateral INO almost always results from MS. The functional result of these deficits is diplopia. Diplopia is often subtle and represents an unstable competition between the eyes to display a clear image. The patient interprets this as blurred vision. Unstable eye movements are sometimes seen as oscillopsia in which images oscillate, producing a severe functional deficit in visual function. Many of these problems with vision and its coordination improve with time, with or without treatment. Some patients are left with severe diplopia, blurred vision, or "dizziness." Vertical nystagmus is an indication of involvement of cerebellar pathways. Alcohol, benzodiazepines, and hypnotics will cause horizontal nystagmus, but a brainstem lesion usually causes vertical nystagmus. Many patients will have better functional vision if they occlude one eye with a patch, an opaque contact, or glasses with one lens covered with a plastic clip. In some instances, symptomatic nystagmus may be improved with memantine. The alleged disadvantage of monocular vision has to relent to acknowledge that approximately 10% of people passing you on the freeway have monocular vision. The author finds it helpful to look for vertical saccades on rapid upgaze. Another useful test is to examine the ability to stop the eyes in the midline when bringing them back from lateral or vertical gaze. Many normal individuals will fail to stop and go through the stop sign, but they quickly learn to correct this. Patients with MS often do not improve and may get worse on further testing. The oculomotor disorders that can occur in MS are worthy of an entire textbook. Various forms of nystagmus and difficulties with up or down gaze, lateral gaze, and oscillopsia are described. Vertical nystagmus is common and regarded as a sign of intrinsic disease associated with the cerebellum and its pathways. Isolated fourth nerve lesions are rare, but they do occur.

The trigeminal nerve and its connections are a common source of symptoms in MS. Facial dysesthesias, tingling, numbness, steady pain, and typical trigeminal neuralgia are seen. Bilateral facial numbness is a troublesome sign and reminds one of Sjögren's syndrome. Trigeminal neuralgia in persons under the age of 50 years usually results from MS but obviously can have other causes as well.

Disturbance of the seventh cranial nerve is sometimes the first symptom of MS. The nerve has a fairly long course inside the brain before it emerges. A demyelinating lesion can affect the nerve, producing a Bell's palsy. It is often difficult to confidently say that this particular Bell's palsy results from an acute viral illness, whereas another one is more typical of MS. Accompanying symptoms, such as ataxia and sensory complaints, may provide a clue. As with classic Bell's palsy, regeneration may be misdirected. This may result in fibers intended for the orbicularis oculi to penetrate the orbicularis oris or mentalis, producing a dimple on that side that appears with each blink of the eye on that side. This is a reliable sign of previous injury to the seventh nerve. Occasionally, regeneration may cause fibers bound for the lachrimal gland to find a salivary gland and vice versa, producing some interesting symptoms sometimes called crocodile tear syndrome. Lesions in the brainstem itself often cause a Horner's syndrome. Bilateral lesions of the seventh nerve should cause some concern about another diagnosis, particularly forms of basal meningitis owing to syphillis, sarcoid, tuberculosis, or meningeal malignancies.

The vestibulocochlear nerve and its connections commonly cause quite violent symptoms of vertigo in MS. It is commonly misdiagnosed as an otological entity, such as vestibular neuronitis. The vertigo can be quite disabling and requires the same treatment that any acute attack would require. Dizziness with movement in any direction is common, and specific positional vertigo in a single position may also be seen. It can last for a long time and be the major cause of disability. Careful testing may be required to distinguish between central and peripheral pathology. Vertigo is commonly associated with nausea and vomiting, regardless of the cause. Tinnitus is rare in MS and is common in otologic disease. Abrupt deafness can be an attack of MS. Obviously, other pathology must be excluded. It is rare for the deafness to be total and bilateral deafness resulting from MS is outside of the author's experience. This deafness will be of a central type so that air conduction would be greater than bone conduction and the Rinne test will lateralize to the side of best hearing.

Lesions in the medulla itself may cause severe singultus (hiccup), which can be a troublesome and persistent symptom for as long as 3 years. This usually responds fairly dramatically to baclofen (Lioresal) in modest doses. Adjacent lesions in the medulla and at higher levels produce difficulty swallowing and speaking. Speech in MS is commonly disturbed and usually presents as slurred speech with irregularities of cadence and emphasis. It is both cerebellar and spastic. Aphonia is rare. The speech tends to remain quite rapid and is often difficult to understand. Difficulties with swallowing are commonly present and usually affect water drinking more than solid food. The pseudobulbar affect introduces an emotional quality to the speech, which is not necessarily intended by the speaker. The affect projected is usually a sad one, so that one senses the patient is going to cry *(15)* at any moment. Alternatively, an effort to smile may produce giggling, which must not be misconstrued.

Other lesions in the brainstem will rarely cause some difficulties with ventilation. More commonly, spinal lesions may affect chest wall movement and even the diaphragm. Lesions at many levels of the brainstem may produce orthostatic hypotension. Cardiac arrhythmias are described in MS. The author has seen patients with migraine whose aura consisted of bouts of atrial flutter and occasionally atrial fibrillation. The author has two patients with MS who, after high-dose IV steroids, developed what was interpreted as a classic Wolf-Parkinson-White syndrome. This persisted for days, but in both cases, it disappeared before electrical correction of the defect could be arranged.

CEREBELLAR SYMPTOMS

A common disability in MS comes from lesions in the cerebellar pathways. Normal cerebellar function modulates movements so that the approach to a target is direct and accurate. It may be likened to an automatic pilot, which adjusts the plane from one position to another to keep it in a straight line. In the absence of this modulation, the movements are from side to side, perpendicular to the direction of movement, and most prominent in the proximal muscles. Over time, many patients learn to regulate this by holding the shoulder close to their side and making the movements from finger to nose rapid to hide the dysmetria. They also tend to hit the side of the finger rather than approach the tip. One can often tell that a finger-nose test is abnormal when the strike of the finger against your finger is harder on one side than the other. In the trunk, cerebellar defects cause a truncal ataxia, making standing in a steady posture without support difficult. This produces titubation, which is a vertical oscillation of the body . This moves the head in a direction of one trying to nod "yes." Rapid alternating movements in the hand and foot are slowed and irregular. The heel-shin test must be done when the patient is supine and will demonstrate this perpendicular deviation from the direction sought determined by proximal muscles. It is sometimes difficult to differentiate this from the weakness seen in limb-girdle muscular dystrophy, which produces a similar instability of proximal muscles by a different mechanism. The gait is broad based, and tandem walking is not feasible. Lurching from one side to the other is usual. There is no fundamental difference between cerebellar ataxia and the motor performance of someone who is intoxicated with alcohol.

SPINAL CORD SYMPTOMS

Central and spinal lesions commonly affect bladder and bowel function, sexual function *(16)*, and blood pressure. Frequency of urination is a ubiquitous symptom in MS *(17)*. Occasionally, it is paradoxically associated or replaced by hesitancy. Urgency may demand access to facilities faster than the patient can achieve, resulting in incontinence. Severe depletion of sensory input from the bladder, usually with position sense loss in the limbs, may produce an atonic bladder, which fills and overflows. Many patients with MS are chronically dehydrated in their attempt to minimize voiding *(18)*. Stubborn constipation is also a nearly universal symptom. At the same time these patients are reluctant to use laxatives for fear of incontinence. Usually the best approach is to affect some means of emptying the bowel and then neglect it during most of the day. Miralax and pyridostigmine are the author's major treatment mainstays in this area.

Sexual dysfunction is usually erectile failure in the male, which is often alleviated by Viagra and similar agents *(19)*. In women, it takes the form of insensitivity resulting in poor libido. Clitoral vibrators may be helpful. Segmental disorders of sweating may be seen. Localized piloerection may be seen. Spinal cord lesions may produce dysautonomia with enormous spikes of high blood pressure from a full bladder, full rectum, or a decubitus ulcer.

APPROACHES TO THE NEUROLOGICAL EXAMINATION AND DIAGNOSIS

The neurological examination has to be comprehensive while also dealing with the rigors of modern medicine. Serial 7s or alternating letters and numbers, the eyes, speech, effect of neck flexion, finger-nose test, finger and second toe position sense, plantar responses, and tandem plus Romberg with bare feet are the author's critical elements.

The diagnosis of MS rests on the dissemination of signs and symptoms in time and in anatomic space. Often, one finds that the patient history provides that information. Colleagues in the United Kingdom and Europe believe the criteria used for first and second attacks must be confirmed by examination. That is often difficult to achieve but is included in the current diagnostic criteria *(20)*. The newly adopted criteria are a bit rigid, but they provide good guidelines to highly accurate diagnosis. If one sees a young woman who had difficulties with bladder control for 3 months with tingling feet, which then clears, and a year later she presents with loss of central vision in one eye, the diagnosis is fairly clear without any further diagnostic procedures. Today, it is essential in almost all cases to get a good MRI following the guidelines set by the National Multiple Sclerosis Society, not only for a diagnosis but also to guide treatment. A family history of MS or other autoimmune disease is often helpful *(21,22)*.

Diagnostic errors go in both directions, but they are infrequent in the hands of any experienced neurologist. It is important to share with the patient the working diagnosis of MS before it is fully confirmed. Many career decisions are affected by the diagnosis. The diagnosis should never be withheld. One should always remember never to use the words "always" and "never" in medicine. The author suggests withholding the diagnosis of MS from a patient with psychosis or who is suicidal *(23)* for some time. At the same time, a certain diagnosis of MS that turns out to be wrong can lead to anger and lawsuits. Almost without exception, honesty with patients is imperative but should not be simplified by not making a firm diagnosis when the criteria have not been fully met. Most medical care proceeds on a working diagnosis, and MS is no exception.

Some patients with MS, perhaps 5% with a higher proportion of men, have a slowly progressive course from the onset. It is likely that this group will have limited memory of the early course of their illness and a sizable proportion will believe that "denial" is a river in Egypt. Over time, it is occasionally possible to get acknowledgment that the first stumbling went away for a month and then returned. A few years ago, the author saw a 70-year-old man who had developed tingling in his right hand and thought he might have had a stroke. His MRI showed advanced and rather severe MS. He was referred to the author because the author was the only neurologist in his age group. After detailed questioning, the patient acknowledged that friends had told him he walked like John Wayne for 30 years, that he found it necessary to take a Valium to control his emotions when he went to a wedding or a funeral, and that his mother had suffered from MS.

The large proportion of men with primary progressive MS is consistent with male tendencies to deny and neglect illness for as long as possible. It also reflects that there are more men than women in hospitals, that women see doctors more often, and that those women live longer than men.

Many patients with MS have paroxysmal symptoms, which do not represent a relapse but rather some brief disturbance of circuitry in affected areas of the brain. The most obvious are trigeminal neuralgia and Lhermitte phenomenon. Extensor and flexor spasms are paroxysmal in many patients. Oscillopsia and vertigo are commonly paroxysmal. If these phenomena clear, at least for a time in seconds or hours, they are probably in this category. If they last for more than 24 hours, one needs to presume that this may be a relapse. In some instances, heat or fever can produce dramatic increases in symptoms that will subside with the body temperature's return to normal. Paroxysmal inability to walk, inability to use a limb, inability to write, and paroxysmal dysarthria are examples of the phenomena. Paroxysmal vision disturbances occur but, with a higher proportion of migraineurs, these symptoms may be an aura with or without a headache.

REFERENCES

1. Trapp BD, Peterson J, Ransohoff RM, Rudick R, Mork S, Bo L. Axonal transection in the lesions of multiple sclerosis. N Engl J Med 1998;338:278–285.
2. Joffe RT, Lippert GP, Gray TA, Sawa G, Horvath Z. Mood disorders and multiple sclerosis. Arch Neurol 1987;44:376–378.
3. Rao SM, Leo GJ, Bernandin L, Unverzagt F. Cognitive dysfunction in multiple sclerosis. Neurology 1991;41:685–691.
4. Rao SM, Reingold SC, Ron MA, Lyon-Caen O, Comi G. Workshop on Neurobehavioral Disorders in Multiple Sclerosis. Diagnosis, underlying disease, natural history, and therapeutic intervention, Bergamo, Italy, June 25–27, 1992. Arch Neurol 1993;50:658–662.
5. Freal JE, Kraft GH, Coryell SK. Symptomatic fatigue in multiple sclerosis. Arch Physical Med Rehabil 1984;65:135–138.
6. Goodin DS, Ebers GC, Johnson KP, Rodriguez M, Sibley WA, Wolinsky JS. The relationship of MS to physical trauma and psychological stress: Report of the Therapeutics and Technology Assessment Subcommittee of the American Academy of Neurology. Neurology 1999;52:1737–1745.
7. Anthony JC, Folstein M, Romanoski AJ, et al. Comparison of the lay diagnostic interview schedule and a standardized psychiatric diagnosis. Arch Gen Psychiatry 1985;42:667–675.
8. Minden SL, Orav J, Reich P. Depression in multiple sclerosis. General Hospital Psychiatry 1987;9:424–434.
9. Mohr DC, Goodkin DE, Gatto N, VanDer Wende J. Depression, coping and level of neurological impairment in multiple sclerosis. Multiple Sclerosis 1997;3:254–258.
10. Whetten-Goldstein K, Sloan F, Conover C, Viscusi K, Kulas B, Chessen H. The economic burden of multiple sclerosis. MS Management 1996;May:33–37.
11. Slamovits TL, Rosen CE, Cheng KP, Striph GG. Visual recovery in patients with optic neuritis and visual loss to no light perception. Am J Ophthalmol 1991;111:209–214.
12. Beck RW, Cleary PA, Anderson MM, Jr., et al. A randomized, controlled trial of corticosteroids in the treatment of acute optic neuritis. N Engl J Med 1992;326:581–588.
13. Beck RW, Cleary PA, Trobe JD, et al. The effect of corticosteroids for acute optic neuritis on the subsequent development of multiple sclerosis. N Engl J Med 1993;239:1764–1769.
14. Beck RW, Cleary PA. Optic neuritis treatment trial: one-year follow-up results. Arch Ophthalmol 1993;111:773–775.
15. Feinstein A, Feinstein K, Gray T, O'Connor P. Prevalence and neurobehavioral correlates of pathological laughing and crying in multiple sclerosis. Arch Neurol 1997;54:1116–1121.
16. Chancellor MB, Blaivas JG. Urological and sexual problems in multiple sclerosis. Clin Neurosci 1994;2:189–195.
17. Andrews KL, Husmann DA. Bladder dysfunction and management in multiple sclerosis. Mayo Clin Proc 1997;72:1176–1183.
18. Blaivas JG, Holland NJ, Giesser B, LaRocca N, Madonna M, Scheinberg L. Multiple sclerosis bladder: studies and care. Ann N Y Acad Sci 1984;436:328–346.
19. Derry FA, W.W. D, Fraser M, et al. Efficacy and safety of oral sildenafil (Viagra) in men with erectile dysfunction caused by spinal cord injury. Neurology 1998;51:1629–1633.

20. McDonald WI, Compston A, Edan G, et al. Recommended diagnostic criteria for multiple sclerosis: guidelines from the International Panel on the diagnosis of multiple sclerosis. Ann Neurol 2001;50:121–127.
21. Sadovnick AD, Baird PA, Ward RH. Multiple sclerosis: updated risks for relatives. Am J Med Genet 1988;29:533–541.
22. Sadovnick AD, Ebers GC. Epidemiology in multiple sclerosis: a critical overview. Can J Neurol Sci 1993;20:17–29.
23. Feinstein A. Multiple sclerosis, depression, and suicide [editorial]. Bmj 1997;315:691–692.

Differential Diagnosis, Clinical Features, and Prognosis of Multiple Sclerosis

Michael J. Olek, DO

INTRODUCTION

The diagnosis and prognosis of multiple sclerosis (MS) has changed dramatically over the years from the first descriptions from St. Lidwina of Schiedam (1380–1433) and Augustus D'Este (grandson of George III) between 1822 and 1848 to the pathological descriptions of Cruveilhier (1829–1842) and Carswell (1838). Serious study and synthesis of clinical and pathological human MS began with the work of Jean Martin Charcot at the Salpetriere in Paris in the last three decades of the 19th century. Recently, there has been a trend to classify MS as an immune-mediated demyelinating disease of the central nervous system (CNS). This classification is useful as a diagnostic tool, as demonstrated by Schumacher (1962) and Poser (1983). The new diagnostic criteria *(1)*, which is discussed in detail in the remainder of this chapter, has changed the diagnosis, prognosis, and treatment of MS.

DIAGNOSIS

The cornerstone of the MS diagnosis remains the neurological history and physical examination. There are no clinical findings that are unique to this disorder, but some are highly characteristic (Table 1). Common presenting MS symptoms are listed in Table 2. The typical patient presents as a young Caucasian adult female with two or more clinically distinct episodes of CNS dysfunction, with at least partial resolution. The history and physical examination are most important for diagnostic purposes, although numerous laboratory tests support the diagnosis (Table 3). To improve the homogeneity of MS patient groups being studied, the Schumacher Committee on Diagnostic Criteria for MS *(2)* elaborated six items that are required to diagnose clinically definite MS: objective CNS dysfunction, involvement of white-matter structures, two or more sites of CNS involvement, relapsing-remitting or chronic (more than 6 months) progressive course, age 10–50 years at onset, and no better explanation of symptoms as assessed by a competent

From: *Current Clinical Neurology: Multiple Sclerosis*
Edited by: M. J. Olek © Humana Press Inc., Totowa, NJ

Table 1
Common Clinical Features of Multiple Sclerosis

Clinical features suggestive of multiple sclerosis	Clinical features not suggestive of multiple sclerosis
Onset between ages 15 and 50	Onset before age 10 or after 60
Relapses and remissions	Steady progression
Optic neuritis	Early dementia
Lhermitte sign	Rigidity, sustained dystonia
Internuclear ophthalmoplegia	Cortical deficits, such as aphasia, apraxia, alexia, and neglect
Fatigue	Deficit developing within minutes
Worsening with elevated body temperature	

Table 2
Presenting Symptoms in Multiple Sclerosis Patients

Symptom	Males (%)	Females (%)	Total (%)
Sensory disturbance–limbs	25.1	33.2	30.7
Visual loss	15.1	16.3	15.9
Motor (subacute)	10.4	8.3	8.9
Diplopia	8.5	6.0	6.8
Gait disturbance	8.3	3.2	4.8
Motor (acute)	4.2	4.4	4.3
Balance problems	4.0	2.5	2.9
Sensory disturbance–face	2.5	2.9	2.8
Lhermitte's phenomenon	2.3	1.6	1.8
Vertigo	1.5	1.8	1.7
Bladder disturbance	1.1	0.9	1.0
Limb ataxia	1.3	0.9	1.0
Acute transverse myelopathy	0.6	0.8	0.7
Pain	0.8	0.3	0.5
Unclassified	2.5	2.6	2.5
Polysymptomatic onset	11.9	14.5	13.7

Adapted from refs. *68* and *69*.

Table 3
Comparison of Sensitivity of Laboratory Testing in Multiple Sclerosis

	Visual evoked response (%)	Brainstem auditory evoked response (%)	Somato-sensory evoked potentials (%)	Oligo-clonal bands (%)	Magnetic resonance imaging (%)
Clinically definite multiple sclerosis*	80–85	50–65	65–80	85–95	90–97

*Numbers show the percentage of patients with abnormal study results.

neurologist. These criteria made no use of laboratory studies. Such stringent criteria would exclude some patients with MS; for example, they were fulfilled in only 95% of a group of patients who came to autopsy study. The criteria were modified for diagnosis in 1983 by Poser et al. *(3)*, expanding the age at onset to 59 years and using data derived from laboratory studies, including analysis of cerebrospinal fluid (CSF), evoked potentials (EP), and neuroimaging. These criteria were developed to ensure that only patients with MS were included in research studies. Recently, McDonald et al. *(1)* have proposed new diagnostic criteria, which include stringent guidelines for magnetic resonance imaging (MRI) and timing intervals to determine possible or definite multiple sclerosis. The outcomes are classified as:

- The diagnosis of MS is given if diagnostic criteria are fulfilled.
- The diagnosis of possible MS is given if the criteria are not completely met.
- The diagnosis of not MS is given if the criteria are fully explored and not met.

Another significant change with the newer criteria (sometimes referred to as the McDonald criteria) is the incorporation of MRI findings. The new diagnostic criteria are shown in Table 4 and in the next section. The new criteria consider CSF analysis, EPs, and neuroimaging, as well as creating a category for patients with clinically isolated syndromes. This information allows patients to be treated at an earlier phase in their disease and will provide the greatest effect on the long-term prognosis of the disease for most patients.

Magnetic Resonance Imaging Demonstration of Space Dissemination for McDonald Diagnostic Criteria for Multiple Sclerosis (4,5)

Three out of four of the following:

1. One gadolinium-enhancing lesion OR nine T2-hyperintense lesions if there is no gadolinium-enhancing lesion;
2. At least one infratentorial lesion;
3. At least one juxtacortical lesion; and/or
4. At least three periventricular lesions.

If the first scan is performed less than 3 months after the onset of the clinical event, a second scan done 3 months or more after the clinical event showing a new gadolinium-enhancing lesion provides sufficient evidence for dissemination in time. However, if no enhancing lesion is seen at this second scan, a further scan, not less than 3 months after the first scan that shows a new T2 lesion or an enhancing lesion, will suffice.

RADIOLOGICAL STUDIES

MRI is the test of choice to support the clinical diagnosis of MS. The characteristic lesion demonstrated on MRI is the cerebral or spinal plaque. Pathologically, plaques consist of a discrete region of demyelination with relative preservation of axons, although spectroscopic and pathological studies suggest axonal loss may be an integral part of the demyelinating process *(6)*. Histological examination of active

Table 4
McDonald Diagnostic Criteria for Multiple Sclerosis (1)

Clinical presentation	Additional data needed for multiple sclerosis (MS) diagnosis
Two or more attacks; objective clinical evidence of two or more lesions	None
Two or more attacks; objective clinical evidence of one lesion	Dissemination in space, demonstrated by MRI OR Two or more MRI-detected lesions consistent with MS plus positive CSF OR Await further clinical attack implicating a different site
One attack; objective clinical evidence of two or more lesions	Dissemination in time, demonstrated by MRI OR Second clinical attack
One attack; objective clinical evidence of one lesion (monosymptomatic presentation; clinically isolated syndrome)	Dissemination in space, demonstrated by MRI OR Second clinical attack OR Two or more MRI-detected lesions consistent with MS plus positive CSF and dissemination in time, demonstrated by MRI
Insidious neurological progression suggestive of MS	Positive CSF and dissemination in space, demonstrated by: (1) Nine or more T2 lesions in: brain, (2) Two or more lesions in spinal cord, or, (3) Four to eight plus one spinal cord lesion OR Abnormal visual evoked response (VER) associated with four to eight brain lesions, or with fewer than four brain lesions plus one spinal cord lesion demonstrated by MRI AND Dissemination in time, demonstrated by MRI OR Continued progression for 1 year

Notes: Positive CSF-oligoclonal bands (detected preferably by isoelectric focusing) or raised immunoglobulin-G index.

plaques reveals perivascular infiltration of lymphocytes (predominantly T-cells) and macrophages with occasional plasma cells. Perivascular and interstitial edema may be prominent.

Plaques suggestive of MS are typically found on MRI in the periventricular region, corpus callosum, centrum semiovale, and, to a lesser extent, deep white-matter structures and basal ganglia. MS plaques usually have an ovoid appearance, and lesions are arranged at right angles to the corpus callosum as if radiating from this area. The plaques appear hyperintense on proton density and T2-weighted studies and are hypointense (if visible at all) on T1-weighted images.

MRI detects many more MS lesions than computed tomography (CT) and is able to detect plaques in regions that are rarely abnormal on CT, such as the brain stem, cerebellum, and spinal cord. Most lesions seen on MRI correlate with pathologic lesions *(7)*. However, some lesions that are extensive on MRI show only small plaques on pathological examination, suggesting that much of the abnormal MRI signal may be a result of increased water content of the brain around such plaques resulting from presumed disruption of the blood–brain barrier.

Patients with clinically definite MS have typical white-matter lesions on MRI in more than 90% of cases. However, CNS lesions resulting from other disorders (e.g., ischemia, systemic lupus erythematosus [SLE], Behçet's disease, other vasculitides, human T-cell lymphotropic virus [HTLV]-1, and sarcoidosis) may appear similar to MS lesions on MRI. This is particularly true for ischemic lesions, which make MRI criteria much less reliable for the diagnosis of MS in patients older than 50 years *(8)*.

In contrast, the frequency of abnormal signals on spinal cord MRI in normal individuals is only 3%, because the non-MS hyperintense signal seen in older patients on cranial MRI does not occur in the spinal cord. Newer technology MRI detects lesions in the spinal cord in 75% of patients with definite MS *(9)*.

The overall sensitivity and specificity of MRI depend on the diagnostic criteria employed. In one study of 1500 brain MRI scans that included 134 scans of patients with a clinical diagnosis of MS, using the criteria of three or four areas of increased signal intensity resulted in a high sensitivity for the diagnosis of MS (90 and 87%, respectively) but a low specificity (71 and 74%, respectively) and positive predictive value (23 and 25%, respectively) *(8)*. Accuracy was improved with criteria that included at least three areas of increased signal intensity plus two of the following features: lesions abutting body of lateral ventricles, infratentorial lesion location, and size >5 mm. Using these criteria, specificity improved to 96%, positive predictive value increased to 65%, and sensitivity decreased slightly to 81%.

MRI scanning is more sensitive and specific for predicting evolution to clinically definite MS than other studies, such as CT scans, CSF parameters, or EPs *(10)*. This was illustrated in a 2-year follow-up of 200 patients referred for suspected MS that found 30% (50% of those under age 50 years) had developed clinically definite MS, of whom 84% had initial MRI scans that were strongly suggestive of MS *(11)*. In contrast, the number of patients who had CSF oligoclonal bands, abnormal visual EPs, or an abnormal CT when initially studied were 69, 69, and 38%, respectively. In a second, 5-year study of 89 patients, progression to clinically definite MS occurred in 37 out of 57 (65%) with an initially abnormal MRI, and only 1 of 32 (3%) with a normal MRI *(12)*. Again, MRI was a better predictor of progression to clinically definite MS than CSF analysis.

Patients who progress to clinically definite MS have a higher lesion load at presentation than those who do not progress *(13)*. Increasing initial lesion load also correlates with a decreasing time to development of MS clinically. Lesion load may also have implications for long-term prognosis.

However, the extent of cranial MRI abnormalities does not necessarily correlate with the degree of clinical disability. Patients with small numbers of lesions may be quite disabled, whereas others can function well despite a large burden of disease detected by MRI. There are several possible explanations for this observation: lesions may occur in areas that are clinically silent, small lesions in the spinal cord can cause major disability in the absence of cerebral lesions, MRI may miss lesions that are clinically relevant *(1)*, such as those in cortex, basal ganglia, and brain stem, and large plaques detected by MRI may not have functional correlates but reflect increased tissue water without impairment of neural function.

The amount of ongoing MRI activity (new or enlarging lesions and/or gadolinium-enhancing lesions) exceeds the observed clinical activity by a factor of 2 to 10 *(14)*. This not only may reflect the factors discussed above but also may result, in part, from underreporting of minor symptoms and underrecognition of minor signs in patients with MS. However, it does suggest that MS is a much more dynamic and active disease than is clinically apparent and that MRI is essential to studies of therapy in MS.

Efforts continue to delineate differences in the MRI appearance of acute or active lesions and chronic lesions. Acute lesions tend to be larger with somewhat ill-defined margins and become smaller with sharper margins as resolution occurs. This presumably reflects resolution of edema and inflammation present at the time of acute plaque formation, leaving only residual areas of demyelination, gliosis, and enlarged extracellular space with remission. The MRI appearance of primary progressive MS shows a smaller total disease burden, a greater preponderance of small lesions, fewer gadolinium-enhancing new lesions, and acquisition of fewer lesions per unit time than the secondary progressive form of MS.

Gadolinium-DTPA, a paramagnetic contrast agent that can cross only disrupted blood–brain barrier, has been used to assess plaque activity *(15)*. Gadolinium increases signal intensity on T1-weighted images. The accumulation of gadolinium in plaques is associated with new or newly active plaques and with pathologically confirmed acute inflammation in MS. Gadolinium enhancement usually remains for <1 month but may persist up to 8 weeks in acute plaques. Gadolinium enhancement diminishes or disappears after treatment with corticosteroids, a therapy believed to restore integrity of the blood–brain barrier permeability.

It is difficult to distinguish the edema of an acute plaque from the gliosis and demyelination of a chronic plaque with conventional MRI technology. Phosphorus MR spectroscopy can provide information on phospholipid metabolism, and proton spectroscopy can generate information about other metabolic components, such as *N*-acetylaspartate (NAA), an exclusively neuronal marker, creatine phosphate (Cr) (energy), choline (membrane component), and lactic acid (LA). Chronic MS brains have a reduced amount of NAA in comparison to C and Cr; a reduced NAA/Cr ratio is the common means of expressing such reduction. This reduced ratio implies loss of neurons or axons, which is consistent with pathological studies and appears to parallel disability in MS *(16)*.

CEREBROSPINAL FLUID

CSF findings alone cannot make or exclude the diagnosis of MS, but they can be useful adjuncts to clinical criteria. The CSF is grossly normal in MS; it is clear, colorless, and under normal pressure. Total leukocyte count is normal in two-thirds of patients, exceeding 15 cells/µL in fewer than 5% of patients and only rarely exceeding 50 cells/µL (a finding that should raise suspicion of another etiology). The predominant cell type is the lymphocyte, the majority of which are T-cells. CSF protein (or albumin) level is normal in the majority of patients with MS. Albumin determinations are preferable because albumin is not synthesized in the CNS and thus gives a better indication of blood–brain barrier disruption than does total protein, some of which may be synthesized within the CNS (i.e., immunoglobulin [Ig]). Albumin levels are elevated in 20–30% of patients, although less than 1% of patients have a level twice that of normal (Table 5). A common finding in MS is an elevation of CSF immunoglobulin level relative to other protein components, implying intrathecal synthesis. The immunoglobulin increase is predominantly IgG, but the synthesis of IgM and IgA is increased also. The IgG shows an excess of IgG λ and κ light chains. The IgG level may be expressed as a percentage of total protein (normal <11%), as a percentage of albumin (normal <27%), by use of the IgG index (normal value <0.66), or by use of a formula for intra-blood–brain barrier synthesis of IgG. An abnormality of CSF IgG production as measured by the IgG index or IgG synthesis rate is found in more than 90% of patients with clinically definite MS, and different formulas have differing sensitivity and specificity. The sensitivity of IgG as a percentage of protein or albumin is slightly lower (Table 5) *(17)*.

Linked to the elevation of IgG is the finding of oligoclonal bands (OCBs) in the cathodal region of an electrophoretic analysis of CSF. When normal CSF is electrophoresed, the cathodal region shows only a homogeneous blur of immunoglobulin. In MS and other conditions usually associated with inflammation, electrophoretic analysis reveals numerous discrete bands distinct from the background; these bands represent excess antibody produced by one or more clones of plasma cells. In subacute sclerosing panencephalitis, the majority of these OCBs represent antibody directed against the causative agent, measles virus. However, in MS, there is no disease-specific antigen yet identified against which the majority of bands are directed. The pattern of banding remains relatively consistent in individual patients during the disease course, although bands may be added over time. Occasionally, patients with definite autopsy-proved MS do not have OCBs.

A common method for electrophoresis uses agarose gels, but a more sensitive assay is the use of isoelectric focusing on polyacrylamide gels. OCBs are found in 85–95% of patients with clinically definite MS (Table 5). Up to 8% of CSF samples

Table 5
Cerebrospinal Fluid Abnormalities in Multiple Sclerosis

	Albumin (%)	IgG/TP (%)	IgG/ Albumin (%)	IgG Index (%)	Oligoclonal Banding of Ig (%)
Clinically definite multiple sclerosis (MS)	23	67	60–73	70–90	85–95
Normal controls	3		36	3	7*

Abbr: IgG/TP, immunoglobulin (Ig) G value/total protein.
*Other neurological diseases.

from patients without MS show OCBs and most are from cases of chronic CNS infections, viral syndromes, and autoimmune neuropathies. The presence of OCBs in patients who are monosymptomatic predicts a significantly higher rate of progression to MS than the absence of bands: 25 vs 9% at a 3 year follow-up *(18)*. However, one must not assume that the presence of OCBs is equivalent to a diagnosis of MS, given the number of false-positive results that can occur and the variability in technique and interpretation in different laboratories.

The presence of myelin components and antimyelin antibodies in CSF and other body fluids has been used to a limited extent as a measure of CNS myelin destruction and presumed demyelinating activity in the CNS *(19)*.

EVOKED POTENTIALS

Evoked potentials (EPs) are the CNS electrical events generated by peripheral stimulation of a sensory organ. The use of EPs is the detection of a CNS abnormality of function that may be clinically undetectable. In the case of MS, detection of a subclinical lesion in a site remote from the region of clinical dysfunction supports a diagnosis of multifocal disease. The EPs also may help define the anatomical site of the lesion in tracts not easily visualized by imaging (optic nerves and dorsal columns). The three most frequently used EPs are somatosensory EP (SSEP) both upper and lower extremities, visual (VER), and brainstem auditory-evoked responses (BAER). MRI technology has largely eliminated the use of EPs, given the much greater anatomical information obtained and the much higher sensitivity of MRI in the diagnosis of MS (Table 3).

Patients with clinically definite MS have abnormal VERs in 85% of cases. The VER is particularly useful in patients who lack clear clinical evidence of dysfunction above the level of the foramen magnum, such as those with a chronic progressive myelopathy. Ocular or retinal disorders must be excluded before attributing abnormal VERs to demyelination in the optic pathways.

Table 6
Summary of Ancillary Testing in Multiple Sclerosis

Test	Percentage abnormal with definite multiple sclerosis (%)
Brainstem auditory evoked response	50–65
Somatosensory evoked potentials	65–80
Visual evoked response	80–85
Cerebrospinal fluid (CSF) Immunoglobulin (Ig) G Index	70–90
CSF oligoclonal bands	85–95
Brain magnetic resonance imaging	90–97

SSEPs are abnormal in 77% of patients with MS, including approximately one-half of those who do not have sensory signs or symptoms. Some patients with clinical evidence of posterior column dysfunction may have abnormal SSEPs.

BAER abnormalities are less frequent in MS than VER or SSEP abnormalities, being present in 67% of patients with MS.

Consistent with these findings, guidelines from the American Academy of Neurology state that VERs are probably useful to identify patients with clinically definite MS, SSEPs are possibly useful, and there is insufficient evidence at this time to recommend BAER as a useful test for diagnostic purposes *(20)*.

Synthesis of the previous data on ancillary testing is presented in Table 6.

AGE OF ONSET

Most studies agree that the median age of onset is 23.5 years of age. The peak age of onset is approximately 5 years earlier for women than for men. The mean age of onset is 30. Relapsing-remitting MS tends to have an earlier onset, averaging 25–29 years, compared with the relapsing-remitting progressive type with an average of onset of 25–29 years, and a mean age of conversion to progressive MS of 40–44 years. Primary progressive MS has a mean age of onset of 35–39 years. The onset of MS can occur as late as the seventh decade, although rarely. Mean age of onset is 30.6 years, median is 27 years, and peak incidence is 25 years.

SEX DISTRIBUTION

Autoimmune diseases in general and MS in particular affect more women than men. In a summary of 30 incidence and prevalence studies, a cumulative ratio of female to male subjects was 1.77:1.00.

MORTALITY

Mortality caused by MS is difficult to ascertain because of poor data collection and reporting. The US Department of Health and Human Services report of deaths in 1992 indicates that 1900 US citizens died of MS in that year, giving MS a US mortality of 0.7 per 100,000. The mean age of death of all patients with MS was 58.1 years, compared with a national average of 70.5 for all causes of death. The life expectancy of patients with MS was therefore calculated to be 82.5% of the normal life span. In Denmark, in an exceptionally complete survey of the country, median survival after diagnosis for men was 28 years and for women 33 years, compared with matched population death rates of 37 and 42 years, respectively. In another study, MS mortality figures were calculated for England and Wales from 1963 to 1990. During this time, there was a steady and consistent decline in the death rate attributable to MS compared with the overall death rate. Patients with MS tended to live longer, and other diseases were more likely to be the cause of death. Current estimates indicate that about half of the deaths in MS patients directly result from their disease, slightly more than half if accidents, and suicide are included as indirect causes.

ROLE OF IMMUNE SYSTEM STIMULI

Because the pathogenesis of MS is believed to involve the immune system, it has been hypothesized that a stimulus of the immune system (e.g., a vaccine) may trigger the disease. However, two well-designed studies have refuted this theory, one finding no association between hepatitis B vaccination and the development of MS *(21)*, and the other finding no association between several different vaccines and disease relapse in patients with MS *(22)*.

On the other hand, a possible infectious stimulus of the immune system has received more support in the literature. Many viruses have been associated with MS, although none has been conclusively linked to the disease *(23)*. A role for Epstein-Barr virus (EBV), which causes infectious mononucleosis, is supported by observations that there is an increased risk of MS after infectious mononucleosis *(24)* and that MS is rare among people without serum anti-EBV antibodies *(25)*. Furthermore, a prospective serologic study of women in the Nurses' Health Study found significant elevations in anti-EBV antibody titers before the onset of MS, particularly antibody to the EBV nuclear antigen 2 (EBNA-2) *(26)*. Although these findings do not confirm that EBV is an etiologic agent, they are suggestive and warrant further study. For further information on the immune response and the role of B-cells in MS, please refer to Chapter 6.

GEOGRAPHIC AND RACIAL DISTRIBUTION

More than 250 prevalence surveys have been conducted, serving as the basis for the delineation of geographic risk for MS. High-frequency areas of the world, with current prevalence of 60 per 100,000 or more, include all of Europe, including Russia, southern Canada, the northern United States, New Zealand, and the southeastern portion of Australia. In many of these areas, the prevalence is more than 100 per 100,000, with the highest reported rate of 300 per 100,000 occurring in the Orkney Islands. In the United States, the prevalence is 0.1%, or a total of 250,000 persons with MS.

Low-risk areas include most of South America, Mexico, most of Asia, and all of Africa. One possible conclusion is that MS is a place-related illness, with a latitude gradient. However, notable exceptions then need to be explained. Japan, situated at the same latitude as areas of high prevalence in Europe, is a low-risk area. Second-generation Japanese in the United States retain their parents' low risk of MS. The white population of South Africa, of medium MS prevalence, is surrounded by a black population in which the disease is uncommon. Native North Americans, especially of pure Amerindian background, have a low prevalence, but they are surrounded by a white population with a medium or high MS risk.

It seems plausible then that race is a determinant of MS risk, with populations of white extraction, especially from Northern Europe being the most susceptible. People of Asian, African, or Amerindian origin have the lowest risk, whereas other groups are variably intermediate. Migration data have often been used to support the view that a transmissible agent is involved in the pathogenesis of MS. The data indicate that persons migrating from an area of high risk to an area of low risk after the age of puberty carry their former high risk with them. With migration during childhood, the risk seems to be that of the new area to which the person has migrated. The data are not always clear-cut. Japanese in Japan are at low risk for MS. People of Japanese extraction who are living in the United States have a higher risk, although this risk is less than their neighbors of Northern European extraction. However, those Japanese who migrate to this country do not acquire the risk of their new area. Comparable data are available for persons moving to Israel from Europe (high risk).

The frequency of familial occurrence of MS has varied from 3 to 23% in different studies. The studies with the higher percentages are those in which ascertainment was more intense; that is, the more one looks, the more one finds. An overall risk in first-, second-, and third-degree relatives of at least 15% seems a reasonable estimate. The risk is highest for siblings and decreases progressively for children, aunts, uncles, and cousins (Table 7). For genetic counseling purposes, it may be stated that the sibling risk is 3–5%, approximately 30–50 times the background risk for this same population. In some studies, unaffected family members have had abnormalities on MRI, implying that the risk may be even higher. The risk applies to blood relatives; only a few studies of adopted children have been done, but they show no increased risk. One unexplained finding is the marked deficiency of transmission from father to son.

Twin studies have shown the familial nature of MS in dramatic fashion. The risk for dizygotic twin pairs is the same as that for siblings; that is, 3–5%. The risk for monozygotic twins is at least 20%, and if the subjects are followed for long periods of time and if various nonclinical data are included, the risk may reach 38.5% *(27)*. Because the highest rates for the genetic basis of MS are less than 50%, there must be a contribution by nongenetic factors. There are several candidate genes for MS, including human leukocyte antigen, T-cell receptor, MBP, portions of the immunoglobulin chain, and mitochondrial genes. Three entire genomic scans for MS susceptibility genes have been reported, without an identifiable region of major interest *(26–28)*. The data argue for nonmendelian polygenic inheritance.

Table 7
Risk of Developing Multiple Sclerosis in Family Members

A. Parent with multiple sclerosis (MS)	Son	Daughter
Mother	3.8%	3.7%
Father	0.8%	2.0%
B. Sibling with MS sister brother		
Female	5.6%	2.2%
Male	3.5%	4.1%
C. Twin with MS either sex		
Identical	25–40%	
Nonidentical	4%	

Source: Modified from ref. *70.*

CLINICAL SYMPTOMS AND PHYSICAL FINDINGS

Although the clinical syndrome of MS is classically described as a relapsing-remitting disorder that affects multiple white-matter tracts within the CNS, with usual onset in young adults, the disorder displays marked clinical heterogeneity. This variability includes age of onset, mode of initial manifestation, frequency, severity and sequelae of relapses, extent of progression, and cumulative deficit over the course of time. The varied clinical features reflect the multifocal areas of CNS myelin destruction (MS plaques), although discrepancies occur between the extent of clinical and pathological findings.

There are no clinical findings that are unique to MS, but some are highly characteristic of the disease. Common presenting symptoms of MS are listed in Table 2. The typical patient presents as a young adult with two or more clinically distinct episodes of CNS dysfunction with at least partial resolution.

CRANIAL NERVE DYSFUNCTION

Impairment of the Visual Pathways

Optic neuritis (ON) is the most frequent type of involvement of the visual pathways, usually presenting as an acute or subacute unilateral syndrome characterized commonly by pain in the eye accentuated by ocular movements, which is then followed by a variable degree of vision loss (scotoma) affecting mainly central vision. Bilateral ON does occur, but one needs to distinguish whether it is truly simultaneous or sequential. Bilateral simultaneous ON is rare in MS, and its occurrence in isolation may suggest another diagnosis, such as Leber's hereditary optic atrophy or toxic optic neuropathy. In bilateral ON in MS cases, the impairment begins asymmetrically and is usually more severe in one eye. Recurrence is highly variable. In a large ON treatment trial, 15% of placebo-treated patients developed recurrent (ipsilateral or contralateral eye) ON within 6 to 24 months after the initial bout of ON *(31)*. Mapping of visual fields reveals a central or cecocentral scotoma (central scotoma involving the physiological blind spot). The finding of a bitemporal hemianopia is rare in MS; if present, it should raise the suspicion of a mass lesion compressing the optic chiasm. Although uncommon, homonymous field defects can be seen in MS caused by involvement of the optic radiations.

Patients with ON have a relative afferent pupillary defect (Marcus Gunn pupil). The afferent pupillary defect is tested by shining a bright light alternately in each eye (the swinging flashlight test), and in the case of unilateral optic nerve dysfunction the abnormal pupil paradoxically dilates when the light is shifted from the normal to the affected eye. The interpretation of this sign becomes difficult when the degree of optic nerve impairment is similar in the two eyes. When the acute ON lesion involves the head of the optic nerve, one observes disc edema (papillitis), a finding more commonly seen in children than in adults. More often, the lesion of the optic nerve is retrobulbar, and funduscopic examination is normal in the acute stage. Later, the optic disc becomes pale as a result of axonal loss and resultant gliosis. This pallor predominates in the temporal segment of the disc (temporal pallor). After an attack of acute ON, 90% of patients regain normal vision, typically during a 2- to 6-month period. Desaturation of bright colors, particularly red, is often reported by patients who have recovered from ON; some also report a mild nonspecific dimming of vision in the affected eye.

Uhthoff's phenomenon refers to a decrease in visual acuity after an increase in body temperature. This can occur after exercise, a hot bath, or fever. This phenomenon, which reflects subclinical demyelination or preexistent injury to the optic nerve, may occur without a history of clinical involvement of the optic nerve. A similar phenomenon can occur at other sites of CNS dysfunction with an increase in body temperature.

Bitemporal hemianopia is rare in MS and, if present, should raise the suspicion of a mass lesion compressing the visual pathways. Homonymous field defects are uncommon but can be seen in MS resulting from involvement of the optic radiations.

Because many patients with MS present with ON as their first neurologic event, it is interesting to consider how many patients who have ON go on to develop MS. The reported risk of progression to clinically diagnosed MS ranges from 15 to 75%. In one population-based study, 39% of 95 patients with isolated ON progressed to clinically definite MS by 10 years of follow-up, 49% by 20 years, 54% by 30 years, and 60% by 40 years *(32)*. There was no difference in the risk of developing MS between men and women. The presence of oligoclonal bands in the CSF of such patients has been associated with an increased risk of developing MS.

MRI can help differentiate groups of patients with ON who are likely or unlikely to develop MS *(31)*. Between 50 and 72% of patients with ON have cranial MRI appearances consistent with MS. Of those with lesions on MRI, there is a 55 to 70% risk of developing clinically definite MS or laboratory-supported definite MS within 5 years *(12)*. In contrast, patients with isolated ON and no evidence of disseminated lesions on MRI have only a 6 to 16% risk of developing MS after 4 years or more of follow-up. The incidence of MRI abnormalities in children with ON is less than in adults; this observation, coupled with clinical experience, suggests that the rate of progression to MS in children with isolated ON may be less than in adults.

IMPAIRMENT OF THE OCULAR MOTOR PATHWAYS

Impairment of individual ocular motor nerves is infrequent in MS. When present, the involved nerves are, in decreasing order of frequency, Cranial Nerves VI, III, and, rarely, IV. More frequent findings are those that reflect lesions of vestibulo-ocular connections and internuclear connections. Nystagmus is a common finding in MS. One form of nystagmus particularly characteristic of MS is acquired pendular nystagmus, in which there are rapid, small amplitude pendular oscillations of the eyes in the primary position resembling quivering jelly. Patients frequently complain of oscillopsia (subjective oscillation of objects in the field of vision). This type of nystagmus usually is seen in the presence of marked loss of visual acuity. Internuclear ophthalmoplegia, defined as abnormal horizontal ocular movements with lost or delayed adduction and horizontal nystagmus of the abducting eye, is secondary to a lesion of the medial longitudinal fasciculus on the side of diminished adduction. Convergence is preserved. When present bilaterally, it is usually coupled with vertical nystagmus on upward gaze. Although most suggestive of MS, a bilateral internuclear ophthalmoplegia can be observed with other intraaxial brainstem lesions, including brainstem glioma, vascular lesions, Arnold-Chiari malformations, and Wernicke's encephalopathy. Ocular pursuit movements are frequently saccadic rather than smooth. Ocular dysmetria may coexist with other signs of cerebellar dysfunction and other ocular oscillations, such as intrusive saccadic movements (square wave jerks).

IMPAIRMENT OF OTHER CRANIAL NERVES

Impairment of facial sensation, subjective or objective, is a relatively common finding in MS. The occurrence of trigeminal neuralgia in a young adult is frequently an early sign of MS. Facial myokymia, a fine undulating wavelike facial twitching, and hemifacial spasm can be caused by MS, but other causes of a focal brainstem lesion must be excluded. Unilateral facial paresis can occur, but taste sensation is almost never affected. In these syndromes, as with acute oculomotor palsy, the nerve is affected in its course within the neuraxis, rather than peripherally. Vertigo is a reported symptom in 30 to 50% of patients with MS and is commonly associated with dysfunction of adjacent cranial nerves. Resulting symptoms include hyperacusis or hypoacusis, facial numbness, and diplopia. Complete hearing loss, usually unilateral, is an infrequent complaint. Malfunction of the lower cranial nerves is usually of the upper motor neuron type (pseudobulbar syndrome).

IMPAIRMENT OF THE SENSORY PATHWAYS

Sensory manifestations are a frequent initial feature of MS and are present in almost every patient at some time during the course of disease. The sensory features can reflect spinothalamic, posterior column, or dorsal root entry zone lesions. The sensory symptoms are commonly described as numbness, tingling, pins and needles, tightness, coldness, or swelling of limbs or trunk. Radicular pains, unilateral or bilateral, can be present, particularly in the low thoracic and abdominal regions, or a band-like abdominal sensation may be described. An intensely itching sensation, especially in the cervical dermatomes, usually unilateral, suggests MS.

The most frequent sensory abnormalities on clinical examination are the following: varying degrees of impairment of vibration and joint position sense, decrease of pain and light touch in a distal distribution in the four extremities, and patchy areas of reduced pain and light touch perception in the limbs and trunk. A bilateral sensory level is a more frequent finding than a hemisensory (Brown-Séquard) syndrome. Patients commonly report that the feeling of pinprick is increased or feels like a mild electric shock or that the stimulus spreads in a ripple fashion from the point at which it is applied. The sensory useless hand is a characteristic but uncommon feature, consisting of an impairment of function secondary to a pronounced alteration of proprioception, without loss of power. A lesion of the relevant root entry zones in the spinal cord is postulated in such cases.

IMPAIRMENT OF MOTOR PATHWAYS

Corticospinal tract dysfunction is common in MS. Paraparesis, or paraplegia, is a much more common occurrence than is significant weakness in the upper extremities. With severe spasticity, extensor or flexor spasms of the legs and sometimes the trunk may be provoked by active or passive attempts to rise from a bed or wheelchair. The physical findings include spasticity, usually more marked in the legs than in the arms. The deep tendon reflexes are exaggerated, sustained clonus may be elicited, and extensor plantar responses are observed. All of these manifestations are commonly asymmetrical. Occasionally, deep tendon reflexes may be decreased because of lesions interrupting the reflex arc at a segmental level, and one may observe an inverted reflex wherein one reflex, such as the triceps, is lost and the efferent component is represented by a contraction of a muscle below the lesion, such as the triceps muscle. The Achilles' reflex can be absent in lesions of the sacral segments of the spinal cord with or without concomitant sphincter and sexual problems. Occasionally, reduced reflexes reflect hypotonia resulting from cerebellar pathway lesions. Amyotrophy, when observed, most frequently affects the small muscles of the hand; lesions of the motor root exit zones may produce muscle denervation caused by axon loss. Secondary entrapment neuropathies are also a cause of muscle atrophy in patients with MS. A common pattern of disease evolution seen in the spinal form of MS is an ascending pattern of weakness that begins with involvement of the lower extremities and spreads to involve first one upper extremity and then the other, beginning in the intrinsic hand muscles. Frequently, there is an associated weakness of the trunk muscles with abnormal posture and involvement of respiratory muscles.

IMPAIRMENT OF CEREBELLAR PATHWAYS

Cerebellar pathway impairment results in gait imbalance, difficulty in performing coordinated actions with the arms, and slurred speech. Examination reveals the usual features of cerebellar dysfunction, such as dysmetria, decomposition of complex movements, and hypotonia, most often observed in the upper extremities. An intention tremor may be noted in the limbs and head. Walking is impaired by truncal ataxia. Ocular findings of nystagmus, ocular dysmetria, and frequent refixation saccades suggest cerebellar or cerebellovestibular connection dysfunction. Speech can be scanning or explosive. In severe cases of MS, there is complete astasia (inability to stand), inability to use the arms because of a violent intention tremor, and virtually incomprehensible speech. Cerebellar signs are usually mixed with pyramidal (corticospinal) tract signs.

IMPAIRMENT OF BLADDER, BOWEL, AND SEXUAL FUNCTIONS

The extent of sphincter and sexual dysfunction often parallels the degree of motor impairment in the lower extremities. The most common complaint related to urinary bladder dysfunction is urgency, usually the result of uninhibited detrusor contraction, reflecting a suprasegmental lesion. As the disease progresses, urinary incontinence becomes more frequent. With involvement of sacral segments of the spinal cord, symptoms of bladder hypoactivity may evolve, such as decreased urinary flow, interrupted micturition, and incomplete bladder emptying. An atonic dilatated bladder that empties by overflow results from loss of perception of bladder fullness and is usually associated with urethral, as well as anal and genital hypoesthesia, and sensory deficits in the sacral dermatomes. A dysynergic voluntary sphincter, interrupting bladder emptying, will lead to frequent small volume urinations, combined with a large postvoiding residual. When evaluating bladder incontinence or urgency in patients with MS, one must exclude other causes, particularly in multiparous women. Urinary tract infections are common in MS, especially in women. These infections usually do not cause fever and back pain and may increase the extent of bladder dysfunction.

Constipation is more common than fecal incontinence and can reflect both upper and lower motor neuron impairment in addition to decreased general mobility. Almost all patients with paraplegia require special measures to maintain regular bowel movements.

Sexual dysfunction, although frequently overlooked, is a common occurrence in MS. Approximately 50% of patients become completely sexually inactive secondary to their disease, and an additional 20% become sexually less active. Men experience various degrees of erectile dysfunction, often with rapid loss of erection at attempted intercourse, whereas loss of ejaculation is less common. Most women preserve their orgasmic capabilities, sometimes even in the presence of complete loss of bladder and bowel function. Sexual dysfunction can be the result of multiple problems, including the direct effects of lesions of the motor and sensory pathways within the spinal cord in addition to psychological factors involved with self-image, self-esteem, and fear of rejection from the sexual partner. Mechanical problems created by spasticity, paraparesis, and incontinence further aggravate the problem.

COGNITIVE IMPAIRMENT

Data from formal neuropsychological studies indicate that cognitive involvement has been underreported in MS. Neuropsychological test results have shown that 34–65% of patients with MS have cognitive impairment. The most frequent abnormalities are with abstract conceptualization, recent memory, attention, and speed of information processing. Patients refer to memory loss or frustration. The abnormalities are usually not apparent during a routine office visit. In a fast-paced environment with multiple stimuli, the cognitive deficit of the MS patient is most obvious. Aphasia, neglect syndrome, cortical blindness, or marked behavioral problems are rare.

Two kinds of recent data have added urgency to the need to assess cognitive deficits: the demonstration by Trapp and colleagues *(6)* of ongoing axon loss in central white matter beginning at the earliest stages of MS and the demonstration that thinning of the corpus callosum, enlargement of the ventricular system, and other evidences of brain atrophy can be measured accurately by MRI and also begin earlier than previously believed.

Cross-sectional studies have shown some degree of affective disturbance in up to two-thirds of patients with MS *(33)*. Depression is the most common manifestation and is, in part, secondary to the burden of having to cope with a chronic, incurable disease. Some data suggest that depression is more common in patients with MS than in others with chronic medical conditions, in whom the lifetime risk of depression was 12.9% in one study. This contrasts with a study of 221 patients with MS, in whom the risk for depression was 34% *(32)*. Some data indicate a comorbid association, presumably genetic, between bipolar illness and MS. Frontal or subcortical white-matter disease may also be a contributory causative factor. Euphoria is usually associated with moderate or severe mental impairment. Patients may manifest a dysphoric state with swings from depression to elation. On occasion, acute cerebral lesions can manifest as a confusional state.

EPILEPSY

Epilepsy is more common in patients with MS than in the general population, occurring in 2 to 3% of patients *(33)*. Convulsions may be either tonic-clonic or partial complex. They generally are benign and transient and respond well to antiepileptic drug therapy or require no therapy. The prevalence of cortical syndromes, such as aphasia, apraxia, and agnosia, is low. As an example, in a study of 5715 patients with MS, 51 (0.89%) experienced seizure activity *(36)*. Generalized tonic-clonic seizures were most common (35 patients, 69%), followed by simple or complex partial seizures (11 patients, 22%). Of the 45 patients who received antiepileptic drug therapy, 35 (78%) became seizure free, whereas 5 (11%) had intractable seizures.

CLINICAL FEATURES DISTINCTIVE OF MULTIPLE SCLEROSIS

Although there are no clinical phenomena that are unique to MS, some are highly characteristic of the disease (Table 1). Bilateral internuclear ophthalmoplegia has been mentioned. Lhermitte's phenomenon is a transient sensory symptom described as an electric shock radiating down the spine or into the limbs on flexion of the neck. It may be infrequent or occur with the least movement of the head or neck. Although most frequently encountered in MS, this symptom can be seen with other lesions of the cervical cord, including tumors, cervical disc herniation, postradiation myelopathy, and after trauma.

Paroxysmal attacks of motor or sensory phenomena may arise as a manifestation of demyelinating lesions. Within the brainstem, lesions can cause paroxysmal diplopia, facial paresthesia, trigeminal neuralgia, ataxia, and dysarthria. Motor system involvement results in painful tonic contractions of muscles of one or two (homolateral) limbs, trunk, and occasionally the face, but these rarely occur in all four limbs or the trunk. These paroxysmal attacks usually respond to low doses of carbamazepine and frequently remit after several weeks to months, usually without recurrence.

Heat sensitivity is a well-known occurrence in MS (Uhtoff's phenomenon); small increases in the body temperature can temporarily worsen current or preexisting signs and symptoms. This phenomenon is encountered in other neurological diseases but to a lesser extent and is presumably the result of conduction block developing in nerves as the body temperature increases. Normally, the nerve conduction safety factor decreases with increasing temperature until a point is reached at which conduction block occurs; this point of conduction block is reached at a much lower temperature in demyelinated nerves.

Fatigue is a characteristic finding in MS, usually described as physical exhaustion that is unrelated to the amount of activity performed. Many patients complain of feeling exhausted on waking, even if they have slept soundly. Fatigue can appear also during the day but may be partially or completely relieved by rest. There is a poor correlation between fatigue and the overall severity of disease or with the presence of any particular symptom or sign. Unlike cognitive deficit, no MRI findings correlate with fatigue, or with depression *(37–40)*. Fatigue is often seen in association with an acute attack and may precede the focal neurological features of the attack and persist long after the attack has subsided.

DIAGNOSTIC CRITERIA

The new McDonald criteria (Table 4) has several advantages. The former categories of possible, probable, and definite MS have become obsolete. The MRI criteria are based on extensive data of Barkof and Tintore and are designed to retain sensitivity while enhancing specificity. They will have little usefulness in patients with clear-cut demyelinating syndromes, such as ON or a brainstem syndrome; in such cases, many clinicians will be satisfied with less stringent MRI criteria. In patients with obscure symptoms, the criteria will help avoid premature diagnosis and treatment. In addition, criteria for primary progressive MS are proposed. Revisions to the McDonald criteria have been proposed. For example, the role of spinal cord lesions must be evaluated and included. It may take some time before the final criteria are decided on and accepted as the standard for diagnosis.

There remains the clinical problem, distinct from research criteria, of the patient early in the course who does not meet such diagnostic criteria. In the setting of a monophasic neurological illness that is clinically consistent with MS and in the presence of multifocal white-matter lesions on MRI consistent with demyelinating plaques, the diagnosis of MS is almost certain. In Brex et al.'s long-term study *(41)*, which followed patients with initial demyelinating episodes for up to 14 years, in practical terms, no diagnoses were encountered other than suspected MS or definite MS. In addition, follow-up studies have shown that a significant percentage of patients with MRI lesions detected at onset do not progress to clinically symptomatic MS, after many years of follow-up. The issue of the monophasic demyelinating disease is discussed in the section on Clinically Isolated Syndromes. Such patients may be classed as suspected MS; they may in fact represent particularly benign forms of the disease.

A common error is to overinterpret multiple hyperintense lesions on MRI as equivalent to MS. Clinical symptoms must be consistent with MS. A few white-matter lesions in T2-weighted MRI scans are not infrequent, particularly in the elderly, and do not indicate a diagnosis of MS. CNS vasculitides, such as SLE, Sjögren's disease, polyarteritis nodosa, syphilis, retroviral diseases, and Behçet's disease, may all produce multifocal lesions with or without a relapsing-remitting course. SLE can present as a recurrent neurological syndrome before the systemic manifestations of this disease declare themselves. Behçet's syndrome is characterized by buccogenital ulcerations in addition to the multifocal neurological findings. Although rare, acute disseminated encephalomyelitis (ADEM) must be considered in the differential diagnosis. An MS-like phenotype associated with mitochondrial gene defects has been described, cerebral autosomal-dominant arteriopathy with subcortical infarcts and leukoencephalopathy (CADASIL); it is of note that when there are multiple MS cases in a family, maternal transmission is more frequent than paternal transmission.

More important than features characteristic for MS are features that should prompt the clinician to reconsider the diagnosis of MS. Many physicians fail to pursue further diagnostic steps when a patient is diagnosed with MS. Features that should alert the clinician to the possibility of other diseases include:

- Family history of neurological disease.
- A well-demarcated spinal level in the absence of disease above the foramen magnum.
- Prominent back pain that persists.
- Symptoms and signs that can be attributed to one anatomical site.
- Patients who are over 60 years of age or younger than 15 years at the onset of disease.
- Progressive disease.

None of these features excludes the diagnosis of MS, but in these situations, one should explore the possibility of other etiologies before accepting the diagnosis.

The differential diagnosis of MS is limited in the setting of a young adult who has had two or more clinically distinct episodes of CNS dysfunction with at least partial resolution. Diagnostic difficulties arise in patients who have atypical presentations, monophasic episodes, or progressive illness.

- The unusual nature of some sensory symptoms and the difficulty patients experience in describing such symptoms may result in a misdiagnosis of hysteria.
- A monophasic illness with symptoms attributable to one site in the CNS creates a large differential that includes neoplasms, vascular events, or infections.
- The most trouble arises with progressive CNS dysfunction; great care must be taken in these patients to exclude treatable etiologies (compressive spinal cord lesions, arteriovenous malformations, cavernous angiomas, and Arnold-Chiari malformation), infection (HTLV-1), HIV, or hereditary disorders (adult metachromatic leukodystrophy, adrenomyelo-leukodystrophy, and spinocerebellar disorders).

COURSE

The most characteristic clinical course of MS is the occurrence of relapses (Fig. 1), which can be defined as the acute or subacute onset of clinical dysfunction that usually reaches its peak from days to several weeks, followed by a remission during which the symptoms and signs resolve partially or completely. The minimum duration for a relapse has been arbitrarily established at 24 hours. Clinical symptoms of shorter duration are less likely to represent what is considered as a true relapse (i.e., new lesion formation or extension of previous lesion size). Worsening of previous clinical dysfunction can occur concurrently with fever, physical activity, or metabolic upset and last for hours to a day or more. Such worsening is believed to reflect conduction block in previously demyelinated axons. Relapses of MS vary markedly regarding CNS site involved, the frequency of attacks (the free interval between relapses ranges from weeks to years), the mode of onset (from quite sudden to subacute), and the duration, severity, and quality of remission. The frequency of relapses is highly variable and depends on the population studied and the closeness of observation and recording by patients and physicians. Summaries of many studies provide an average figure of 0.4–0.6 relapses per year. Patients followed closely in clinical trials have higher relapse rates, probably reflecting self-selection and closer reporting and examinations in such studies. The attack rate in the placebo group in clinical studies ranges from 0.8 to 1.2 attacks per year. In

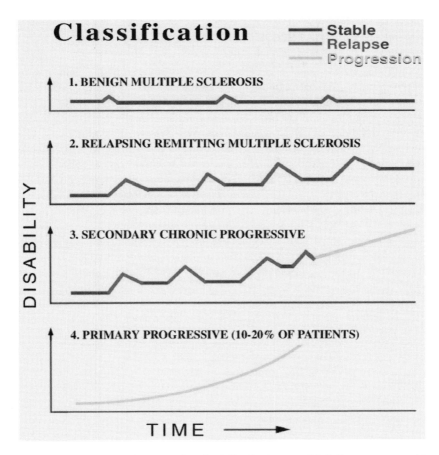

Fig. 1. Relapsing-remitting MS: Clearly defined relapses with full recovery or with sequelae and residual deficit on recovery. The periods between disease relapses are characterized by a lack of disease progression. Primary-progressive MS: Disease progression from onset with occasional plateaus and temporary minor improvements allowed. Secondary-progressive MS: Initial relapsing-remitting disease course followed by progression with or without occasional relapses, minor remissions, and plateaus. Two severity outcomes are also described.

general, relapses are more frequent during the first years of the disease and tend to wane in later years. A course marked by relapses, interspersed by periods during which the disease seems relatively dormant, is termed relapsing-remitting.

The course of MS can be expressed in patients as follows:

1. Severe relapses, increasing disability, and early death.
2. Many short attacks, tending to increase in duration and severity.
3. Slow progression from onset, superimposed relapses, and increasing disability.

4. Slow progression from onset without relapses.
5. Abrupt onset with good remission followed by long latent phase.
6. Relapses of diminishing frequency and severity, slight residual disability only.
7. Abrupt onset, few if any relapses after first year, no residual disability *(42)*.

Approximately 15% of patients never experience a second relapse. The exact frequency of such benign MS is unknown, however, because many such individuals never come to medical attention. Autopsy studies found significant numbers of cases with CNS pathology consistent with MS and yet no documented clinical evidence of such disease. Similarly, MRI studies have shown MS-like plaques in T2-weighted scans in patients who have never had a neurological episode. Asymptomatic relatives of patients with MS have MRI lesions consistent with demyelination in up to 15% of these relatives *(43)*. The use of MRI may expand the spectrum of MS by detecting milder cases that previously were not included in prognosis studies.

A standardization of terms has been agreed on to determine the pattern and course of the illness *(44)*. Four categories of disease are described:

- *Relapsing-remitting MS:* Clearly defined relapses with full recovery or with sequelae and residual deficit on recovery. The periods between disease relapses are characterized by a lack of disease progression.
- *Primary-progressive MS:* Disease progression from onset with occasional plateaus and temporary minor improvements allowed.
- *Secondary-progressive MS:* Initial relapsing-remitting disease course followed by progression with or without occasional relapses, minor remissions, and plateaus.
- *Progressive-relapsing MS:* Progressive disease from onset, with clear acute relapses, with or without full recovery. The periods between relapses are characterized by continuing progression.

Two severity outcomes are also described:

1. Benign MS is a disease in which the patient remains fully functional in all neurological systems 15 years after the disease onset.
2. Malignant MS is a disease with a rapid progressive course, leading to significant disability in multiple neurological systems or death in a relatively short time after disease onset.

Data from a clinic-based study of 1100 patients *(45)* who represented the population of the region found that 66% of patients at onset had relapsing and remitting disease, 15% had relapsing-progressive, and 19% had progressive disease from the onset. Patients evolved from a relapsing-remitting course to a progressive course; 85% of patients began with a relapsing course, but the proportion continuing as relapsing disease decreased steadily, so that by 9 years from onset, only 50% were still relapsing. Likewise, the probability of reaching 6 on the Kurtzke disability score was 50% 16 to 17 years after onset. The course of MS with onset after the age of 40 was progressive in more than 60% of patients.

The rate of clinical progression of MS is variable. The commonly used index of clinical disability, the Kurtzke disability status score (DSS), or the expanded version called the expanded disability status score (EDSS), uses numbers ranging from

0, for normal examination and function, to 10, for death caused by MS. This scale is nonlinear, with great emphasis on ambulation capabilities with scores above 4.

Most MS populations have bimodal distributions of EDSS scores, with peaks at values of 1 and 6 (ambulation with unilateral assistance). The time spent by a patient at a given level of disability varies with the score. Thus, for patients with DSS scores of 4 or 5, median time spent at these levels was 1.2 years, whereas for those at DSS 1, median time to stay at that level was 4 years, and at DSS 6, 3 years. These results have powerful implications for the conduct of clinical studies with respect to patient selection, stratification, and duration of follow-up: if many patients of DSS 1 or 6 are included, little movement is seen in a group followed for 1 or 2 years. The rate of progression with chronic progressive disease in the placebo groups of three clinical trials ranged from 0.5 to 0.7 points per year on the DSS scale.

In a cohort of 308 patients followed for 25 years, the following data emerged *(46)*:

- 80% of the patients had reached the progressive phase by 25 years.
- 15% of the patients had died.
- 65% of the patients had reached EDSS 6 (requiring aids for walking).
- 50% of the patients reached EDSS 6 within 16 years of onset.

The EDSS, although universally used in clinical trials, has numerous serious limitations. Even with special training and examiner blinding, interrater and intrarater variations in scoring are common. EDSS scores of 4 and higher depend almost entirely on the ability to walk. Developing dementia, vision loss, or weakness of hands may pass undetected by the scoring. An obvious implication of these facts is that other outcome measures should be used as well, and that minor changes in EDSS alone should not be overinterpreted.

The Multiple Sclerosis Functional Composite Scale (MSFC) is a more recent clinical tool designed to avoid the problems encountered with the EDSS. The MSFC consists of three parts: (1) Paced Auditory Serial Addition Test (PASAT), (2) 9-Hole Peg Test (9HPT), and (3) Timed 25-Foot Walk (T25FW). These three measures take into account cognition, upper extremity, and lower extremity functions. A z-score is obtained for each measure, and a combined z-score is then derived. The MSFC has been validated in several clinical trials. The tests can be performed by a nonphysician and are highly reproducible and predictable *(47–49)*.

EFFECT OF EXOGENOUS FACTORS ON THE COURSE

The role of several exogenous factors either influencing the development of MS or inducing disease exacerbations has been examined using epidemiological techniques. A disproportionately high number of relapses occur in patients with MS who have suffered recently from viral infections, and a high number of infections are followed by acute attacks. Increased interferon (IFN)-γ and tumor necrosis factor (TNF)-α produced by cells of the immune system during viral infections may play a role in this increased relapse rate by increasing expression of major histocompatibility complex class II antigens and adhesion molecules on cells of the immune system and CNS, with a resultant increase in the number of activated T-cells being attracted to the CNS. Controversy exists about a link between occurrence of stressful events and exacerbation of MS. Trauma is not implicated in disease induction or relapse, although in the experimental animal model EAE, lesions are most prominent at sites of preexistent traumatic lesions. Performance of neurological diagnostic procedures, such as myelography and lumbar puncture, has not been linked with aggravation of the MS disease course, neither has administration of local or general anesthetics. Recent data do not establish a link between vaccination and disease exacerbations, and few clinicians withhold immunization programs, for example, for influenza or hepatitis.

EFFECT OF PREGNANCY ON THE COURSE

MS is a disease that predominantly affects women and has a maximum incidence during childbearing years. The influence of pregnancy on MS has been repeatedly examined, with evidence that relapses are reduced late in pregnancy and are more frequent than expected in the 3-month postpartum period. However, this is not the finding in all studies. There is general agreement that the overall prognosis is no different in women who have been pregnant compared with those who have not. Studies of women with MS reveal no increase in stillbirths, ectopic pregnancies, or spontaneous abortions. These data would suggest that pregnancy has no ill effect on MS and that MS has no negative effect on the fetus or the course of pregnancy. In a study of postmenopausal women, there *(50)*. An important issue in the pregnant woman with MS is to avoid exposing the fetus to toxic drugs (Table 8).

PROGNOSIS

Although great individual variability exists regarding disease prognosis, several factors have been identified as possible prognostic indicators. The rate of clinical progression of MS is variable. The commonly used index of clinical disability, the DSS, or the expanded version (EDSS), uses numbers ranging from 0 for normal examination and function to 10 for death caused by MS. This scale is nonlinear, with great emphasis on ambulation capabilities with scores higher than 4. Most MS populations have bimodal distributions of EDSS scores, with peaks at values of 1 and 6 (ambulation with unilateral assistance). The time spent by a patient at a given level of disability varies with the score. Thus, for patients with DSS scores of 4 or 5, median time spent at these levels was 1.2 years, whereas for those at DSS 1, median time to stay at that level was 4 years, and at DSS 6, 3 years. These results have powerful implications for the conduct of clinical studies with respect to patient selection, stratification, and duration of follow-up: if many patients of DSS 1 or 6 are included, little movement is seen in a group followed for 1 or 2 years. The rate of progression with chronic progressive disease in the placebo groups of three clinical trials ranged from 0.5 to 0.7 points per year on the DSS scale.

A large database of 1844 MS patients was analyzed to determine predictors of disability. This study concluded that it takes longer to reach landmarks of irreversible disability in younger female patients with relapsing disease, patients present-

Table 8
Safety in Pregnancy of Drugs Used in the Treatment of Multiple Sclerosis

Category B: Animal data showing no harm to the fetus; no human data available
Glatiramer acetate (Copaxone)
Pemoline
Oxybutynin
Fluoxetine (and other selective serotonin reuptake inhibitors)
Desmopressin

Category C: Animal data shows harm to the fetus; no human data available
Corticosteroids
Interferon (IFN)-β-1a (Avonex/Rebif)
IFN-β-1b (Betaseron)
Baclofen
Amantadine
Tizanidine
Carbamazepine

Category D: Known to cause fetal harm when administered to pregnant women
Azathioprine
Cladribine
Cyclophosphamide
Mitoxantrone (Novantrone)

Category X: Contraindicated for use during pregnancy
Methotrexate

Source: Modified from ref. *50*.

ing with ON, and patients with fewer relapses in the first years of the disease. The study also showed that these good prognostic clinical variables held true for patients up to an EDSS of 4 but did not seem to remain predictive of the time course of disability past 4 to landmarks 6 and 7 *(51)*.

Another MS study between 1976 and 1987 in Norway verified these results and also evaluated primary progressive (PP) patients. The probability of being alive after 15 years was 94.8%. The probability of managing without a wheelchair was 75.8%, of walking without assistance was 60.3%, and of not being awarded a disability pension was 46%. The probability of still having a relapsing remitting (RR) course after 15 years was 62%. Analysis of the total MS population showed that patients with PPMS had more than 7.5 times higher risk of reaching EDSS = 6 than patients with RRMS *(52)*.

Between 1990 and 1998, 98 newly diagnosed patients were evaluated for prognosis using six risk factors:

1. Age at onset (<40 vs >40)
2. Symptoms at onset (isolated sensory or cranial nerve vs motor or sensory plus motor)
3. MRI (at first attack vs CDMS)

4. Interval between first and second attack (>2.5 or <2.5 years)
5. Attack frequency in first 2 years (<2 or >2)
6. Completeness of recovery from initial attack (good vs poor)

Analysis showed 17% with low risk of progression (0–1 risk factors) and 24% with high of progression (4–6 risk factors). The high-risk group did significantly worse in terms of final EDSS and progression to higher EDSS. At the time of diagnosis of CDMS, MRI findings suggestive of MS were seen in 84%, suspicious in 13%, and negative in 3% *(53)*.

Sex: MS appears to follow a more benign course in women than in men.

Age at onset: The average age at onset of MS is 29 years. Onset at an early age is seemingly a favorable factor, whereas onset at a later age carries a less favorable prognosis. As previously stated, the pattern of disease varies in different age groups, with the relapsing-remitting form being more common in younger patients and the progressive form being more common in the older age group. Data are lacking regarding whether prognosis differs as a function of age in patients with similar patterns of disease.

Initial disease course: The relapsing form of the disease is associated with a better prognosis than progressive disease. A high rate of relapses early in the course of illness may correlate with shorter time to reach EDSS 6, as does a short first interval between attacks.

Initial complaints: Among initial symptoms, impairment of sensory pathways or cranial nerve dysfunction, particularly ON, are found in several studies to be favorable prognostic features, whereas pyramidal and particularly brainstem and cerebellar symptoms carry a poor prognosis. Both benign and fulminant forms of MS are recognized. There is no agreement among workers in the field as to the meaning of these terms. It is the general experience that a patient whose disease has had a benign course for 15 years only rarely develops a more severe course. Patients with mild disease (EDSS score 0–3) 5 years after diagnosis only uncommonly progress to severe disease (EDSS score 6) by 10 years (7.5% of patients) and 15 years (11.5% of patients) *(46)*. The term malignant MS is variably used by different workers; some use it to imply a rapid course, others to a clinical course in which there are frequent severe relapses with little recovery. Clues to etiology, susceptibility, and resistance factors must be present in such extremes of the clinical spectrum, but they remain elusive at present. Entities such as Devic's disease, Baló's concentric sclerosis, and particularly Marburg's disease are more fulminant variants of MS with early disability and even death.

OPTIC NEURITIS

The incidence of MRI abnormalities in children with ON is less than that in adults, which, when coupled with clinical experience, suggests that the rate of progression to MS in children with isolated ON may well be less than that in adults. Five-year data from the original Optic Neuritis Treatment Trial revealed that the 5-year cumulative probability of developing clinically definite MS was 30% and did not differ by treatment group (oral prednisone, IV methylprednisolone, and placebo). However, MRI was a strong predictor; the 5-year risk of developing clinically definite MS was 16% in patients with no brain MRI lesions and 51% in patients with three or more lesions *(31)*.

MYELOPATHIC SYNDROMES

Acute Myelopathy

Patients presenting with acute complete transverse myelitis have a cited risk of MS of only 5–10%. However, partial or incomplete myelitis is a much more common clinical entity and bears more relevance to MS. Studies examining the issue of acute partial myelitis as an initial presentation of MS found that 57–72% of such patients had cranial MRI abnormalities consistent with MS. Follow-up from 3 to 5 years found that 60–90% of these patients developed MS, whereas 10–30% of those with normal MRI developed MS *(12)*. CSF studies suggest that patients with monosymptomatic disease with positive OCBs have a higher risk of evolution to MS than those without OCBs, although CSF results do not help further in prognosis when compared with MRI alone. CSF analysis would be most useful in a situation in which MRI is not available.

Chronic Myelopathy

In patients with chronic progressive myelopathy, 60–70% have cranial MRI abnormalities consistent with MS in the absence of clinical evidence of disease above the level of the spinal cord. What remains unclear is whether the remaining 30% have a disease other than MS or whether MS can manifest as a purely spinal disorder. Probably both situations apply; improved spinal neuroimaging should help resolve this issue.

VARIANTS OF MULTIPLE SCLEROSIS

Diseases affecting CNS myelin can be classified on the basis of whether a primary biochemical abnormality of myelin exists (dysmyelinating) or whether some other process damages the myelin or oligodendroglial cell (demyelinating). Demyelinating diseases in which normal myelin is disrupted include autoimmune, infectious, toxic and metabolic, and vascular processes (Table 9). Dysmyelinating diseases in which a primary abnormality of the formation of myelin exists include several hereditary disorders (Table 9), infectious demyelinating disease (progressive multifocal leukoencephalopathy), toxic and metabolic demyelinating diseases, and vascular demyelinating disease (Binswanger's disease). A list of differential diagnoses can be found in Table 10.

MS is a condition with many variable forms, but in most cases the common signs and symptoms described are readily apparent, and with proper laboratory confirmation, the diagnosis is not difficult. Some patients have their entire clinical illness confined to the optic nerves. One optic nerve may be affected sequentially

Table 9
Diseases of Myelin

Autoimmune
Acute disseminated encephalomyelitis
Acute hemorrhagic leukoencephalopathy
Multiple sclerosis

Infectious
Progressive multifocal leukoencephalopathy

Toxic/metabolic
Carbon monoxide
Vitamin B_{12} deficiency
Mercury intoxication (Minamata disease)
Alcohol/tobacco amblyopia
Central pontine myelinolysis
Marchiafava-Bignami syndrome
Hypoxia
Radiation

Vascular
Binswanger's disease

Hereditary disorders of myelin metabolism
Adrenoleukodystrophy
Metachromatic leukodystrophy
Krabbe's disease
Alexander's disease
Canavan-van Bogaert disease
Pelizaeus-Merzbacher disease
Phenylketonuria

after another, or there can be simultaneous bilateral visual loss, a state that is uncommon in classic MS. In some instances, a head MRI will show scattered intracerebral lesions in addition to lesions of the optic nerves or CSF examination will show OCB, attesting to some degree of dissemination of the lesions. Children and preadolescent patients are more likely than adults to have recurrent or simultaneous optic neuropathy. The distinction from an MS variant can be challenging. Sarcoidosis is commonly a diagnostic consideration in patients with bilateral ON. However, there are several inflammatory demyelinating disorders that bear an unknown relationship to MS. They are listed here as variants of MS, rather than as separate illnesses, because it is often found, after long follow-up, that the disease has reverted to a more standard variety of MS.

Recurrent Optic Neuropathy

There are patients whose entire clinical illness is confined to the optic nerves. They may have sequential affection of one nerve, then the other, or they may have

Table 10
Differential Diagnosis in Multiple Sclerosis

Inflammatory diseases
Granulomatous angiitis
Systemic lupus erythematosus
Sjögren's disease
Behçet's disease
Polyarteritis nodosa
Paraneoplastic encephalomyelopathies
Acute disseminated encephalomyelitis/postinfectious encephalomyelitis

Infectious diseases
Lyme neuroborreliosis
Human T-cell lymphotropic virus type 1 infection*
Human immunodeficiency virus infection
Progressive multifocal leukoencephalopathy*
Neurosyphilis*

Granulomatous diseases
Sarcoidosis
Wegener's granulomatosis
Lymphomatoid granulomatosis

Diseases of myelin
Metachromatic leukodystrophy (juvenile and adult)*
Adrenomyeloleukodystrophy*

Miscellaneous
Spinocerebellar disorders*
Arnold-Chiari malformation
Vitamin B_{12} deficiency*

*Indicates disorders that are predominantly important to differentiate in the setting of progressive disease.

simultaneous bilateral vision loss, a state that is quite uncommon in classic MS. In some instances, MRI of the head shows (in addition to lesions of the optic nerves) scattered intracerebral lesions, or a CSF examination shows OCB, attesting to some degree of dissemination of the lesions. Children and preadolescent patients are more likely than adults to have recurrent or simultaneous optic neuropathy. Rarely there is slowly progressive optic neuropathy, similar to that seen with optic nerve sheath tumors, such as meningioma. The distinction from an MS variant can be challenging. In bilateral ON, sarcoidosis is commonly a diagnostic consideration.

Devic's Disease (Neuromyelitis Optica)

A combination of bilateral optic neuropathy and cervical myelopathy comprise this condition, which most authorities now classify as a variant of MS. Reported cases indicate that the myelopathy tends to be more severe, with less likelihood of recovery, and that the neuropathological features at autopsy are those of a much more severe necrotic lesion of the cord rather than incomplete demyelination *(54)*. In some patients, the optic neuropathy and the myelopathy occur at the same time; in others, one or the other component is delayed. The longer the interval, the more like typical MS is the pathology. Because the optic nerve and the cervical spinal cord are two of the locations in the nervous system in which MS lesions are typically found, many patients could be classified as having Devic's disease or syndrome. Little is to be gained by this nomenclature, because Devic's syndrome can be a manifestation of acute disseminated encephalomyelitis (ADEM) (*see* Acute Disseminated Encephalomyelitis), or rarely of other autoimmune disease, such as SLE. This is especially true of patients with relapsing Devic's syndrome, comprising approximately one-half of the patients. In a few patients, the distinction between an MS variant and SLE (so-called lupoid sclerosis) is essentially impossible to make, and some of these are patients with neuromyelitis optica (NMO). A study of 80 patients with NMO revealed that predictors of a relapsing course were longer interattack interval between the first two clinical events, older age at onset, female sex, and less severe motor impairment with the sentinel myelitis event. A history of other autoimmune disease, higher attack frequency during the first 2 years of disease, and better motor recovery after the index myelitis event were associated with mortality resulting from relapsing NMO with almost one-third of the deaths secondary to recurrent myelitis with respiratory failure and concomitant medical complications *(55)*.

Slowly Progressive Myelopathy

A syndrome of slowly progressive spinal cord dysfunction can present a major diagnostic challenge. If there are no sensory signs or symptoms, the entity known as primary lateral sclerosis, one of the group of motor neuron disease, may be the cause. HTLV-1 infection, vitamin B_{12} deficiency, and human immunodeficiency virus infection all can be excluded by appropriate testing. Spinal dural arteriovenous fistula can cause a steadily or stepwise progressive myelopathy, usually in the lower spinal segments. Adrenomyeloneuropathy should be considered. Numerous patients remain who do not fit into these categories and whose spinal MRI results are repeatedly negative. VERs, CSF OCBs, and MRI of the head show no sign of demyelination elsewhere. No firm diagnosis is possible. Minor clues that MS is present may be furnished by a Lhermitte's sign that has come and gone or by undue sensitivity to elevated temperature. The degree of compression of the cervical cord by intervertebral disc disease is often an issue in the middle-aged patient, because a majority of persons have some degree of disc disease. There is little doubt that some laminectomies have been carried out for cervical spondylosis where MS was the final correct diagnosis. Progressive myelopathy caused by MS is part of the primary progressive MS group and carries the poor prognosis typical of that group. The choice of therapy is difficult. Some patients do better for a time with monthly IV corticosteroid therapy.

Acute Tumor-Like Multiple Sclerosis (Marburg Variant)

Some patients with demyelinating disease present with a large acute lesion of one hemisphere or rarely other locations, such as the spinal cord. Mass effect may occur, with compression of the lateral ventricle and shift across the midline. The clinical abnormalities in such patients are variable: they may be slight even in a patient with a massive lesion, whereas confusion, hemiparesis, or neglect syndrome may be seen in another patient with a lesion that appears no different. Much of the T2 bright lesion volume is often caused by edema and may be rapidly responsive to corticosteroids. (This change with corticosteroids also may occur with glioma or CNS lymphoma and is, therefore, not a useful diagnostic criterion.) Biopsy is often required.

In a series of 31 patients with Marburg variant, the prognosis was good, most patients recovered well clinically, and their lesion volume rapidly cleared *(56)*. In 24 of the patients, the demyelinating lesion was solitary, whereas in the others there were one or more satellite nodules. Six of the patients were older than 57 years. At follow-up, 28 of the patients did not develop additional evidence of demyelinating activity during a 9-month to 12-year period. Others have reported a higher rate of recurrent disease, particularly a conversion to more ordinary types of MS, both clinically and by scan criteria *(57)*.

Acute Disseminated Encephalomyelitis (ADEM)

This variant is classically described as a uniphasic syndrome occurring in association with an immunization or vaccination (postvaccination encephalomyelitis) or systemic viral infection (parainfectious encephalomyelitis). Pathologically, perivascular inflammation, edema, and demyelination within the CNS are present. Clinically, patients present with the rapid development of focal or multifocal neurological dysfunction. Prototypical illness arises after acute measles infection or rabies vaccine administration. Uncertainty regarding the diagnosis occurs when patients with clinical features of ADEM occur on the background of viral infections or vaccine administration not significantly linked with the syndrome by epidemiological criteria.

Neurological sequelae complicate 1 in 400 to 1 in 1000 cases of measles infection *(58)*. Multiple subgroups of patients have been described, including those with diffuse cerebral features, focal or multifocal cerebral findings, cerebellar dysfunction, and spinal cord abnormalities; patients do not develop peripheral nerve damage or relapses of disease.

In addition to measles, an array of other viral and bacterial infections have tentatively been associated with ADEM, including rubella, mumps, herpes zoster, herpes simplex, influenza, EBV, coxsackievirus, Borrelia burgdorferi, mycoplasma, and leptospira. Acute encephalomyelitis occurring in the background of nonspecific viral illness is difficult to diagnose with certainty and to distinguish from episodes of MS.

The occurrence of neuroparalytic accidents as a consequence of the Pasteur rabies vaccine prepared from spinal cords of rabbits inoculated with fixed rabies virus was recorded soon after introduction of the treatment: the incidence of encephalomyelitis associated with the original Pasteur rabies vaccine prepared in rabbit brain has been estimated at 1 per 3000 to 35,000 vaccinations. Similar neurological complications were observed as a consequence of the Jenner vaccine used for the prevention of smallpox. Postvaccination ADEM does not result from the direct cytopathic effects of the virus but rather to immune-mediated mechanisms directed against specific components of the CNS *(59)*.

ADEM also has been associated with other vaccines, including pertussis, rubella, diphtheria, and measles. The association between influenza vaccination, particularly the swine flu vaccine, and ADEM has been the subject of medicolegal controversy.

ADEM has been reported after the administration of some drugs. These drugs include sulfonamides and paraaminosalicylic acid (PAS)/streptomycin.

All of these associations can only be substantiated by strong epidemiological evidence or by the development of a pathognomonic laboratory finding for ADEM. However, neither of these circumstances currently exists.

Clinical features of the postvaccination and parainfectious syndromes are similar, except that the postrabies vaccination complications frequently involve the peripheral nervous system as well as the CNS. Many patients with postrabies immunization illness have only mild clinical features of fever, headache, or myalgia without CSF pleocytosis.

The hallmark clinical feature of the disorder is the development of a focal or multifocal neurological disorder after exposure to virus or receipt of vaccine. In some, but not all cases, a prodromal phase of several days of fever, malaise, and myalgias occurs. The onset of the CNS disorder is usually rapid (abrupt or up to several hours), reaching peak dysfunction within several days. Initial features include encephalopathy ranging from lethargy to coma, seizures, and focal and multifocal signs reflecting cerebral (hemiparesis), brain stem (cranial nerve palsies), and spinal cord (paraparesis) involvement. Other reported findings include movement disorders and ataxia. Each of these findings may occur as isolated features or in various combinations.

Features deemed characteristic of ADEM include simultaneous bilateral ON, loss of consciousness, meningismus, loss of deep tendon reflexes and retained abdominal reflexes in the presence of Babinski's reflexes, central body temperature of >100°F (37.8°C), and severe shooting limb pains. By comparison, features characteristic of MS are unilateral ON, diplopia, hyperactive reflexes, and preserved awareness. Headache is an equivocal feature.

Recovery can begin within days, with complete resolution noted on occasion within a few days but more often over the course of weeks or months. Relapses are rare. Recovery from ADEM is more rapid compared to MS and usually more complete.

The mortality rate varies among reported series but is usually estimated at 10 to 30%, with complete recovery rates of 50% cited. Poor prognosis is correlated with severity and abruptness of onset of the clinical syndrome. Measles virus-associated ADEM may carry a worse prognosis than vaccine-associated disease. In earlier series, the occurrence of acute hemiplegias, which were interpreted as vascular occlusions and akin to the syndrome of acute hemiplegia of childhood, carried a particularly unfavorable prognosis regarding recovery.

Multifocal CNS lesions are generally evident on MRI that are initially indistinguishable from those observed in MS *(60)*. Pathologically, ADEM produces scattered small perivenous lesions, often uniform in size, but this feature is not reliably detected by MRI. After several weeks, ADEM lesions show at least partial resolution without the appearance of new lesions, unlike MS. In some cases, lesions can persist. MRI in ADEM, as with MS, is more sensitive than CT scanning, which may, in some cases, reveal enhancing lesions.

The usual CSF formula is normal pressure, little or no (<100 cells/μL) increase in cell count, and a modest increase in protein. Well-documented cases exist with totally normal CSF pressure, cell counts, and protein content. Cases with high cell counts, including some polymorphonuclear cells and high protein values, represent a more necrotizing disease process. The high counts usually return to normal within a few days. The CSF Ig content is not usually increased, and OCB patterns are not usually observed. The content of myelin basic protein (MBP) in the CSF may be increased, as it can be in many conditions in which myelin destruction occurs, as in MS, or as part of more widespread tissue destructive process, such as cerebral infarction.

In many patients with postrabies vaccination and postmeasles ADEM, systemic blood lymphocyte sensitivity to MBP can be demonstrated in vitro, even though generalized cellular reactivity is depressed in patients with systemic measles virus infection. Although technically difficult to assess, CSF lymphocyte sensitivity to MBP may be even more marked than is systemic lymphocyte sensitivity. The occurrence of cases without MBP sensitivity indicates that this assay is insufficiently sensitive to establish or exclude the diagnosis of ADEM.

The diagnosis of ADEM can usually be made with confidence in the setting of a clear-cut antecedent event strongly associated with the disorder, such as measles infection or vaccination. The occurrence of an acute focal or multifocal CNS syndrome subsequent to a more nonspecific viral illness or vaccination in which the epidemiological link with ADEM is weak creates a wider differential diagnosis:

- An initial episode of what will prove to be MS: The presence of increased CSF IgG levels may favor MS. Follow-up MRI may be needed to distinguish the two disorders because the initial MRI scans can appear similar *(60)*. The occurrence of a nonspecific viral illness before the onset of the clinical neurological syndrome does not distinguish between MS and ADEM because the incidence of exacerbations of MS is increased after such infections.
- CNS vasculitis with or without systemic features (such as disseminated intravascular coagulation or serum sickness)

- Multiple cerebral infarcts, particularly embolic from infected cardiac valves
- Chronic meningitis or granulomatous disease (sarcoidosis).

In addition, encephalitis, abscess, or tumor needs to be excluded if the main clinical feature is unifocal.

ACUTE HEMORRHAGIC LEUKOENCEPHALITIS

Acute hemorrhagic leukoencephalitis is a rare entity that represents a hyper-acute form of ADEM *(61)*. The most frequent antecedent history is that of an upper respiratory infection. Given the nonspecific nature of the antecedent event and the lack of a specific diagnostic clinical laboratory test, the exact incidence and full clinical spectrum of the disorder can only be estimated and is based largely on descriptions of autopsy-proved cases.

The clinical manifestations, including focal or multifocal signs, seizures, and obtundation, mimic ADEM but develop more abruptly and are more severe. Relapse after initial recovery has been described. Fever is common.

The CSF usually demonstrates increased pressure, protein, and both white and red cells. The peripheral white blood cell count also is usually increased.

CT scans in suspected clinical cases show an initially normal scan followed by low-density white-matter lesions developing within 72 hours of the first symptoms. With improvement, the lesions on CT may largely resolve. MRI may yield additional information on lesion evolution.

The differential diagnosis of this syndrome includes entities that present as rapidly evolving focal cerebral disorders with fever and obtundation. These include brain abscess and encephalitis, particularly resulting from herpes simplex, in addition to those syndromes considered in the section on ADEM (*see* Acute Disseminated Encephalomyelitis).

ACUTE AND SUBACUTE TRANSVERSE MYELITIS

Acute and subacute transverse myelitis is defined as the development of isolated spinal cord dysfunction over hours or days in patients in whom there is no evidence of a compressive lesion. In the combined experience of several series reviewing complete transverse myelitis, 37% of patients reported a preceding febrile illness. The initial symptoms are paresthesias, back pain, or leg weakness; 37% of patients had the maximal deficit within 1 day, 45% in 1 to 10 days, and 18% in more than 10 days *(62)*.

Patients presenting with acute complete transverse myelitis have a cited risk of MS of only 5–10%. However, partial or incomplete myelitis is a much more common clinical entity and bears more relevance to MS; 57–72% of patients with acute partial myelitis as an initial presentation have cranial MRI abnormalities consistent with MS *(12,63)*. Over 3 to 5 years, 60 to 90% of these patients develop MS, whereas 10–30% of those with a normal MRI developed MS. CSF studies suggest that patients with monosymptomatic disease and positive OCBs have a higher risk of evolution to MS than those without OCBs, although CSF results do not help further in prognosis when compared to MRI alone. CSF analysis is most useful in the situation where MRI is not available.

CEREBELLITIS

Acute, isolated ataxia has been observed after many different viral illnesses, but most frequently in association with varicella infections. Cerebellar ataxia accounts for 50% of the postvaricella neurological syndromes, which overall occur in 1 in 1000 cases of childhood varicella *(64)*.

The prognosis for recovery is excellent, although the duration of symptoms varies from a few days up to 3 to 4 weeks. That most cases remit spontaneously and the etiology (direct invasion vs autoimmune) is unresolved leaves the issue of corticosteroid therapy unsettled.

CLINICALLY ISOLATED SYNDROMES (CIS)

Clinically isolated syndromes (CISs) are single, monosymptomatic attacks compatible with MS (e.g., ON) that can create a diagnostic and therefore therapeutic, dilemma. More than 80% of patients with a CIS and MRI lesions go on to develop MS, whereas approximately 20% have a self-limited process *(41)*. Identifying those 80% may have particular importance because some studies suggest that starting disease modifying therapies early in the course of MS improves outcomes.

The newer McDonald criteria incorporate MRI findings, potentially allowing for earlier diagnosis of patients with clinically isolated syndromes because two clinical events are not necessary. However, it is not clear that these criteria are sufficiently accurate in patients with CIS to make decisions regarding disease modifying therapy.

At least two studies have evaluated the ability of the McDonald criteria to predict which patients with clinically isolated syndromes will go on to develop MS *(65,66)*. One study prospectively evaluated 50 patients with CIS by clinical and MRI examinations at 3 months, 1 year, and 3 years of follow-up. At 1 year, fulfillment of the newer criteria had a sensitivity, specificity, and accuracy of 83% *(65)*. The second study was an analysis of 139 patients that is limited by a retrospective design and that MRI was performed at 1 year rather than 3 months and inconsistently used contrast *(66)*. Nevertheless, the sensitivity, specificity, and accuracy in predicting conversion to MS were similar to the previous report (74%, 86%, and 80%, respectively).

The conversion rate from a clinically isolated syndrome to clinically definite multiple sclerosis, defined as the patient's development of a second clinical attack, was evaluated by several investigators (Table 11). The conversion rate with an initially normal brain MRI was 6% after 5 years, 11% after 10 years, and 19% after 14.1 years. Only 4% of the patients with an initially normal brain MRI followed for 10 years reached an EDSS greater than 5.5, whereas patients with > 10 MRI lesions at onset had a conversion rate from 80 to 88% and up to 73% reached a score >5.5 on the EDSS.

Table 11
Risk of Multiple Sclerosis After Monosymptomatic Episodes*

Investigator (Ref)	Follow-up	Patients	MRI lesions (initial)	Conversion rate to CDMS	EDSS > 3	EDSS > 5.5
Morrissey	5 years	32	0	6%	0	
1993 *(12)*		6	1	17%	0	
		18	2–3	67%	17%	
		13	4–10	92%	30%	
		16	>10	80%	56%	
O'Riordan	10 years	27	0	11%	0	4%
1998 *(71)*		3	1	33%	0	0
		16	2–3	87%	31% 27%	13%
		15	4–10	87%	75%	20%
		20	>10	85%		35%
Brex	14.1 years	21	0	19%	0	0
2002 *(41)*		18	1–3	89%	31% 53%	12.5%
		15	4–10	87%	80%	38%
		17	>10	88%		73%

* The conversion rate to clinically definite MS (CDMS) indicates that the patient had a second clinical episode.
Adapted from refs. *12, 41,* and *71.*

Recently, patients with CIS were tested for serum antibodies to myelin oligo-dendrocyte protein (MOG) and MBP to predict time to definite MS. A second relapse occurred in 95% seropositive for both antibodies, 83% seropositive for MOG antibodies, and only 23% of seronegative patients *(67)*. Thus, additional prospective studies demonstrating greater accuracy in patients with clinically isolated syndromes are necessary before diagnosis based on the new criteria alone can be used to begin disease-modifying therapy. Assessment of B-cell measurements in the CSF may be more accurate as discussed in Chapter 6. In either case, early detection can lead to early treatment which has been shown to slow the disease progression.

REFERENCES

1. McDonald WI, Compston A, Edan G, et al. Recommended diagnostic criteria for multiple sclerosis: guidelines from the International Panel on the diagnosis of multiple sclerosis. Ann Neurol 2001;50:121–127.
2. Schumacher GA, Beebe G, Kibler RF, et al. Problems of experimental trials of therapy in multiple sclerosis: report by the panel on the evaluation of experimental trials of therapy in multiple sclerosis. Ann N Y Acad Sci 1965;122:552–568.
3. Poser CM, Paty DW, Scheinberg L, et al. New diagnostic criteria for multiple sclerosis: guidelines for research protocols. Ann Neurol 1983;13:227–231.

4. Barkhof F, Filippi M, Miller DH, et al. Comparison of MRI criteria at first presentation to predict conversion to clinically definite multiple sclerosis. Brain 1997;12:2059–2069.
5. Tintore M, Rovira A, Martiniez MJ, et al. Isolated demyelinating syndrome: comparison of different MRI criteria to predict conversion to clinically definite multiple sclerosis. Am J Neuroradiol 2000;1:702–706.
6. Trapp BD, Peterson J, Ransohoff RM, et al. Axonal transection in the lesions of multiple sclerosis. N Engl J Med 1998;338:278–285.
7. Newcombe J, Hawkins CP, Henderson CL, et al. Histopathology of multiple sclerosis lesions detected by magnetic resonance imaging in unfixed postmortem central nervous system tissue. Brain 1991;114(Pt 2):1013–1023.
8. Offenbacher H, Fazekas F, Schmidt R, et al. Assessment of MRI criteria for a diagnosis of MS. Neurology 1993;43:905.
9. Kidd D, Thorpe JW, Thompson AJ, et al. Spinal cord MRI using multi-array coils and fast spin echo. II. Findings in multiple sclerosis. Neurology 1993;43:2632–2637.
10. Paty DW, Oger JJ, Kastrukoff LF, et al. MRI in the diagnosis of MS: a prospective study with comparison of clinical evaluation, evoked potentials, oligoclonal banding, and CT. Neurology 1988;38:180.
11. Lee KH, Hashimoto SA, Hooge JP, et al. Magnetic resonance imaging of the head in the diagnosis of multiple sclerosis: a prospective 2-year follow-up with comparison of clinical evaluation, evoked potentials, oligoclonal banding, and CT. Neurology 1991;41:657.
12. Morrissey SP, Miller DH, Kendall BE, et al. The significance of brain magnetic resonance imaging abnormalities at presentation with clinically isolated syndromes suggestive of multiple sclerosis. A 5-year follow-up study. Brain 1993;116(pt 1):135–146.
13. Filippi M, Horsfield MA, Morrissey SP, et al. Quantitative brain MRI lesion load predicts the course of clinically isolated syndromes suggestive of multiple sclerosis. Neurology 1994;44:635.
14. Miller DH, Barkhof F, Nauta JJ. Gadolinium enhancement increases the sensitivity of MRI in detecting disease activity in multiple sclerosis. Brain 1993; 116(pt 5):1077.
15. Tortorella C, Codella M, Rocca MA, et al. Disease activity in multiple sclerosis studied by weekly triple-dose magnetic resonance imaging. J Neurol 1999;246:689.
16. Arnold DL, Riess GT, Matthews PM, et al. Use of proton magnetic resonance spectroscopy for monitoring disease progression in multiple sclerosis. Ann Neurol 1994;36:76.
17. Rudick RA, Whitaker JN. Cerebrospinal fluid tests for multiple sclerosis. In: Scheinberg P, ed. Neurology/Neurosurgery Update Series, Vol. 7. CPEC, Princeton, NJ, 1987, p 1.
18. Avasarala JR, Cross AH, Trotter JL. Oligoclonal band number as a marker for prognosis in multiple sclerosis. Arch Neurol 2001;58:2044.
19. McLean BN, Luxton RW, Thompson EJ. A study of immunoglobulin G in the cerebrospinal fluid of 1007 patients with suspected neurological disease using isoelectric focusing and the Log IgG-Index. A comparison and diagnostic applications. Brain 1990;113(pt 5):1269.
20. Gronseth GS, Ashman EJ. Practice parameter: the usefulness of evoked potentials in identifying clinically silent lesions in patients with suspected multiple sclerosis (an evidence-based review): Report of the Quality Standards Subcommittee of the American Academy of Neurology. Neurology 2000;54:1720.
21. Ascherio A, Zhang SM, Hernan MA, et al. Hepatitis B vaccination and the risk of multiple sclerosis. N Engl J Med 2001;344:327.
22. Confavreux C, Suissa S, Saddier P, et al. Vaccinations and the risk of relapse in multiple sclerosis. N Engl J Med 2001;344:319.
23. Hernan MA, Zhang SM, Lipworth L, et al. Multiple sclerosis and age at infection with common viruses. Epidemiology 2001;12:301.
24. Marrie RA, Wolfson C, Sturkenboom MC, et al. Multiple sclerosis and antecedent infections: a case-control study. Neurology 2000;54:2307.
25. Wandinger K, Jabs W, Siekhaus A, et al. Association between clinical disease activity and Epstein-Barr virus reactivation in MS. Neurology 2000;55:178.

26. Ascherio A, Munger KL, Lennette ET, et al. Epstein-Barr virus antibodies and risk of multiple sclerosis: a prospective study. JAMA 2001;286:3083.
27. Sadovnick AD, Armstrong H, Rice GP, et al. A population-based study of multiple sclerosis in twins: update. Ann Neurol 1993;33:281.
28. Sawcer S, Jones HB, Feakes R, et al. A genomic screen in multiple sclerosis reveals susceptibility loci on chromosome 6p21 and 17q22. Nat Genet 1996;13:464–468.
29. The Multiple Sclerosis Genetics group. A complete genomic screen for multiple sclerosis underscores a role for the major histocompatability complex. Nat Genet 1996;13:469–471.
30. Ebers GC, Kukay K, Bulman DE, et al. A full genomic search in multiple sclerosis. Nat Genet 1996;13:472–476.
31. The 5-year risk of MS after optic neuritis. Experience of the optic neuritis treatment trial. Optic Neuritis Study Group. Neurology 1997;49:1404–1413.
32. Rodriguez M, Siva A, Cross SA, et al. Optic neuritis: a population-based study in Olmsted County, Minnesota. Neurology 1995;45:244.
33. Rao SM, Reingold SC, Ron MA, et al. Workshop on Neurobehavioral Disorders in Multiple Sclerosis. Diagnosis, underlying disease, natural history, and therapeutic intervention, Bergamo, Italy, June 25–27, 1992. Arch Neurol 1993;50:658.
34. Mohr DC, Goodkin DE, Gatto N, Van der Wende J. Depression, coping and level of neurological impairment in multiple sclerosis. Mult Scler 1997;3:254.
35. Olafsson E, Benedikz J, Hauser WA. Risk of epilepsy in patients with multiple sclerosis: a population-based study in Iceland. Epilepsia 1999;40:745.
36. Nyquist PA, Cascino GD, Rodriguez M. Seizures in patients with multiple sclerosis seen at Mayo Clinic, Rochester, Minn, 1990–1998. Mayo Clin Proc 2001;76:983.
37. Bakshi R, Miletich RS, Henschel K, et al. Fatigue in multiple sclerosis: cross-sectional correlation with brain MRI findings in 71 patients. Neurology 1999;53:1151.
38. Hohol MJ, Guttmann CR, Orav J, et al. Serial neuropsychological assessment and magnetic resonance imaging analysis in multiple sclerosis. Arch Neurol 1997;54:1018.
39. Rao SM, Leo GJ, Haughton VM, et al. Correlation of magnetic resonance imaging with neuropsychological testing in multiple sclerosis. Neurology 1989;39:161.
40. Franklin GM, Heaton RK, Nelson LM, et al. Correlation of neuropsychological and MRI findings in chronic/progressive multiple sclerosis. Neurology 1988;38:1826.
41. Brex PA, Ciccarelli O, O'Riordan JI, Sailer M, Thompson AJ, Miller DH. A longitudinal study of abnormalities on MRI and disability from multiple sclerosis. N Engl J Med 2002;346:158–164.
42. McAlpine D, Compston A, Ebers G, et al. McAlpine's Multiple Sclerosis (3rd ed). Churchill Livingstone, London, 1999.
43. Sadovnick AD, Ebers GC. Epidemiology of multiple sclerosis: a critical overview. Can J Neurol Sci 1993;20:17.
44. Lublin FD, Reingold SC. Defining the clinical course of multiple sclerosis: results of an international survey. National Multiple Sclerosis Society (USA) Advisory Committee on Clinical Trials of New Agents in Multiple Sclerosis. Neurology 1996;46:907–911.
45. Weinshenker BG. Natural history of multiple sclerosis. Ann Neurol 1994;36(Suppl):S6.
46. Runmarker B, Andersen O. Prognostic factors in a multiple sclerosis incidence cohort with twenty-five years of follow-up. Brain 1993;116(Pt 1):117–134.
47. Cutter GR, Baier ML, Rudick RA, et al. Development of a multiple sclerosis functional composite as a clinical trial outcome measure. Brain 1999;122:871–882.
48. Cohen JA, Cutter GR, Fischer JS, et al. Use of the MSFC as an outcome measure in a phase III clinical trial. Arch Neurol 2001;58:961–967.
49. Kalkers NF, Bergers L, de Groot V, et al. Concurrent validity of the MSFC using MRI as a biological disease marker. Neurology 2001;56:215–219.
50. Damek DM, Shuster EA. Pregnancy and multiple sclerosis. Mayo Clin Proc 1997;72:977–989.
51. Confavreux C, Vukusic S, Adeleine P. Early clinical predictors and prognosis of irreversible disability in multiple sclerosis: an amnestic process. Brain 2003;126;770–782.

52. Myhr KM, Riise T, Vedeler C, et al. Disability and prognosis in multiple sclerosis: demographic and clinical variables important for the ability to walk and awarding of disability pension. Mult Scler 2001;7:59–65.
53. Scott TF, Schramke CJ, Novero J, Chieffe C. Short-term prognosis in early relapsing-remitting multiple sclerosis. Neurology 2000;55:689–693.
54. Mandler RN, Davis LE, Jeffery DR, Kornfield M. Devic's neuromyelitis optica: a clinicopathological study of 8 patients. Ann Neurol 1993;34:162.
55. Wingerchuk DM, Weinshenker BG. Neuromyelitis optica: clinical predictors of a relapsing course and survival. Neurology 2003;60:848–853.
56. Kepes JJ. Large focal tumor-like demyelinating lesions of the brain: Intermediate entity between multiple sclerosis and acute disseminated encephalomyelitis? A study of 31 patients. Ann Neurol 1993;33:18–27.
57. Johnson MD, Lavin P, Whetsell WO Jr. Fulminant monophasic multiple sclerosis, Marburg's type. J Neurol Neurosurg Psychiatry 1990;53:918–921.
58. Johnson RT, Griffin DE, Hirsch RL, et al. Measles encephalomyelitis—clinical and immunologic studies. N Engl J Med 1984;310:137–141.
59. Olek MJ, Dawson DM. Multiple Sclerosis and Other Inflammatory Demyelinating Diseases of the Central Nervous System. Butterworth-Heinemann, 1999.
60. Kesselring J, Miller DH, Robb SA, et al. Acute disseminated encephalomyelitis. MRI findings and the distinction from multiple sclerosis. Brain 1990;113(Pt 2):291–302.
61. Lieberman AP, Grossman RI, Lavi E. Case of the month: April 1997—a 32-year-old man with mental status changes and a severe occipital headache. Brain Pathol 1998;8:229.
62. Knebusch M, Strassburg HM, Reiners K. Acute transverse myelitis in childhood: nine cases and review of the literature. Dev Med Child Neurol 1998;40:631.
63. Ford B, Tampieri D, Francis G. Long-term follow-up of acute partial transverse myelopathy. Neurology 1992;42:250–252.
64. de Fraiture DM, Sie TH, Boezeman EH, Haanen HC. Cerebellitis as an uncommon complication of infectious mononucleosis. Nether J Med 1997;51:79.
65. Dalton CM, Brex PA, Miszkiel KA, et al. Application of the new McDonald criteria to patients with clinically isolated syndromes suggestive of multiple sclerosis. Ann Neurol 2002;52:47.
66. Tintore M, Rovira A, Rio J, et al. New diagnostic criteria for multiple sclerosis: application in first demyelinating episode. Neurology 2003;60:27.
67. Berger TB, Rubner P, Schautler F, et al. Antimyelin antibodies as a predictor of clinically definite multiple sclerosis after a first demyelinating event. N Engl J Med 2003;349:107–109.
68. Paty D, Studney D, Redekop K, Lublin F. MS COSTAR: a computerized patient record adapted for clinical research purposes. Ann Neurol 1994;36:S134.
69. Studney D, Lublin F, Marcucci L, et al. MS COSTAR: a computerized patient record adapted for clinical research purposes. J Neurol Rehab 1993;7:145.
70. Sadovnick AD, Baird PA, Ward RH, et al. Multiple sclerosis: updated risks for relatives. Am J Med Genet 1988;29:533–541.
71. O'Riordan JI, Thompson AJ, Kingsley DP, et al. The prognostic value of brain MRI in clinically isolated syndromes of the CNS: a 10-year follow-up. Brain 1998;121:495–503.

Role of Magnetic Resonance Imaging in the Diagnosis and Prognosis of Multiple Sclerosis

Robert Zivadinov, PhD, MD, and Rohit Bakshi, MD

INTRODUCTION

Multiple sclerosis (MS) is an inflammatory disease of the central nervous system (CNS) characterized by demyelination and axonal loss for which the exact immunopathogenic mechanisms underlying disease initiation and progression are unknown. In the last two decades, magnetic resonance imaging (MRI) has become the most important laboratory diagnostic and monitoring tool in MS *(1)*. Moreover, MRI is 5 to 10 times more sensitive than clinical data in the assessment of disease activity *(2)*. The sensitivity of T2-weighted images (T2-WI) in detection of MS lesions, together with the ability of gadolinium (Gd)-enhanced T1-WI to reflect increased blood–brain barrier (BBB) permeability associated with active inflammatory activity, allows the demonstration of spatial and temporal dissemination of MS lesions earlier than is possible from clinical assessments. Therefore, in the last decade, metrics derived from conventional MRI have been widely employed in therapeutic clinical trials *(3–6)*. Several conventional MRI protocols, in conjunction with clinical assessment, are now routinely used to detect therapeutic effects and extend clinical observations *(7)*.

USE OF MRI IN MULTIPLE SCLEROSIS

Recently, several cross-sectional and longitudinal studies *(8,9)* have shown that conventional and nonconventional MRI techniques can be used as surrogate markers in monitoring the destructive pathological processes that most likely are related to disease activity and clinical progression. These MRI techniques are able to reveal a range of pathological substrates of MS lesions that include edema, inflammation, demyelination, and axonal loss *(10)*. Therefore, in a disease with a high degree of longitudinal variability of clinical signs and symptoms within and between patients

From: *Current Clinical Neurology: Multiple Sclerosis*
Edited by: M. J. Olek © Humana Press Inc., Totowa, NJ

and with no current adequate biological markers of disease progression, MRI techniques provide a powerful tool to noninvasively study disease pathology *(11)*. However, although conventional MRI has substantially contributed to the diagnosis and prognosis of MS, the sensitivity and specificity of nonconventional MRI is limited *(12)*. For example, hyperintense lesions on T2-WI show pathological non-specificity, are not sensitive to disease affecting normal-appearing gray and white matter, show an unreliable correlation with clinical measures of disability, and provide incomplete assessments of therapeutic outcomes. Hyperintensity on T2-WI of MS lesions is related primarily to increased water content and thus cannot distinguish inflammation, edema, demyelination, Wallerian degeneration, and axonal loss *(13)*. Although the presence of Gd-enhancing lesions on T1-WI indicates disruption of the BBB, it does not provide sufficient information about the extent and severity of the inflammatory phase, the constitution of its cellular components, or resultant tissue damage *(12)*. In addition, conventional MRI is unable to detect and quantify the extent and severity of tissue damage occurring in so called normal appearing brain tissue, including normal appearing gray and white matter, which probably contributes to short-term and long-term clinical impairments *(14–18)*.

In the past few years, a host of nonconventional MRI techniques, which are able to monitor disease evolution, have been introduced for the assessment of MS. Measurement of brain and spinal cord atrophy, hypointense lesions on T1-WI ("black holes"), hypointensity on T2-WI (T2 hypointensity), magnetization transfer imaging (MTI), diffusion-weighted imaging (DWI), proton MR spectroscopy (MRS), functional MRI (fMRI), cell-specific MRI, perfusion MRI, and ultra-high-field MRI are emerging as promising tools for improving our understanding of the pathophysiology of MS.

The aim of this chapter is to review the role of conventional and nonconventional MRI techniques in the diagnosis and prognosis of MS.

ROLE OF MAGNETIC RESONANCE IMAGING IN THE DIAGNOSIS OF MULTIPLE SCLEROSIS

Conventional Magnetic Resonance Imaging in the Diagnosis of Multiple Sclerosis

Involvement of the Brain

In clinical practice, the diagnosis of MS is usually based on the principle of dissemination in time and space of a neurologic illness compatible with MS in the absence of other causes *(19)*.

MS lesions ("plaques") may be seen practically anywhere in the brain, including white matter or gray matter. However, the most typical sites are in white matter such as the periventricular region (Fig. 1A), corpus callosum (Fig. 1B), and posterior fossa (Fig. 1C). When involving the periventricular white matter, lesions typically make contact with the ependymal surface of the ventricles. Corpus callosum involvement is characteristically seen on the inner surface adjacent to the lateral ventricles. Typical sites of posterior fossa involvement include the brain stem,

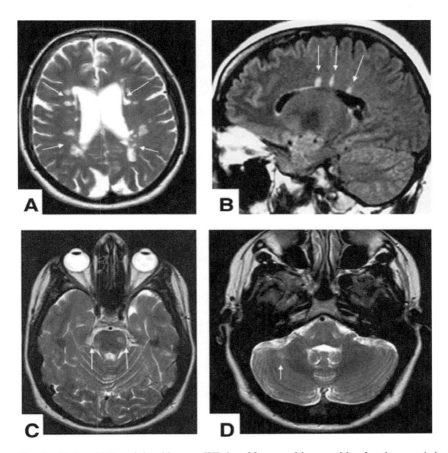

Fig. 1. (A) Axial T2-weighted image (WI) in a 33-year-old man with relapsing-remitting MS (RRMS) showing multiple hyperintense lesions in the periventricular white matter (*arrows*). Note the classic oval/ovoid appearance of lesions, the size of each is generally ±5 mm and many directly contact the ventricular ependyma. **(B)** Sagittal fluid-attenuated inversion recovery (FLAIR) in a 44-year-old man with relapsing-remitting MS (RRMS) showing multiple pericallosal lesions (*arrows*) with a classic perivenular orientation (Dawson's fingers); **(C,D)** Axial T2-WI of a 26-year-old woman with RRMS demonstrating typical hyperintense lesions in the pons (**C**, *arrows*) and right cerebellum (**D**, *arrow*).

middle cerebellar peduncles, and cerebellar white matter (Figs. 1C,D). Although axial images are more sensitive for posterior fossa lesions (Fig. 1C), sagittal images are clearly superior in identifying callosal and pericallosal lesions (Fig. 1B). The long-axis of periventricular lesions is frequently perpendicular to the long-axis of the lateral ventricles resulting from perivenular demyelination (Dawson's fingers) (Fig. 1B). MS lesions are commonly oval or ovoid (Fig. 1), isointense to hypointense on T1-WI (Fig. 2), and hyperintense on T2-WI and proton density-

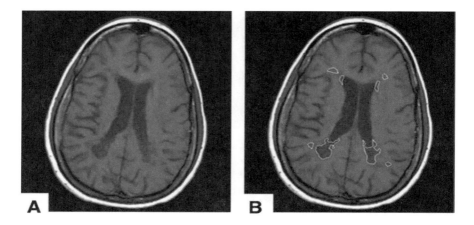

Fig. 2. (A) Axial T1-weighted image (WI) in a 39-year-old man with secondary progressive MS (SPMS) with severe disability (Expanded Disability Status Scale [EDSS] score of 6.5) and multiple hypointense lesions (black holes) in the periventricular white matter. **(B)** Hypointense T1 lesions are segmented for volumetric analysis at the edges of the anterior and posterior horns of the lateral ventricles using an edge finding computerized analysis technique.

weighted images (PD-WI) (Figs. 1 and 3) and fluid-attenuated inversion recovery (FLAIR) images (Figs. 3 and 4), and are usually >5 mm in diameter. These hyperintensities become confluent as the disease progresses (Fig. 5).

Conventional spin-echo (CSE) images of the brain are routinely used for MS diagnosis because of their high sensitivity in the detection of MS lesions *(11)*. CSE T2-WI are also used to monitor short-term MS activity (the number of new and enlarging lesions on serial scans) *(20)* and to monitor long-term disease evolution by assessing the changes of total T2 lesion volume (T2LV) *(21)* over time. Changes in lesion size and T2LV are believed to be related to disease activity *(22)*. However, small periventricular lesions may be indistinguishable from the adjacent high signal cerebrospinal fluid (CSF) on T2-WI. Better lesion to CSF contrast is achieved with PD-WI because of the relatively lower signal intensity of CSF on this sequence and improved lesion to tissue contrast (Fig. 3). T2-WI and PD-WI can be acquired in a single sequence by using either a conventional dual spin-echo technique or a rapid acquisition relaxation enhanced (RARE) dual spin-echo sequence *(23)*.

In the last several years, continuous technical improvements of MRI hardware and software have led to the development of new pulse sequences with more efficiency and sensitivity. Among them, turbo or fast spin-echo (TSE or FSE) *(24)* and fast-FLAIR *(25)* (Figs. 3 and 4) have already demonstrated their use in a variety of neurologic diseases, including MS. FSE showed greater sensitivity than CSE in the detection of areas of T2 prolongation in MS *(24)*. Fast FLAIR sequences are especially helpful in evaluating periventricular and cortical lesions where CSF signal may mask these plaques on T2-WI *(20,25)* (Fig. 3). In a study of 84 patients with

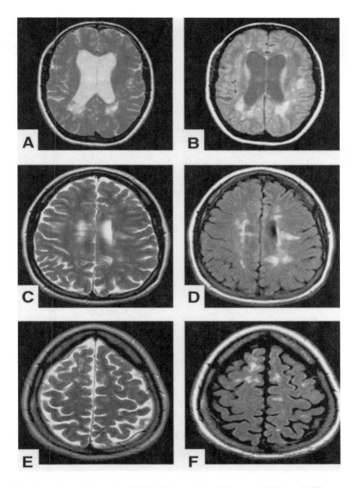

Fig. 3. (**A**)Axial fast spin-echo (FSE) T2-weighted image (WI) and (**B**) proton density-WI (PD-WI) in a 42-year-old woman with relapsing-remitting multiple sclerosis (RRMS) show typical hyperintense confluent periventricular lesions. Note the improved lesion contrast achieved with PD-WI because of the relatively lower signal intensity of cerebrospinal fluid (CSF) vs lesions. Axial images of 28-year-old woman with RRMS show clear evidence how fluid-attenuated inversion recovery (FLAIR) (**D,F**) is superior to FSE T2-WI (**C,E**) in the detection of periventricular (**C,D**) and cortical/juxtacortical (**E,F**) lesions.

MS, 810 cortical or juxtacortical lesions were identified by fast FLAIR while only 26% of these lesions were seen on T2-WI *(25)*. However, in the posterior fossa (Fig. 1C) and spinal cord, FLAIR detects significantly fewer lesions than T2-WI *(26)*. Areas of T2 prolongation can also be detected using short tau inversion recovery (STIR) sequences. This sequence may be superior to T2-WI in detecting spinal cord lesions in MS when using certain scanning platforms *(27)*. Because of fat

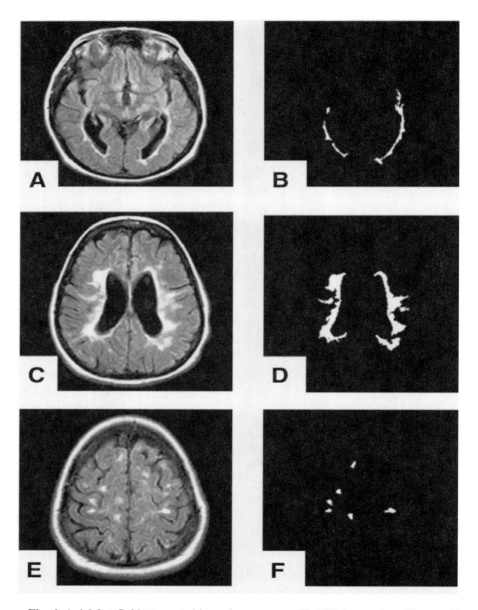

Fig. 4. Axial fast fluid-attenuated inversion recovery (FLAIR) images in a 32-year-old man with relapsing-remitting multiple sclerosis (RRMS) showing hyperintense lesions (**A,C,E**) and the output resulting from computer-assisted segmentation showing lesions only (**B,D,F**). FLAIR sequences are especially helpful in evaluating supratentorial periventricular (**A–D**) and juxtacortical (**E,F**) lesions where cerebrospinal fluid (CSF) signal may mask these plaques on T2-WI (*see also* Fig. 3).

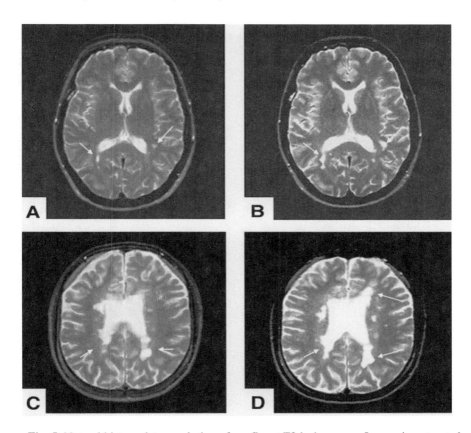

Fig. 5. Natural history data: evolution of confluent T2 lesions over 5 years in untreated patients. **(A)** Baseline scan and **(B)** 5-year follow-up scan show the enlargement and development of confluence of T2 lesions (*white arrows*) in a 31-year-old man with relapsing-remitting multiple sclerosis (RRMS). **(C)** Baseline scan and **(D)** 5-year follow-up scan show increasing confluence of T2 lesions (*white arrows*) in a 35-year-old man with RRMS.

suppression, the STIR sequence is an added advantage when imaging the optic nerves because the contrast between lesions and the surrounding retrobulbar fat is increased *(28)*.

Gd-enhancing lesions on T1-WI (Figs. 6A,B) often correspond to areas of high signal on T2-WI and low-signal intensity on unenhanced T1-WI, probably owing to edema. Approximately 10–20% of lesions on T2-WI will show contrast enhancement at any one time. Gd enhancement is a transient phenomenon in MS and usually disappears after 30 to 40 days; persistence of enhancement should caution against the diagnosis of MS *(29)*. It is not completely clear if inflammation is the triggering event that causes demyelination and axonal degeneration, although previous longitudinal studies demonstrated that the presence of active lesions on serial

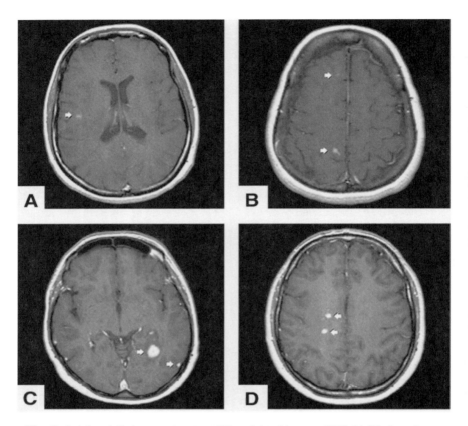

Fig. 6. Axial gadolinium postcontrast T1-weighted images (WI) (**A,B**) show homogeneously enhancing (hyperintense) lesions, indicating disruption of the blood–brain barrier and acute inflammation in a 33-year-old woman with relapsing-remitting multiple sclerosis (RRMS). Axial postcontrast T1-WI in a 28-year-old man shows how a double dose of contrast is useful to increase the sensitivity in detecting active areas of inflammation (**C,D**).

scans carries a high risk of continuous disease activity *(30,31)*. A meta-analysis by Kappos et al. *(32)* demonstrated that Gd enhancement predicts the occurrence of relapses, but it is not a strong predictor of the development of cumulative impairment or disability. There are several methods that can be used to increase the sensitivity of Gd-enhanced MRI for the detection of active MS lesions, which leads to increased statistical power of patient samples and the follow-up duration needed to show a treatment effect *(33)*. This increased sensitivity may be obtained with higher doses of Gd (Fig. 6C,D) *(34,35)* (e.g., a triple dose instead of a standard 0.1 mmol/ kg dose) *(36)*, MTI *(37)*, thinner slices, or delayed imaging *(38)*. Wolansky et al. *(36)* were the first to show that triple-dose Gd is more sensitive than single-dose Gd in detecting MS lesions. At the authors' centers, they use a 5-minute delay after

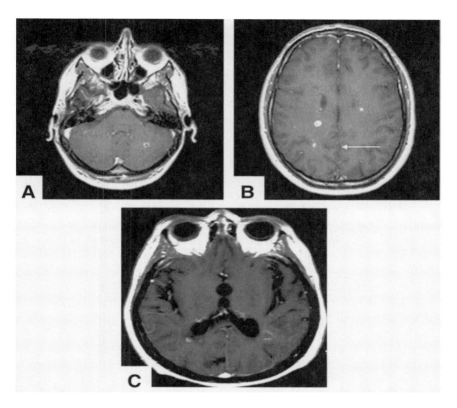

Fig. 7. Axial postcontrast T1-weighted image (WI) demonstrates concentric ring-enhancing lesions (*arrows*) in the infratentorial (**A**) and periventricular (**B**) regions in a 27-year-old woman with relapsing-remitting multiple sclerosis (RRMS). Characteristic open-ring-enhancing lesion with increased specificity for MS (*arrow*) in 52-year-old women scanned during an MS relapse (**C**).

single-dose Gd infusion to increase the sensitivity, which they believed is cost effective and practical. The majority of enhancing plaques are clinically asymptomatic, although the presence of ongoing enhancement suggests continuing disease activity, which likely contributes to cumulative pathophysiology.

Gd-enhancement patterns may provide some specificity of the underlying pathology of lesions (Fig. 7). Concentric ring-enhancing lesions with central contrast pallor (Fig. 7) arise in previously damaged areas or in areas of accelerated local inflammation *(39–45)*. They are larger and of longer duration than homogeneously enhancing lesions *(39,40,42)*. Magnetization transfer ratios (MTRs) *(41,43)* and apparent diffusion coefficients (ADCs) *(44)* are lower in ring-enhancing than in homogeneously enhancing lesions. Moreover, ring-enhancing lesions weakly predict the development of persisting hypointense lesions on T1-W1 *(46)*. Therefore, ring-enhancing lesions are believed to be related to accelerated disease activity and extensive tissue damage *(39,45,46)* and may mark a type of inflammation in more aggressive forms of disease. Ring enhancement may also occur in an incomplete (open) ring pattern, which is somewhat more specific for MS than infections or neoplastic diseases (Fig. 7).

On noncontrast T1-WI, the authors have observed that plaques frequently possess an outer ring of hyperintensity (T1 shortening), which may represent paramagnetic effects of free radicals, lipid-containing macrophages, or proteinaceous accumulation (unpublished data). This phenomenon has been poorly characterized in the literature and only mentioned anecdotally. The authors are in the process of completing a formal study on this phenomenon.

MRI findings in patients with MS are not disease specific. A number of conditions can cause multiple T2 hyperintense white-matter abnormalities appearing similar to MS. The MRI pattern of MS is usually relatively specific when age, clinical information and the full range of MRI abnormalities (including lesion number, topography, size, and shape) are considered. However, clinical correlation remains the cornerstone of diagnosing MS. Table 1 lists the most common conditions to be considered in the differential diagnosis when confronted with multifocal lesions on MRI scans suggestive of MS or clinical entities suggesting MS *(11,19,47,48)*.

In particular, lesions of ADEM *(49)*, a monophasic illness, may resemble those of early MS. ADEM is typically triggered by a viral infection or vaccination, although idiopathic cases may also occur. MRI typically shows multifocal white-matter lesions involving the cerebral hemispheres, cerebellum, and brain stem that may or may not be distinguishable from MS; however, involvement of the subcortical gray-matter nuclei and large size and early confluence of lesions favor ADEM (Fig. 8) *(49)*. Nonetheless, ADEM is a clinical diagnosis that is only supported by imaging findings and a follow-up scan after 3 months, which has been suggested for identifying new lesions suggestive of MS *(50)*.

Involvement of the Spinal Cord

Spinal cord hyperintensities on T2-WI have been detected in 50 to 90% of patients with MS *(51–53)* (Fig. 9). Several MRI studies demonstrated that the frequency of Gd-enhancing lesions is higher in the spinal cord than in the brain *(54,55)*. The enhancement may become more apparent when scanning the entire cord *(55)* or using a triple dose of Gd *(56)*. The presence of characteristic cord lesions may increase the confidence in diagnosing MS *(51)*. In addition, cord lesions may be seen in approximately 5–15% of patients with a clinical picture suggestive of MS but a normal brain MRI scan *(57)*, and in 30% of those presenting with clinically isolated syndromes (CIS) of the brain or optic nerve suggestive of MS *(58)*. Moreover, spinal cord lesions appear to be symptomatic more often than brain lesions *(59)* and correlate better with the degree of physical disability *(60)*. Proper sensitivity for the detection of cord involvement requires optimization of MRI hardware and pulse sequences. We prefer 1.5 T closed bore systems with fast-spin echo sag-

Table 1
Principal Conditions Mimicking Multiple Sclerosis on Magnetic Resonance Imaging Scans or Considered in the Clinical Differential Diagnosis of Multiple Sclerosis

Multiple sclerosis (MS) variants
Acute malignant MS (Marburg variant)   ·
Charcot type
Clinically isolated syndromes
Neuromyelitis optica (Devic's disease)
Schilder's disease
Solitary inflammatory masses (leukoencephalitis)

Normal aging

Migraine

Cerebrovascular diseases
Collagen vascular disease
Diabetes
Hypertension
Periventricular leukomalacia
Primary central nervous system vasculitis
Subcortical atherosclerotic encephalopathy (Binswanger's disease)
Susac syndrome

Infectious and inflammatory diseases
Abscesses
Acute disseminated encephalomyelitis
Human immunodeficiency virus encephalitis
Lyme disease
Progressive multifocal leukoencephalopathy
Sarcoidosis
Subacute sclerosing panencephalitis
Syphilis
Tuberculosis

Toxic/metabolic diseases
Chemotherapy or radiotherapy effects
Leukodystrophies
Mitochondrial diseases
Osmotic myelinolysis
Toluene toxicity
Vitamin B_{12} deficiency

Neoplastic disease
Metastases
Primary brain or intravascular lymphoma

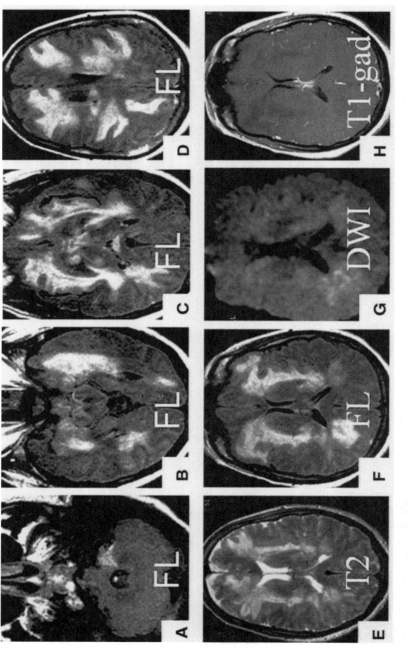

Fig. 8. Fatal acute disseminated encephalomyelitis (ADEM) in a 51-year-old woman after an upper respiratory infection. (**A–F**) Note the multiple hyperintensities in the infratentorial and supratentorial region on fluid-attenuated inversion recovery (FLAIR) (FL) and T2-weighted image (WI). (**G**) Diffused WI (DWI) shows slight hyperintensity of the lesions resulting from T2 shinethrough. (**H**) The lesions are isointense to mildly hypointense on T1WI and nonenhancing after gadolinium infusion (T1-gad). Minimal or no mass effect is noted. The large size of lesions, confluence, and involvement of the thalamus and globus pallidus favors ADEM instead of multiple sclerosis.

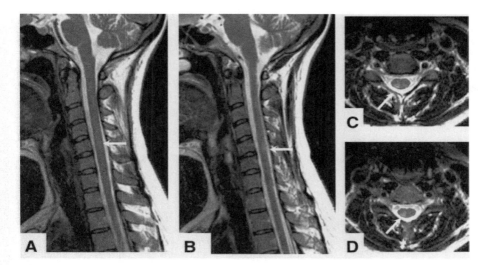

Fig. 9. Spinal fast-spin echo (FSE) T2-weighted image (WI) of a 30-year-old man with RRMS. **(A,B)** Contiguous sagittal T2-WI show hyperintense lesions *(arrows)* in cervical spinal cord. **(C,D)** Contiguous axial T2-WI demonstrate a hyperintense lesion *(arrows)* in the cervical cord (C5-6 level). The lesion is classic for MS, involving less than one spinal level and less than one-half of the cord diameter.

ittal and axial T2-WI with 3–4 mm slice thickness for detection of hyperintense intramedullary lesions (Fig. 9). On some scanning platforms, PD-WI or STIR may also be useful.

The diagnosis of MS can be easily made in subjects with acute spinal cord symptoms when MRI of the brain shows typical white-matter lesions and CSF demonstrates intrathecal immunoglobulin (Ig) G synthesis and oligoclonal bands. However, when MRI of the brain is normal or atypical, the CSF is normal, or other concomitant factors are present (e.g., cord-compressive lesion), alternative causes must be considered. MRI is sensitive in detecting focal demyelinating syndromes, such as myelitis *(61)*, leukoencephalitis *(62)*, and optic neuritis (ON) *(63)*. Myelitis, an inflammatory syndrome associated with intramedullary dysfunction of the spinal cord, is often associated with an identifiable etiology, such as infectious, postinfectious, postvaccination, collagen vascular disease, toxic, paraneoplastic, sarcoidosis, or MS-related myelitis (Fig. 9) *(61)*. Diagnosing myelitis promptly and accurately and distinguishing these various etiologies has therapeutic and prognostic value but may be difficult with routine clinical and laboratory testing. MRI plays a central role in the differential diagnosis of myelitis.

Acute transverse myelitis (ATM) is a focal inflammatory disorder of the spinal cord, resulting in motor, sensory, and autonomic dysfunction. A set of uniform diagnostic criteria and nosology for ATM has been proposed to avoid the confusion that inevitably results when investigators use differing criteria *(64)*. This has ensured a common language of classification, reduced diagnostic confusion, and laid the groundwork for multicenter clinical trials. In addition, a framework is suggested for evaluation of individuals presenting with ATM signs and symptoms. The best treatment often depends on a timely and accurate diagnosis. Because ATM is relatively rare, delayed and incomplete workups often occur. Identification of etiologies may suggest medical treatment, whereas no clearly established medical treatment currently exists for idiopathic ATM. Bakshi et al. *(61)* studied brain and spinal MRI findings in 22 consecutive patients with various forms of myelitis, including non-MS-related ATM and myelitis associated with preexisting or subsequent MS (MS-myelitis). They compared non-MS-related ATM ($n = 9$), to myelitis associated with MS (MS-myelitis, $n = 13$). Several major differences between ATM and MS-myelitis patients were found:

1. The patients with ATM were significantly older than patients with MS at the time of the myelitis diagnosis (mean age 46 vs 35, $p > 0.05$).
2. ATM appeared as a "longitudinal myelitis," with fusiform cord expansion on T1-WI and intramedullary increased signal on T2-WI, each involving multiple spinal levels (mean = 7–8). However, MS-myelitis lesions appeared focal, involving significantly fewer spinal levels (mean = 1–2, $p > 0.001$).
3. Brain MRI was more likely to be normal in ATM (78%) than in MS-myelitis (15%, $p < 0.001$).

The most striking MRI finding was that ATM appeared tumor-like as a "longitudinal" lesion that included fusiform spinal cord swelling on T1-WI and hyperintense intramedullary lesions on T2-WI. Thus, MRI findings in ATM, although suspicious for a primary spinal cord neoplasm and suggesting the need for a biopsy, may reflect an inflammatory disorder. The MRI features of ATM in the Bakshi et al. series were readily distinguishable from MS-myelitis. However, MRI findings were similar in ATM because of vaccination, infection, sarcoidosis, and collagen vascular disease. The differential diagnosis of these lesions on MRI studies also includes infarction or vascular malformation of the spinal cord, which may require exclusion by clinical and laboratory findings. MS-myelitis is most common in the cervical cord and appears focal (involving one to two levels or less), well circumscribed, and hyperintense on T2-WI *(61)*. Spinal cord expansion associated with MS may reflect a more acute or subacute myelopathy rather than clinically silent or chronic myelopathies. Axial MRI may also be helpful in distinguishing ATM and MS-myelitis. ATM is typically located in the central aspect of the cord and occupies more than one-half of the cord diameter, whereas MS-myelitis is typically more peripheral and involves less than one-half of the cross-sectional cord area.

Role of MRI in New Diagnostic Criteria for Multiple Sclerosis

No single clinical feature or diagnostic test is sufficient for the diagnosis of MS. A formal review of diagnostic criteria occurred in 1983, at which time degrees of diagnostic certainty were identified by categories ranging from clinically definite to laboratory-supported definite, clinically probable, and laboratory-supported

Table 2
Magnetic Resonance Imaging Diagnostic Criteria for Multiple Sclerosis

Authors (Ref.)	Features
Paty et al. (1988) *(66)*	Either four lesions or three lesions present with one being in periventricular region
Fazekas et al. (1988) *(67)*	Three or more lesions with two of them presenting at least one of the following lesion characteristics: • Size of a lesion no. 6 mm • A lumpy-bumpy ventricular interface • An infratentorial lesion
Barkhof et al. (1997) *(68)*	At least one lesion with gadolinium-enhancement At least one lesion in juxtacortical region At least one lesion in infratentorial region At least three lesions in periventricular region

probable MS *(65)*. An international panel has recently revised the diagnostic criteria (McDonald criteria) *(50)*. The panel aimed to create criteria that could be used by a practicing physician and adapted for clinical trials and would integrate MRI, include the diagnosis of primary progressive (PP) disease, clarify definitions used in the diagnosis of MS, and simplify the diagnostic classification and descriptions. The McDonald criteria reaffirmed the concept of "dissemination in time and space."

To use MRI to support the diagnosis of MS, multiple characteristic lesions should be present. Several authors have proposed MRI criteria to help differentiate between MS and other causes of hyperintense lesions in the brain *(66–68)* (Table 2). In 1997, Barkhof et al. *(68)* suggested that contrast-enhanced and juxtacortical and infratentorial T2 lesions are more specific for MS than the more commonly seen periventricular lesions. In a prospective comparison with earlier sets of criteria proposed by Paty et al. *(66)* and Fazekas et al. *(67)*, Barkhof et al. demonstrated that their criteria achieved the highest accuracy in predicting conversion to MS in patients presenting with CIS (Table 3) *(68)*. Based on these findings, the McDonald panel maintained that stringent MRI criteria should be followed in making a diagnosis of MS. The panel chose the guidelines of Barkhof et al. *(68)* and Tintore et al. *(69)* for the definition of dissemination in space, which requires at least three of the following:

1. At least one Gd-enhancing lesion or nine T2 hyperintense lesions if no Gd-enhancing lesion.
2. At least one or more infratentorial lesion.
3. At least one or more juxtacortical lesion.
4. At least three or more periventricular lesions.
5. Note: one cord lesion can substitute for one brain lesion.

The following MRI criteria may be used to demonstrate dissemination in time (Table 4):

1. Gd-enhancing lesion demonstrated in a scan done at least 3 months after the initial clinical attack at an anatomic site different from the first attack;

Table 3
**Predictive Value of Magnetic Resonance Imaging Developing
a Second Attack Indicative of Clinically Definite Multiple Sclerosis
in Patients with Clinically Isolated Syndromes (Barkhof et al.) (68)**

Magnetic resonance imaging criteria	Sensitivity (%)	Specificity (%)	NPV (%)	PPV (%)	Accuracy (%)
Paty et al. (1988) (66)	88	54	86	60	69
Fazekas et al. (1988) (67)	88	54	86	60	69
Barkhof et al. (1997) (68)	82	78	85	75	80

Abbr: NPV, negative predictive value; PPV, positive predictive value.

Table 4
**Magnetic Resonance Imaging Criteria
for Dissemination of Lesions in Time (50)**

- If a first scan occurs 3 months after the onset of clinical event, the presence of a gadolinium-enhancing lesion is sufficient to demonstrate dissemination in time, provided that it is not at the site implicated in the original clinical event. If there is no enhancing lesion at this time, a follow-up scan is required. The timing of this follow-up scan is not crucial, but 3 months is recommended (70). A new T2- or gadolinium-enhancing lesion at this time then fulfills the criterion of dissemination in time.
- If the first scan is performed <3 months after the onset of the clinical event, a second scan done 3 months or more after the clinical event showing a new gadolinium-enhancing lesion provides sufficient evidence for dissemination in time. However, if no enhancing lesion is seen at this second scan, a further scan not <3 months after the first scan that shows a new T2 lesion or an enhancing lesion will suffice.

2. In the absence of Gd-enhancing lesions at the 3-month scan, a follow-up scan after an additional 3 months showing a new Gd or T2-lesion.

Although the McDonald MRI criteria were generally regarded as difficult to apply, they allow MRI to be used to define dissemination in space and (with a repeat MRI) dissemination in time. The McDonald criteria accept the occurrence of new T2 lesions or new Gd-enhancing lesions appearing after a minimum interval of 3 months as acceptable evidence for dissemination in time. This minimum interval should be further validated. In addition, the optimal interval that provides the maximum yield in the most cost-effective manner needs to be defined. Emerging data from serial MRI studies that have been done might provide additional information to make such recommendations (71–75).

The McDonald criteria included new diagnostic criteria for PP MS (76). However, the diagnosis of PP MS remains difficult. The McDonald MRI criteria for the diagnosis of PP MS are probably insensitive, and it is clear that some clinically typical cases will not meet the formal MRI criteria *(77)*. Additional information is likely to become available as results of current PP MS clinical trials are published *(77)*.

As mentioned, MS has many mimics. The McDonald criteria consider the differential diagnosis. Although it is possible to diagnose MS without MRI, the number of errors in diagnosis is reduced markedly when both clinical and MRI studies are available to the physician.

The authors believe that formal diagnostic criteria have a role in selecting patients for research trials to ensure uniformity but that for routine clinical practice, these criteria may be too restrictive and require long-term validation (*see* Validation of New Diagnostic Criteria).

VALIDATION OF NEW DIAGNOSTIC CRITERIA

Data on the sensitivity, specificity, and reliability of MRI in supporting a diagnosis of MS are limited. The McDonald guidelines cite the Barkhof et al. *(68)* and Tintore et al. *(69)* MRI criteria, even though they have not been validated longitudinally in MS populations. In the Barkhof et al. study *(68)*, MRI scans of 33 patients who converted from clinically isolated syndromes (CIS) to clinically definite MS were evaluated. In the Tintore et al. study *(69)*, 22 converting patients were studied for an average of 28 months. These numbers may not be sufficient to establish standards, and, therefore, such criteria (and those modified by the McDonald panel) should be validated for accuracy in the diagnosis of MS and not only for the predictive value of short-term conversion to clinically definite MS in CIS.

Four studies *(71,73–75)* have recently evaluated the ability of the new McDonald criteria to predict which clinically isolated syndrome (CIS) patients will develop clinically definite MS *(65)*. In a recently published study of 50 patients with CIS, Dalton et al. *(73)* examined the value of MRI in predicting conversion to clinically definite MS within 3 years. At 3 months, 20 of 95 (21%) patients had developed MS according to the McDonald criteria, whereas only 7 of 95 (7%) had developed clinically definite MS. After 1 year, the corresponding figures were 38 of 79 (48%) and 16 of 79 (20%), and after 3 years, they were 29 of 50 (58%) and 19 of 50 (38%). The development of MS with the McDonald criteria after 1 year had a high sensitivity (83%), specificity (83%), positive predicative value (75%), negative predictive value (89%), and accuracy (83%) for clinically definite MS at 3 years (Table 5). The authors concluded that the use of the McDonald criteria more than doubled the rate of diagnosis of MS within a year of presentation with a CIS and that therefore the high specificity, positive predictive value, and accuracy of the new criteria for predicting clinically definite MS support their clinical relevance. In another study, Tintore et al. *(71)* reported the predictive value of the McDonald criteria in 139 patients who presented with CIS and who were followed for a median of 3 years. At 12 months, 11% had clinically definite MS according to the Poser criteria, compared to 37% with the McDonald criteria. Eighty percent of patients fulfilling these new criteria developed a second clinical episode within a mean follow-up of 49 months. The new criteria showed a sensitivity of 74%, specificity

Table 5
**Ability to Predict the Conversion of Clinically Isolated
Syndromes to Clinically Definite Multiple Sclerosis:
Validation of the McDonald Criteria *(50)***

Magnetic resonance imaging criteria	Sensitivity (%)	Specificity (%)	Accuracy (%)
Dalton et al. (2002) *(73)*	83	83	83
Tintore et al. (2003) *(71)*	74	86	80

of 86%, and accuracy of 80% in predicting conversion to clinically definite MS (Table 5). The authors emphasized that 1 year after symptom onset, more than three times as many patients with CIS were diagnosed with MS using McDonald criteria vs previous criteria. These two studies *(71,73)* retrospectively examined data collected for other reasons and used them to evaluate the McDonald criteria. In particular, the Tintore et al. study *(71)* is limited by the study design, the timing of the scans, and the inconsistent use of Gd. In both studies, the McDonald criteria were not strictly applied and they failed to show that these criteria can guide routine clinical practice *(72)*. The results of these two studies are consistent with earlier studies suggesting that MRI has important limitations as a surrogate marker in clinical trials, especially in patients with CIS.

In CIS, the McDonald criteria require new Gd-enhancing lesions for dissemination in time at a 3-month follow-up scan. The diagnosis of MS in patients with a new lesion on T2-WI that appears at the 3-month follow-up scan is not permitted by the current criteria. However, it has been demonstrated that new T2 lesions are detected more often than new Gd-enhancement lesions after 3 months *(70)*. Dalton et al. *(74)* addressed the accuracy of new T2 lesions at a 3-month follow-up scan in making the diagnosis of MS. In a cohort of 56 patients, these criteria were highly specific (95%) but poorly sensitive (58%) for clinically definite MS at 3 years. If new T2 lesions were allowed as an alternative for dissemination in time, sensitivity increased (74%) with a high specificity preserved (92%), enabling an accurate diagnosis of MS in more patients. The authors proposed that in adults aged 16 to 50 years presenting with CIS, the McDonald MRI criteria for dissemination in time should be expanded to include new T2 lesions seen on a 3-month follow-up scan when the first scan is obtained within 3 months of symptom onset.

Disease-modifying therapies, such as interferon (IFN)-β, often show a discordant effect on clinical vs MRI disease effects, reducing MRI activity by greater than 70% *(3–6)* and the relapse rate by approximately 30%. In a recently published study *(68)*, the predictive value of the modified Barkhof criteria for progression to clinically definite MS, as evidenced by the occurrence of a new clinical episode, has been examined *(75)*. In addition, the predictive response to treatment with once-weekly subcutaneous IFN-β-1a has been evaluated. Conversion to clinically definite MS within 2 years of follow-up, as evidenced by a new clinical episode, occurred (independent of treatment) in 41% of patients with Gd enhancement or nine or more T2 lesions vs 11% of those without either finding ($p = 0.017$); similarly, proportions converting were 44 vs 31% for infratentorial lesions ($p = 0.026$), 40 vs 35% for juxtacortical lesions ($p = 0.413$), and 41 vs 17% for three or more periventricular lesions ($p = 0.034$). The rate of conversion to clinically definite MS based on the modified Barkhof criteria *(50)* was 22% for two or fewer positive criteria, increasing to 47% with four positive criteria. For a cutoff of three positive criteria, the hazard ratio for time to clinically definite MS was 2.3 (95% confidence interval, 1.17–4.55; $p = 0.016$). The results of validation of the modified McDonald criteria in the Early Treatment of MS (ETOMS) study *(75)* suggest that meeting the criteria increases the odds of conversion to clinically definite MS, and thus the number of patients needing to be treated to prevent one patient converting to clinically definite MS within 2 years decreases from 50 in patients with two or fewer positive criteria to 5.6 with four positive criteria. On the other hand, the effect of once-weekly IFN-β-1a therapy seems to be stronger in the patients with a high number of positive criteria.

Nonconventional Magnetic Resonance Imaging in the Diagnosis of Multiple Sclerosis

On T1-WI, most MS lesions are isointense to white matter, but some are hypointense or appear as "black holes" (BH) *(8,78–80)*, particularly in the supratentorial region (Fig. 2). These hypointense lesions are nonspecific at a given time because nearly half will revert to normal in a few months, most likely resulting from remyelination and resolution of edema *(81)*. Persistent BH, however, are markers of severe demyelination and axonal loss *(8)*. Therefore, the pathological substrate of the accumulation of persisting BH is predominantly axonal damage *(8,15,78,81)*, as shown in a postmortem histopathology-MRI correlation study *(8)*. Such focal axonal loss most likely contributes to Wallerian degeneration. The correlation between BH volume and clinical disability (Expanded Disability Status Scale-[EDSS]) suggests that these may be clinically relevant for measuring disease progression *(15,78–80)*. However, studies comparing various MRI metrics for their association with physical disability or cognitive dysfunction have shown that markers of global tissue degeneration, such as brain atrophy, have higher clinical predictive value than BH and other lesion assessment measurements *(17,82,83)*. Thus, the utility of BH is not entirely clear and further longitudinal studies are necessary for validation of BH as therapeutic outcome measures. The role of BH in the setting of CIS is not well understood and will await extended subanalysis of the Controlled High-Risk Subjects Avonex MS Prevention Study (CHAMPS) *(84,85)* and ETOMS trial *(75,86)*. For unknown reasons, BH are rarely seen in the posterior fossa or spinal cord, regardless of disease severity or lesion burden on T2-WI.

The presence of brain atrophy in MS has been recognized for many years. The measurement of brain atrophy seems to be of growing clinical relevance as a biomarker of the disease process *(16,17,82,83,87–91)* (Figs. 10 and 11). There is a consensus developing that the assessment of brain atrophy by serial MRI represents a potentially powerful tool for monitoring disease progression and therapeutic efficacy in MS *(16,17,82,83,88,89)*. When compared to conventional MRI lesion measurements, brain atrophy is a better predictor of clinical impairments, such as physical disability *(17,79,83,90,92,93)*, cognitive dysfunction *(82,89,93)*, depression *(94)*, and quality of life *(95)*. The pathophysiology of brain atrophy in MS is unknown but likely represents an epiphenomenon consisting of a combination of the accumulation of focally destructive plaques, axonal injury, neuronal loss, and distal effects of Wallerian degeneration *(16,17,30,78,79)*. Another factor proposed to be related to brain atrophy is hypointensity of gray-matter structures on T2-WI (T2 hypointensity) *(96,97)*. T2 hypointensity, suggestive of iron deposition, has been described early in the course of MS and is related to physical disability, disease course, and brain atrophy *(96,97)*. It is not clear to what extent abnormal iron deposition in the brain contributes to disease pathophysiology or if it is purely an epiphenomenon of neurodegeneration. Although several studies have recognized the presence of brain atrophy in the earliest phases of MS *(17,89,98–102)*, it is unclear whether measurable brain atrophy is present at the time of the first clinical episode and how rapidly it progresses at this early stage (Fig. 10). Several studies have addressed this issue *(100–102)*. Brex et al. *(100)* followed 17 patients with CIS for 1 year, of whom nine developed MS and eight did not. Significant ventricular enlargement occurred after 1 year in the group that developed MS but not in the other group. The authors showed that atrophy, albeit mild, can be detected early in the course of MS. Dalton et al. *(102)* performed MRI of the brain on 55 consecutive patients with CIS, within 3 months of symptom onset and again 1 year later. Clinically definite MS had developed after 1 year in 16 of 40 patients with lesions on baseline T2-WI and 2 of 15 with a normal scan. Significant ventricular enlargement was seen in 27 of 55 patients who fulfilled the McDonald MRI criteria for MS at clinical follow-up. A significant increase in ventricular volume was also seen in 18 of 55 patients who developed clinical MS during the follow-up period. This study indicates that brain atrophy measures have a complementary predictive role in monitoring the course of MS, even in the earliest clinical stages. There is also evidence that spinal cord atrophy *(101)* is detectable in patients at the time of presentation with CIS in those at high-risk for developing MS.

MTI is an advanced MRI technique based on the interactions between protons that are unbound in a free water pool and those where motion is restricted because of binding with macromolecules (Fig. 12). Tissue damage in MS is usually reflected by a reduction in magnetization transfer ability and thus a decreased MTR. These decreases in MTR most likely reflect a reduction in the size of the tissue matrix and an increase in size of the free water pool. MTR is a quantitative measure. Although MTR decreases are not specific to any of the various MS pathologic substrates, a relationship has been shown between MTR and the percentage of residual axons and the degree of demyelination *(103)*. MTR analysis can provide information about

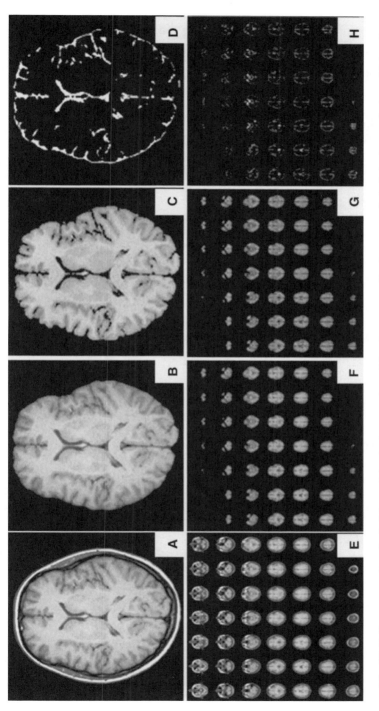

Fig. 10. Fully automated method of determining brain parenchymal fraction, a normalized measure of whole-brain atrophy in multiple sclerosis (MS), at the Buffalo Neuroimaging Analysis Center. (**A–D**) A single axial slice, spin-echo T1-weighted noncontrast, from a 27-year-old woman with clinically isolated syndromes (CIS) showing the raw image (**A**) after masking (removal) of extracranial tissue has been performed to isolate the outer brain contour (**B**) and after thresholding to separate the intracranial volume into brain parenchyma (**C**) and cerebrospinal fluid (CSF) (**D**). (**E–H**) Show that the algorithm is applied to all images from the midcerebellum to the vertex.

75

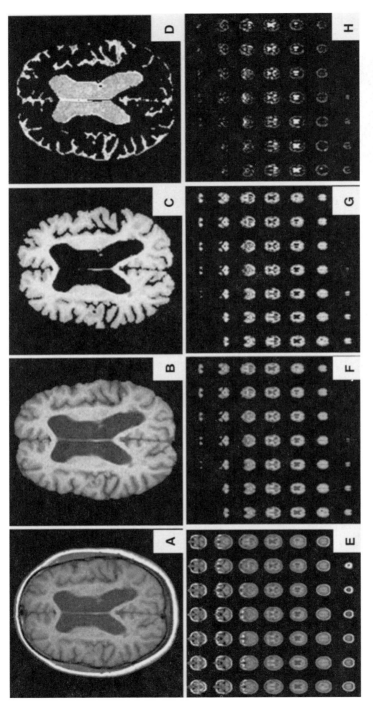

Fig. 11. Fully automated method of determining brain parenchymal fraction, a normalized measure of whole-brain atrophy at the Buffalo Neuroimaging Analysis Center, in a 44-year-old man with secondary progressive MS (SPMS). There is clear evidence of advanced atrophy, including prominence of cortical sulci (suggesting cortical atrophy) and ventriculomegaly (indicating central atrophy) as compared to a patient in the earliest phases of disease (Fig. 10). **(A–D)** A single axial slice, spin-echo T1-weighted noncontrast showing the raw image **(A)** after masking (removal) of extracranial tissue has been performed to isolate the outer brain contour **(B)** and after thresholding to separate the intracranial volume into brain parenchyma (C) and cerebrospinal fluid (CSF) **(D)**. **(E–H)** Show that the algorithm is applied to all images from the midcerebellum to the vertex.

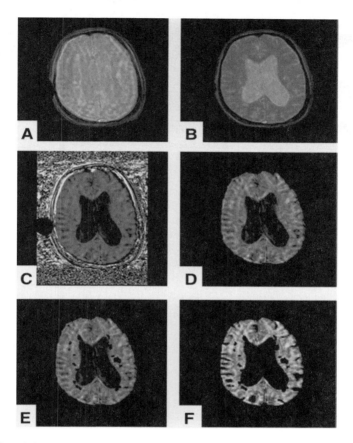

Fig. 12. Axial magnetization transfer (MT) images of the brain obtained by 3 D gradient-echo (GE) pulse PD-weighted images (PD-WI). **(A,B)** The image is shown with **(A)** and without **(B)** the onresonance saturation radio frequency (RF) pulse. **(C–E)** The GE images are coregistered and MT ratio (MTR) maps are created **(C)**. The MTR maps are coregistered with the corresponding masked (deskulled) PD-WI **(D)**, and the lesion tracings on PD-WI are superimposed onto the MTR maps leading to nulling of lesions **(E)**. An automated segmentation algorithm is applied to null the cerebrospinal fluid obtain MTR of the normal-appearing brain tissue **(F)**.

tissue injury occurring in the whole brain (global) and in specific brain structures (regional) *(18,19,104)*. MTI metrics have been correlated with the degree of disability *(18,19,104)*. Recent MTI studies *(105–108)* have revealed clinically relevant pathologic changes in areas of white matter that appear normal on conventional images; such changes in normal appearing white matter (NAWM) occur early in the disease process, including at the time of presentation with CIS and provide prognostic information pertaining to the risk of developing MS.

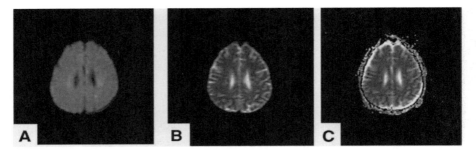

Fig. 13. Example of magnetic resonance imaging (MRI) diffusion weighted images (DWI) in a 35-year-old woman with relapsing-remitting multiple sclerosis (RRMS). Echoplanar DWI is performed generating trace images with a b-factor of 1000 (**A**) and 0 (**B**) s/mm^2 applied in three orthogonal directions. On the b-1000 DWI map (**A**) lesions appear as hyperintense areas compared with the surrounding tissue most likely resulting from T2 shinethrough rather than restricted diffusion. To calculate apparent diffusion coefficients (ADCs), an ADC map (**C**) is generated from images **A** and **B**. The diffusivity was computed separately in the x, y, and z orthogonal directions, and the results averaged to form the mean ADC map (**C**).

MRS provides a quantitative assessment of disease involvement related primarily to two major pathologic aspects of MS, active inflammatory demyelination and axonal/neuronal injury *(109)*. Inflammation and demyelination are represented by increases in choline, lactate, and lipids. Axonal and neuronal injury can be quantified through decreases in *N*-acetylaspartate (NAA). Decreases of NAA in the white matter of patients with MS reflect changes in density, size, or metabolism of axons *(109)*. Decreased NAA levels have been correlated with disability *(110,111)*. Moreover, axonal damage can be detected using MRS in patients with CIS *(112–114)*.

Diffusion is the random translational motion of molecules in a fluid system. In the brain, diffusion is influenced by the microscopic architecture of tissue, including axons, cell membranes, and organelles. Water molecular diffusion can be measured in vivo using MRI, and consequently, DWI is sensitive to pathologic processes that modify tissue integrity and result in changes in the permeability or density of barriers restricting water molecular motion, thereby affecting tissue anisotropy. Thus, measures derived from DWI reflect changes in the size, shape, geometry, and orientation of tissues (Fig. 13) *(115,116)*. DWI also provides quantitative data. MS lesions commonly show hyperintensity on DWI scans resulting from T2 shinethrough, which can be differentiated from true restriction of diffusion using ADC maps (Fig. 13). Tissue damage related to MS is usually reflected on DWI scans as increased diffusivity and increased ADC. Significant cross-sectional correlations between DWI and clinical findings in MS are emerging *(116,117)*. However, the stage at which DWI can detect abnormalities in NAWM is not clear. There is only one study *(118)* demonstrating that DWI did not detect alterations in NAWM of patients with CIS at baseline but that such abnormalities became apparent 1 year later.

Functional MRI (fMRI) is a unique MRI technique that can noninvasively detect activation of brain areas during the performance of tasks. To investigate how early cortical reorganization occurs in the course of MS, fMRI has been used to study the visual and motor systems of patients with CIS *(113,119–122)*. Recently, Pantano et al. *(121)* studied a group of 20 patients with early MS. In 10 patients, the CIS was hemiparesis, and in the other 10 patients, the CIS was ON. The group with hemiparesis showed functional adaptive changes that involved both the symptomatic and the asymptomatic hemisphere during a simple motor task. Moreover, the group with hemiparesis showed a significantly higher EDSS score and T1LV in the corticospinal tract than the group with ON. More severe specific damage to motor pathways in patients with a previous hemiparesis may explain the significantly higher involvement of ipsilateral motor areas observed in the group with hemiparesis than in the group with ON. Filippi et al. *(120)* studied cortical activation related to motor tasks in patients at presentation with CIS and a high risk for subsequently developing MS. Compared with healthy controls, the CIS group had an altered pattern of cortical activation, characterized by activation of the contralateral primary sensorimotor cortex. These data suggest that functional cortical reorganization occurs in response to injury at the earliest stages of MS.

ROLE OF MAGNETIC RESONANCE IMAGING IN THE PROGNOSIS OF MULTIPLE SCLEROSIS

MRI plays a role in determining the risk for developing MS in patients who present with CIS. However, the direct relationship between early MRI findings and subsequent long-term disability is not clear. Usually the first manifestation of MS is CIS, involving the optic nerves, brainstem, or spinal cord. The time between the first clinical attack and subsequent relapses, as well as the rate of accumulation of sustained neurological disability, is highly variable among patients. Baseline clinical and MRI findings are only moderately predictive of these subsequent occurrences. Brain MRI at the time of presentation in patients with CIS is useful for excluding other neurologic conditions and to stratify the risk of developing MS (a high risk is indicated by subclinical evidence of spatial dissemination of lesions) *(50)*. This is important in selecting patients for early disease-modifying treatments to reduce the likelihood of developing further clinical relapses and long-term disability *(84,86,123)*.

Use of Conventional Magnetic Resonance Imaging in the Prognosis of Multiple Sclerosis

Focal areas of high signal, identical to those seen in patients with established MS, have been found on T2-WI in 50 to 80% of the patients at presentation with CIS *(124–126)*. Several longitudinal studies using conventional MRI *(127–132)* showed that the number and volume of T2 lesions at presentation with CIS are associated with an increased risk of developing MS and lead to a higher level of disability at long-term follow-up.

Filippi et al. *(129)* studied 84 patients presenting with acute CIS of the optic nerves, brainstem, or spinal cord. At 5-year follow-up, 38 (45%) had developed probable or definite MS. Patients who developed MS during follow-up had a higher T2LV at presentation than those who did not. There was a strong correlation between baseline T2LV and both the increase in T2LV and accumulation of disability during the next 5 years. Ten year follow-up of this subgroup showed that 45 (83%) developed MS, of whom 11 (20%) had RR disease with at least moderate disability (EDSS > 3), 13 (24%) secondary progressive (SP) and 21 (39%) RR disease but mild disability *(130)*. For those with a normal baseline MRI, progression to MS occurred in only three out of 27 (11%), and all had RR disease with mild disability. The number and volume of baseline T2 lesions correlated moderately with the degree of disability 10 years later ($r = 0.45$, $p = 0.001$) *(131)*. After 14 years, MS developed in 44 of the 50 patients (88%) with abnormal MRI at presentation and in 4 of 21 patients (19%) with normal baseline MRI *(132)*. The EDSS disability score at 14 years correlated moderately with T2LV on MRI at 5 years ($r = 0.60$, $p > 0.001$) and with the increase in T2LV over the first 5 years ($r = 0.61$, $p > 0.001$). Thus, early MRI findings have prognostic value in patients with CIS, in terms of both conversion to MS and the long-term development of disability. However, the relationships were only moderate, indicating that T2LV alone may not be adequate for decisions about the use of disease-modifying treatment.

Kappos et al. *(32)* investigated the prognostic value of Gd-enhanced MRI in a meta-analysis of data from five natural-course studies and four placebo groups of clinical trials of 307 patients, 237 with RRMS, and 70 with SPMS. Neither the initial scan nor monthly scans for 6 months were predictive of change in the EDSS in the subsequent 12 or 24 months. The mean number of Gd-enhancing-lesions in the first 6 monthly scans was weakly predictive of EDSS change after 1 year (odds ratio = 1.34, $p = 0.082$) and 2 years (odds ratio = 1.65, $p = 0.049$). The authors concluded that although Gd enhancement in MRI is a predictor of subsequent relapses, it is not a strong predictor of the development of cumulative impairment or disability. This discrepancy supports the idea that discordant mechanisms are operative in the occurrence of relapses and in the development of sustained disability in MS. Several groups investigated the predictive value of homogeneously- and ring-enhancing lesions vs disability progression *(133–137)*. The findings suggested that the presence and frequency of Gd enhancement and changes in disability during a short period are predictive of future long-term deterioration. In one study *(39)*, the frequency of ring-enhancement did not predict sustained disability 3 years later. However, in a subgroup of patients treated with IFN-β-1b, ring-enhancing lesions were predictive of EDSS worsening after 3 years ($p = 0.01$). Further studies are warranted to test whether the presence of ring-enhancing lesions predicts long-term disability progression.

Use of Nonconventional Magnetic Resonance Imaging in the Prognosis of Multiple Sclerosis

Several studies have used brain atrophy, T1-hypointense LV, MTI, DWI, and MRS to test whether the extent and severity of tissue loss in lesions and in normal-appearing brain tissue at the time of CIS or in the early phase of RR MS may have value in predicting disability progression in the short- and long-term.

Several studies have shown that the development of brain atrophy in the early phase of RR MS is a good predictor of subsequent sustained neurological impairment in the long-term (5 years) *(17,79,90)*. These findings indicate that once brain atrophy is present, irreversible damage has already occurred (Fig. 11). The ability of the CNS to compensate for the loss of axons and neurons likely depends on the location of atrophy and the available brain reserve capacity. The authors believe that once the level of tissue loss reaches a critical threshold, patients are likely to begin to suffer clinical impairments and disease progression.

Several studies showed moderate but significant correlations between the accumulation of BH and long-term disability progression from the earliest stages of RR MS *(78–80,81,89,138–142)*. Results from the Multiple Sclerosis Collaborative Research Group trial *(80)* in placebo vs 80 IFN-β-1a RRMS treated patients with mild to moderate disability showed a modest but significant correlation between T1-hypointense LV and disability at baseline and during the trial. In patients who received the placebo, there was a 29.2% increase in the mean volume of T1-hypointense LV over 2 years, as compared to an 11.8% increase in the patients treated with IFN-β-1a. The development of T1 BH is influenced by prior inflammatory disease activity, as indicated by enhancing lesions, and can be partially prevented by disease-modifying therapy. The role of BH in the longitudinal monitoring of patients with MS is not clear and requires further validation studies.

Recently, four prospective MTI studies *(105–108)* demonstrated that subtle changes occurring in normal-appearing brain tissue are associated with an increased risk of developing MS in patients with CIS. The ability of MTI to predict the clinical evolution of MS has been investigated in a 5-year longitudinal study *(143)*. The authors found significant differences in baseline MTR values in NAWM between clinically stable and worsening patients with MS. A strong correlation was found between baseline MTR and subsequent 5-year change in EDSS disability score. MTR of the NAWM at baseline correctly predicted clinical evolution in 15 out of 18 patients (1 false-positive and 2 false-negatives), yielding a positive predictive value of 77%, a negative predictive value of 88%, and an odds ratio of 28. These data support the belief that MTR abnormalities in NAWM can predict the clinical evolution of MS.

MRS has been used by several groups to predict clinical evolution in RRMS *(14,144–147)*. In a 30-month longitudinal study of 29 patients with RR MS, De Stefano et al. *(146)* assessed NAA from a large central brain volume to evaluate the relationship between axonal/neuronal integrity and the accumulation of clinical disability. Changes in the NAA to creatine ratio correlated strongly with clinical disability suggesting that axonal injury contributes to long-term functional impairment of patients with MS.

DWI has been used to predict the clinical evolution of MS. In a recently published study, water diffusion changes in NAWM of 19 patients with CIS and in 12 healthy controls were compared *(118)*. The MRI scans obtained at baseline and at

12 months were reviewed according to the McDonald criteria for the diagnosis of MS. T2- and T1-LVs in the whole brain and ADCs in NAWM were evaluated. Thirteen patients developed MS during the study and three other patients remained as possible MS. ADCs in NAWM were significantly higher in patients than in controls at the 12-month follow-up but not at baseline. This study suggested that DWI cannot detect alterations in NAWM of patients with CIS. After 1 year, when most patients develop MS, DWI abnormalities in NAWM become apparent. These abnormalities are correlated with T2LV and may contribute to neurological impairment.

ACKNOWLEDGMENT

This study was supported in part by research grants to R. Bakshi from the National Institutes of Health (NIH-NINDS 1 K23 NS42379-01), National Multiple Sclerosis Society (RG 3258A2/1), and National Science Foundation (DBI-0234895). The authors thank Sarah Ludwig, Kelly Watts, Jin Kuwata, Jitendra Sharma, Chris Tjoa, Eve Salczynski, and Mike Dwyer for their technical support.

REFERENCES

1. McFarland HF, Frank JA, Albert PS, et al. Using gadolinium-enhanced magnetic resonance imaging to monitor disease activity in multiple sclerosis. Ann Neurol 1992;32:758–766.
2. Thompson AJ, Miller D, Youl B, et al. Serial gadolinium-enhanced MRI in relapsing/remitting multiple sclerosis of varying disease duration. Neurology 1992;42:60–63.
3. The IFNB Multiple Sclerosis Study Group and the University of British Columbia MS/MRI Analysis Group. Interferon-β-1b in the treatment of multiple sclerosis: Final outcome of the randomized controlled trial. Neurology 1995;45:1277–1285.
4. Simon JH, Jacobs LD, Campion M, et al. Magnetic resonance studies of intramuscular interferon β-1a for relapsing multiple sclerosis. Ann Neurol 1998;43:79–87.
5. Li DKB, Paty DW, the UBC MS/MRI Analysis Research Group and the PRISMS Study Group. Magnetic resonance imaging results of the PRISMS trial: a randomized, double-blind, placebo-controlled study of interferon β-1b in relapsing-remitting multiple sclerosis. Ann Neurol 1999;46:197–206.
6. Miller DH, Molyneaux PD, Barker GJ, et al. and the European Study Group on interferon β-1b in secondary progressive multiple sclerosis. Ann Neurol 1999;46:850–859.
7. Molyenux PD, Miller DH. Magnetic resonance imaging techniques to monitor phase III treatment trials. In: Filippi M, Arnold DL, Comi G, eds. Magnetic Resonance Spectroscopy in Multiple Sclerosis. Springer Verlag, Berlin, 2000, pp. 49–72.
8. van Walderveen MA, Kamphorst W, Scheltens P, et al. Histopathologic correlate of hypointense lesions on T1-weighted spin echo MRI in multiple sclerosis. Neurology 1998;50:1282–1288.
9. Filippi M, Campi A, Dousset V, et al. A magnetization transfer imaging study of normal-appearing white matter in multiple sclerosis. Neurology 1995;45:478–482.
10. Lucchinetti CF, Bruck W, Rodriguez M, Lasmman H. Distinct patterns of multiple sclerosis pathology indicates heterogeneity in pathogenesis. Brain Pathol 1996;6:259–274.
11. Miller DH, Grossman RI, Reingold SC, McFarland HF. The role of magnetic resonance techniques in understanding and managing multiple sclerosis. Brain 1998;121:3–24.
12. Filippi M, Rovaris M, Comi G. Introduction. In: Filippi M, Comi G, eds. New Frontiers of MR-Based Techniques in Multiple Sclerosis. Springer Verlag, Berlin, 2003, pp. 1–3.
13. Markovic-Plese S, McFarland HF. Immunopathogenesis of the multiple sclerosis lesion. Curr Neurol Neurosci Rep 2001;1:257–262.

14. Fu L, Matthews PM, De Stefano N, et al. Imaging axonal damage of normal appearing white matter in multiple sclerosis. Brain 1998;121:103–113.
15. van Wasberghe JHTM, Kamphorst W, De Groot JA, et al. Axonal loss in multiple sclerosis lesions: magnetic resonance imaging insight into substrates of disability. Ann Neurol 1999;46:747–754.
16. Miller DH, Barkhof F, Frank JA, Parker GJM, Thompson AJ. Measurement of atrophy in multiple sclerosis: pathological basis, methodological aspects and clinical relevance. Brain 2002;125:1676–1695.
17. Fisher E, Rudick RA, Simon JH, et al. Eight-year follow-up study of brain atrophy in patients with MS. Neurology 2002;59:1412–1420.
18. Filippi M, Grossman RI. MRI techniques to monitor MS evolution. The present and the future. Neurology 2002;58:1147–1153.
19. Arnold DL, Matthews PM. MRI in the diagnosis and management of multiple sclerosis, Neurology 2002;58(Suppl 4):S23–S31.
20. Filippi M, Mastronardo G, Bastianello S, et al. A longitudinal brain MRI study comparing the sensitivities of the conventional and a newer approach for detecting active lesions in multiple sclerosis. J Neurol Sci 1998;59:94–101.
21. Filippi M, Horsfield MA, Ader HJ, et al. Guidelines for using quantitative measures of brain magnetic resonance imaging abnormalities in monitoring the treatment of multiple sclerosis. Ann Neurol 1998;43:499–506.
22. Miller DH, Albert PS, Barkhof F, et al. Guidelines for the use of magnetic resonance techniques in monitoring the treatment of multiple sclerosis. Ann Neurol 1996;39:6–16.
23. Rovaris M, Rocca MA, Yousry I, et al. Lesion load quantification on fast-FLAIR, rapid acquisition relaxation-enhanced, and gradient spin echo brain MRI scans from multiple sclerosis patients. Mag Res Imaging 1999;17:105–110.
24. Bastianello S, Bozzao A, Paolillo A, et al. Fast spin-echo and fast fluid-attenuated inversion recovery sequences versus conventional spin-echo for MRI quantification of multiple sclerosis lesions. Am J Neuroradiol 1997;18:699–704.
25. Bakshi R, Ariyaratana S, Benedict RHB, Jacobs L. Fluid-attenuated inversion recovery magnetic resonance imaging detects cortical and juxtacortical multiple sclerosis lesions. Arch Neurol 2001;58:742–748.
26. Gawne-Cain ML, O'Riordan JI, Thompson AJ, Moseley IF, Miller DH. Multiple sclerosis lesion detection in the brain: a comparison of fast fluid-attenuated inversion recovery and conventional T2-weighted dual spin echo. Neurology 1997;49:364–370.
27. Campi A, Pontesilli S, Gerevini S, Scotti G. Comparison of MRI pulse sequences for investigation of lesions of the cervical spinal cord. Neuroradiology 2000;42:669–675.
28. Gass A, Moseley IF, Barker GJ, et al. Lesion discrimination in optic neuritis using high-resolution fat-suppressed fast spin-echo MRI. Neuroradiology 1996;38:317–321.
29. Smith ME, Stone LA, Albert PS, et al. Clinical worsening in multiple sclerosis is associated with increased frequency and area of gadopentetate dimeglumine-enhancing magnetic resonance imaging lesions. Ann Neurol 1993;33:480–489.
30. Simon JH. From enhancing lesions to brain atrophy in relapsing MS. J Neuroimmunol 1999;98:7–15.
31. Molyenux PD, Filippi M, Barkhof F, et al. Correlations between monthly enhanced MRI lesion rate and changes in T2 lesion volume in multiple sclerosis. Ann Neurol 1998;43:332–329.
32. Kappos L, Moeri D, Radue EW, et al. Predictive value of gadolinium-enhanced magnetic resonance imaging for relapse rate and changes in disability or impairment in multiple sclerosis: a meta-analysis. Lancet 1999;353:964–969.
33. Molyneux PD, Tofts PS, Fletcher A, et al. Precisions and reliability for measurement of change in MRI lesion volume in multiple sclerosis: a comparison of two computer-assisted techniques. J Neurol Neurosurg Psychiatry 1998;65:42–47.
34. Filippi M, Rocca MA, Rizzo G, et al. A multi-centre longitudinal study comparing the sensitivity of monthly MRI after standard and triple dose gadolinium DTPA for monitoring disease activity in multiple sclerosis. Implications for phase II clinical trials. Brain 1998;21:2011–2020.

35. Filippi M. Enhanced magnetic resonance in multiple sclerosis. Mult Scler 2000;6:320–326.
36. Wolansky LJ, Bardini JA, Cook SD, et al. Triple-dose versus single-dose gadoteridol in multiple sclerosis patients. J Neuroimaging 1994;4:141–145.
37. Silver NC, Good CD, Barker GJ, et al. Sensitivity of contrast enhanced MRI in multiple sclerosis. Effects of gadolinium dose magnetization transfer contrast and delayed imaging. Brain 1997;120:1149–1161.
38. Miller DH, Rudge P, Johnson G, et al. Serial gadolinium enhanced magnetic resonance imaging in multiple sclerosis. Brain 1988;111:927–939.
39. Morgen K, Jeffries NO, Stone R, et al. Ring-enhancement in multiple sclerosis: marker of disease severity. Mult Scler 2001;7:167–171.
40. He J, Grossman RI, Ge Y, Mannon LJ. Enhancing patterns in multiple sclerosis: evolution and persistence. Am J Neuroradiol 2001;22:664–669.
41. Rovira A, Alonso J, Cucurella G, et al. Evolution of multiple sclerosis lesions on serial contrast-enhanced T1-weighted and magnetization-transfer MR images. Am J Neuroradiol 1999;20: 1939–1945.
42. Guttman CR, Ahn SS, Hsu L, Kikinis R, Jolesz FA. The evolution of multiple sclerosis lesions on serial MR. Am J Neuroradiol 1995;16:1481–1491.
43. Petrella JR, Grossman RI, McGowan JC, Campbell G, Cohen JA. Multiple sclerosis lesions: relationship between MR enhancement pattern and magnetization transfer effect. Am J Neuroradiol 1996;17:1041–1049.
44. Roychowdhury S, Maldijian JA, Grossman RI. Multiple sclerosis: comparison of trace apparent diffusion coefficients with MR enhancement pattern of lesions. Am J Neuroradiol 2000;21: 869–874.
45. Leist TP, Gobbibi MI, Frank JA, McFarland HF. Enhancing magnetic resonance imaging lesions and cerebral atrophy in patients with relapsing multiple sclerosis. Arch Neurol 2001;58:57–60.
46. van Wasberghe JH, van Walderveen MA, Castelijns JA, et al. Patterns of lesion development in multiple sclerosis: longitudinal observations with T1-weighted spin-echo and magnetization transfer MR. Am J Neuroradiol 1998;19:675–683.
47. Pretorius PM, Quaghebeur G. The role of MRI in diagnosis of MS. Clin Radiol 2003;58:434–448.
48. O'Connor P on behalf of the Canadian Multiple Sclerosis Working Group. Key issues in the diagnosis and treatment of multiple sclerosis. An overview. Neurology 2002;59(Suppl 3):1–33.
49. Murthy SNK, Faden HA, Cohen ME, Bakshi R. Acute disseminated encephalomyelitis in children. Pediatrics 2002;110(e21-1):1–7.
50. McDonald WI, Compston A, Edan G, et al. Recommended diagnostic criteria for multiple sclerosis: guidelines from the International Panel on the diagnosis of multiple sclerosis. Ann Neurol 2001;50:121–127.
51. Kidd D, Thorpe JW, Thompson AJ, et al. Spinal cord MRI using multi-array coils and fast spin echo. II. Findings in multiple sclerosis. Neurology 1993;43:2632–2637.
52. Tartaglino LM, Friedman DP, Flanders AE, et al. Multiple sclerosis in the spinal cord: MR appearance and correlation with clinical parameters. Radiology 1995;195:725–732.
53. Loseff NA, Webb SL, O'Riordan JI, et al. Spinal cord atrophy and disability in multiple sclerosis. A new reproducible and sensitive MRI method with potential to monitor disease progression. Brain 1996;119:701–708.
54. Thorpe JW, Kidd D, Moseley IF, et al. Serial gadolinium-enhanced MRI of the brain and spinal cord in early relapsing-remitting multiple sclerosis. Neurology 1996;46:373–378.
55. Kidd D, Thorpe JW, Kendall BE, et al. MRI dynamics of brain and spinal cord in progressive multiple sclerosis. J Neurol Neurosurg Psychiatry 1996;60:15–19.
56. Yousry TA, Fesl G, Walther E, Voltz R, Filippi M. Triple dose of gadolinium-DTPA increases the sensitivity of spinal cord MRI in detecting enhancing lesions in multiple sclerosis. J Neurol Sci. 1998;158:221–225.
57. Thorpe JW, Kidd D, Moseley IF, et al. Spinal MRI in patients with suspected multiple sclerosis and negative brain MRI. Brain 1996;119:709–714.

58. O'Riordan JI, Losseff NA, Phatouros C, et al. Asymptomatic spinal cord lesions in clinically isolated optic nerve, brain stem, and spinal cord syndromes suggestive of demyelination. J Neurol Neurosurg Psychiatry 1998;64:353–357.

59. Trop I, Bourgouin PM, Lapierre Y, et al. Multiple sclerosis of the spinal cord: diagnosis and follow-up with contrast-enhanced MR and correlation with clinical activity. Am J Neuroradiol 1998;19:1025–1033.

60. Lycklama a Nijeholt GJ, Barkhof F, et al. MR of the spinal cord in multiple sclerosis: relation to clinical subtype and disability. Am J Neuroradiol. 1997;18:1041–1048.

61. Bakshi R, Kinkel PR, Mechtler LL, et al. Magnetic resonance imaging findings in 22 cases of myelitis: comparison between patients with and without multiple sclerosis. Eur J Neurol 1998;5:35–48.

62. Bakshi R, Glass J, Louis DN, Hochberg FH. Magnetic resonance imaging features of solitary inflammatory brain masses. J Neuroimaging 1998;8:8–14.

63. Wingerchuck DM, Weinshenker BG. Neuromyelitis optica. Clinical predictors of a relapsing course and survival. Neurology 2003;60:848–853.

64. Transverse Myelitis Consortium Working Group. Proposed diagnostic criteria and nosology of acute transverse myelitis. Neurology 2002;59:499–505.

65. Poser CM, Paty DW, Scheinberg L, et al. New diagnostic criteria for multiple sclerosis: guidelines for research protocols. Ann Neurol 1983;12:227–231.

66. Paty DW, Oger JJ, Kastrukoff LF, et al. MRI in the diagnosis of MS: a prospective study with comparison of clinical evaluation, evoked potentials, oligoclonal banding, and CT. Neurology. 1988;38:180–185.

67. Fazekas F, Offenbacher H, Fuchs S, et al. Criteria for an increased specificity of MRI interpretation in elderly subjects with suspected multiple sclerosis. Neurology 1988;38:1822–1825.

68. Barkhof F, Filippi M, Miller DH, et al. Comparison of MR imaging criteria at first presentation to predict conversion to clinically definite MS. Brain 1997;120:2059–2069.

69. Tintoré M, Rovira A, Martinez M, et al. Isolated demyelinating syndromes: comparison of different imaging criteria to predict conversion to clinically definite MS. Am J Neuroradiol 2000;21:702–706.

70. Brex PA, Miszkiel KA, O'Riordan JI, et al. Assessing the risk of early multiple sclerosis in patients with clinically isolated syndromes: the role of a follow up MRI. J Neurol Neurosurg Psychiatry 2001;70:390–393.

71. Tintore M, Rovira A, Rio J, et al. New diagnostic criteria for multiple sclerosis: application in first demyelinating episode. Neurology 2003;60:27–30.

72. Giovannoni G, Bever CT Jr. Patients with clinically isolated syndromes suggestive of MS: does MRI allow earlier diagnosis? Neurology 2003;60:6–7.

73. Dalton CM, Brex PA, Miszkiel KA, et al. Application of the new McDonald criteria to patients with clinically isolated syndromes suggestive of multiple sclerosis. Ann Neurol 2002;52:47–53.

74. Dalton CM, Brex PA, Miszkiel KA, et al. New T2 lesions enable an earlier diagnosis of multiple sclerosis in clinically isolated syndromes. Ann Neurol. 2003;53:673–676.

75. Barkhof F, Rocca M, Francis G, et al., and Early Treatment of Multiple Sclerosis Study Group. Validation of diagnostic magnetic resonance imaging criteria for multiple sclerosis and response to interferon beta1a. Ann Neurol 2003;53:718–724.

76. Thompson AJ, Polman CH, Miller DH, et al. Primary progressive multiple sclerosis. Brain 1997;12:1085–1096.

77. Wolinsky JS, PROMiSe Study Group. The diagnosis of primary progressive multiple sclerosis. J Neurol Sci 2003;206:145–152.

78. Paolillo A, Pozzilli C, Gasperini C, et al. Brain atrophy in relapsing-remitting multiple sclerosis. Relationship with black holes, disease duration and clinical disability. J Neurol Sci 2000; 174:85–91.

79. Zivadinov R, Rudick RA, De Masi R, et al. Effects of intravenous methylprednisolone on brain atrophy in relapsing-remitting multiple sclerosis. Neurology 2001;57:1239–1247.

80. Simon JH, Lull J, Jacobs LD, et al. A longitudinal study of T1 hypointense lesions in relapsing MS: MSCRG trial of interferon beta-1a. Multiple Sclerosis Collaborative Research Group. Neurology 2000;55:185–192.
81. Bitsch A, Kuhlmann T, Stadelmann C, et al. A longitudinal MRI study of histopathologically defined hypointense multiple sclerosis lesions. Ann Neurol 2001;49:793–796.
82. Benedict RHB, Weinstock-Guttman B, Fishman I, Sharma J, Tjoa CW, Bakshi R. Prediction of neuropsychological impairment in multiple sclerosis: a comparison of conventional MRI measures of atrophy and lesion burden. Arch Neurol 2004;61:226–230.
83. Bermel RA, Sharma J, Tjoa CW, Puli SR, Bakshi R. A semiautomated measure of whole-brain atrophy in multiple sclerosis. J Neurol Sci 2003:208;57–65.
84. Jacobs LD, Beck RW, Simon JH, et al. Intramuscular interferon beta-1a therapy initiated during a first demyelinating event in multiple sclerosis. CHAMPS Study Group. N Engl J Med 2000;343:898–904.
85. Beck RW, Chandler DL, Cole SR, et al. Interferon beta-1a for early multiple sclerosis: CHAMPS trial subgroup analyses. Ann Neurol 2002;51:481–490.
86. Comi G, Filippi M, Barkhof F, et al., and Early Treatment of Multiple Sclerosis Study Group Effect of early interferon treatment on conversion to definite multiple sclerosis: a randomised study. Lancet 2001;357:1576–1582.
87. Rovaris M, Filippi M. Interventions for the prevention of brain atrophy in multiple sclerosis: current status. CNS Drugs 2003;17:563–575.
88. Rudick RA, Fisher E, Lee JC, et al., and the Multiple Sclerosis Collaborative Research Group. Use of the brain parenchymal fraction to measure whole brain atrophy in relapsing-remitting MS. Neurology 1999;53:1698–1704.
89. Zivadinov R, Sepcic J, Nasuelli D, et al. A longitudinal study of brain atrophy and cognitive disturbances in the early phase of relapsing-remitting multiple sclerosis. J Neurol Neurosurg Psychiatry 2001;70:773–780.
90. Paolillo A, Pozzilli E, Giugni E, et al. A 6-year clinical and MRI follow-up study of patients with relapsing-remitting multiple sclerosis treated with Interferon-beta. Eur J Neurol 2002;9:1–11.
91. Zivadinov R, Zorzon M. Is gadolinium enhancement predictive of the development of brain atrophy in multiple sclerosis? A review of the literature. J Neuroimaging 2002;12:302–309.
92. Bakshi R, Benedict RHB, Bermel RA, Jacobs L. Regional brain atrophy is associated with physical disability in multiple sclerosis: semiquantitative MRI and relationship to clinical findings. J Neuroimaging 2001;11:129–136.
93. Zivadinov R, De Masi R, Nasuelli D, et al. Magnetic resonance imaging techniques and cognitive impairment in early phase of relapsing-remitting multiple sclerosis. Neuroradiology 2001;43:272–278.
94. Bakshi R, Czarnecki D, Shaikh ZA, et al. Brain MRI lesions and atrophy are related to depression in multiple sclerosis. NeuroReport 2000;11:1153–1158.
95. Janardhan V, Bakshi R. Quality of life and its relationship to brain lesions and atrophy on magnetic resonance images in 60 patients with multiple sclerosis. Arch Neurol 2000;57:1485–1491.
96. Bakshi R, Dmochowski J, Shaikh ZA, Jacobs L. Gray matter T2 hypointensity is related to plaques and atrophy in the brains of multiple sclerosis patients. J Neurol Sci 2001;185:19–26.
97. Bakshi R, Benedict RHB, Bermel RA, et al. T2 hypointensity in the deep gray matter of patients with multiple sclerosis: a quantitative magnetic resonance imaging study. Arch Neurol 2002;59:62–68.
98. Luks TL, Goodkin DE, Nelson SJ, et al. A longitudinal study of ventricular volume in early relapsing-remitting multiple sclerosis. Mult Scler 2000;6:322–327.
99. Chard DT, Griffin CM, Parker GJM, et al. Brain atrophy in clinically early relapsing-remitting multiple sclerosis. Brain 2002;125:327–337.
100. Brex PA, Jenkins R, Fox NC, et al. Detection of ventricular enlargement in patients at the earliest clinical stage of MS. Neurology 2000;54:1689–1691.

101. Brex PA, Leary SM, O'Riordan JI, et al. Measurement of spinal cord area in clinically isolated syndromes suggestive of multiple sclerosis. J Neurol Neurosurg Psychiatry 2001;70:544–547.

102. Dalton CM, Brex PA, Jenkins R, et al. Progressive ventricular enlargement in patients with clinically isolated syndromes is associated with the early development of multiple sclerosis. Ann Neurol 2002;73:141–147.

103. van Buchem MA, McGowan JC, Kolson DL, Polansky M, Grossman RI. Quantitative volumetric magnetization transfer analysis in multiple sclerosis: estimation of macroscopic and microscopic disease burden. Magn Reson Med 1996;36:632–636.

104. Rovaris M, Filippi M. Magnetization transfer imaging. In: Filippi M, Comi G, eds. New Frontiers of MR-Based Techniques in Multiple Sclerosis. Springer Verlag, Berlin, 2003, pp. 11–32.

105. Iannucci G, Tortorella C, Rovaris M, et al. Prognostic value of MR and magnetization transfer imaging findings in patients with clinically isolated syndromes suggestive of multiple sclerosis at presentation. A J Neuroradiol 2000;21:1034–1038.

106. Filippi M, Inglese M, Rovaris M, et al. Magnetization transfer imaging to monitor the evolution of MS: a 1-year follow-up study. Neurology 2000;55:940–946.

107. Brex PA, Larry SM, Plant GT, et al. Magnetization transfer imaging in patients with clinically isolated syndromes suggestive of multiple sclerosis. Am J Neuroradiol 2001;22:947–951.

108. Traboulsee A, Dehmeshki J, Brex PA, et al. Normal-appearing brain tissue MTR histograms in clinically isolated syndromes suggestive of MS. Neurology 2002;59:126–128.

109. Gonen O, Grossman RI. Global brain proton spectroscopy in MS. In: Filippi M, Comi G, eds. New Frontiers of MR-Based Techniques in Multiple Sclerosis. Springer Verlag, Berlin, 2003, pp. 47–71.

110. Davie CA, Barker GJ, Webb S, et al. Persistent functional deficit in multiple sclerosis and autosomal dominant cerebellar ataxia is associated with axon loss. Brain 1995;118:1583–1592.

111. Fu L, Matthews PM, De Stefano N, et al. Imaging axonal damage of normal appearing white matter in multiple sclerosis. Brain 1998;21:103–113.

112. Brex PA, Gomez-Anson B, Parker GJ, et al. Proton MR spectroscopy in clinically isolated syndromes suggestive of multiple sclerosis. J Neurol Sci 1999;166:16–22.

113. Rocca MA, Mezzapesa DM, Falini A, et al. Evidence for axonal pathology and adaptive cortical reorganization in patients at presentation with clinically isolated syndromes suggestive of multiple sclerosis. Neuroimage 2003;18:847–855.

114. Filippi M, Bozzali M, Rovaris M, et al. Evidence for widespread axonal damage at the earliest clinical stage of multiple sclerosis. Brain 2003;126:433–437.

115. Maldjian JA, Grossman RI. Future applications of DWI in MS. J Neurol Sci 2001;186(Suppl 1):55–57.

116. Fabiano AJ, Sharma J, Weinstock-Guttman B, et al. Thalamic involvement in multiple sclerosis: a diffusion-weighted magnetic resonance imaging study. J Neuroimaging 2003;13:307–314.

117. Cercignani M, Ingle M, Pagani E, Comi G, Filippi M. Mean diffusivity and fractional anisotropy histograms in patients with multiple sclerosis. Am J Neuroradiol 2001;22:952–958.

118. Caramia F, Pantano P, Di Legge S, et al. A longitudinal study of MR diffusion changes in normal appearing white matter of patients with early multiple sclerosis. Magn Reson Imaging 2002;20:383–388.

119. Werring DJ, Bullmore ET, Toosy AT, et al. Recovery from optic neuritis is associated with a change in the distribution of cerebral response to visual stimulation: a functional magnetic resonance imaging study. J Neurol Neurosurg Psychiatry 2000;68:441–449.

120. Filippi M, Rocca MA, Falini A, et al. A functional MRI study of patients at presentation with clinically isolated syndromes suggestive of multiple sclerosis. J Neurol 2002;249(Suppl 1):I/20.

121. Pantano P, Iannetti GD, Caramia F, et al. Cortical motor reorganization after a single clinical attack of multiple sclerosis. Brain 2002;125:1607–1615.

122. Pantano P, Mainero C, Iannetti GD, et al. Contribution of corticospinal tract damage to cortical motor reorganization after a single clinical attack of multiple sclerosis. Neuroimage 2002;17:1837–1843.

123. Noseworthy JH, Lucchinetti C, Rodriguez M, Weinshenker BG. Multiple sclerosis. New Engl J Med 2000;343:938–952.

124. Jacobs L, Kinkel PR, Kinkel WR. Silent brain lesions in patients with isolated idiopathic optic neuritis. A clinical and nuclear magnetic resonance imaging study. Arch Neurol 1986;43: 452–455.

125. Ormerod IE, Miller DH, McDonald WI, et al. The role of NMR imaging in the assessment of multiple sclerosis and isolated neurological lesions. A quantitative study. Brain 1987;110: 1579–1616.

126. Jacobs LD, Kaba SE, Miller CM, Priore RL, Brownscheidle CM. Correlation of clinical, magnetic resonance imaging, and cerebrospinal fluid findings in optic neuritis. Ann Neurol 1997;41:392–398.

127. Optic Neuritis Study Group. The 5-year risk of MS after optic neuritis. Experience of the optic neuritis treatment trial. Optic Neuritis Study Group. Neurology 1997;49:1404–1413.

128. Morrisey SP, Miller DH, Kendall BE, et al. The significance of brain magnetic resonance imaging abnormalities at presentation with clinically isolated syndromes suggestive of multiple sclerosis. A 5-year follow-up study. Brain 1993;116:135–146.

129. Filippi M, Horsfield MA, Morrisey MD, et al. Quantitative brain MRI lesion load predicts the course of clinically isolated syndromes suggestive of multiple sclerosis. Neurology 1994;44: 635–641.

130. O'Riordan JI, Thompson AJ, Kingsley DP, et al. The prognostic value of brain MRI in clinically isolated syndromes suggestive of demyelination. Brain 1998;121:495–503.

131. Sailer M, O'Riordan JI, Thompson AJ, et al. Quantitative MRI in patients with clinically isolated syndromes suggestive of demyelination. Neurology 1999;52:599–606.

132. Brex PA, Ciccarelli O, Jonathon I, et al. A longitudinal study of abnormalities on MRI and disability from multiple sclerosis. N Engl J Med 2002;346:158–164.

133. Losseff NA, Miller DH, Kidd D, Thompson AJ. The predictive value of gadolinium enhancement for long-term disability in relapsing-remitting multiple sclerosis—preliminary results. Mult Scler 2001;7:23–25.

134. Losseff NA, Kingsley DP, McDonald WI, Miller DH, Thompson AJ. Clinical and magnetic resonance imaging predictors of disability in primary and secondary progressive multiple sclerosis. Mult Scler 1996;1:218–222.

135. Koudriavtseva T, Thompson AJ, Fiorelli M, et al. Gadolinium enhanced MRI predicts clinical and MRI disease activity in relapsing-remitting multiple sclerosis. J Neurol Neurosurg Psychiatry 1997;62:285–287.

136. Simon JH. Contrast-enhanced MR imaging in the evaluation of treatment response and prediction of outcome in multiple sclerosis. J Magn Reson Imaging 1997;7:29–37.

137. Giovannoni G, Lai M, Thorpe J, et al. Longitudinal study of soluble adhesion molecules in multiple sclerosis: correlation with gadolinium enhanced magnetic resonance imaging. Neurology 1997;48:1557–1656.

138. Truyen L, van Waesberghe JH, van Walderveen MA, et al. Accumulation of hypointense lesions ("black holes") on T1 spin-echo MRI correlates with disease progression in multiple sclerosis. Neurology 1996;47:1469–1476.

139. Koziol JA, Wagner S, Sobel DF, et al. Predictive value of lesions for relapses in relapsing-remitting multiple sclerosis. AJNR Am J Neuroradiol 2001;22:284–291.

140. Wagner S, Adams H, Sobel DF, et al. New hypointense lesions on MRI in relapsing-remitting multiple sclerosis patients. Eur Neurol 2000;43:194–200.

141. Gasperini C, Pozzilli C, Bastianello S, et al. Interferon-beta-1a in relapsing-remitting multiple sclerosis: effect on hypointense lesion volume on T1 weighted images. J Neurol Neurosurg Psychiatry 1999;67:579–584.

142. Bagnato F, Jeffries N, Richert ND, et al. Evolution of T1 black holes in patients with multiple sclerosis imaged monthly for 4 years. Brain 2003;126:1–8.

143. Santos AC, Narayanan S, de Stefano N, et al. Magnetization transfer can predict clinical evolution in patients with multiple sclerosis. J Neurol 2002 ;249:662–668.

144. Arnold DL, Riess GT, Matthews PM, et al. Use of proton magnetic resonance spectroscopy for monitoring disease progression in multiple sclerosis. Ann Neurol. 1994;36:76–82.

145. De Stefano N, Matthews PM, Narayanan S, et al. Axonal dysfunction and disability in a relapse of multiple sclerosis: longitudinal study of a patient. Neurology 1997;49:1138–1141.

146. De Stefano N, Matthews PM, Fu L, et al. Axonal damage correlates with disability in patients with relapsing-remitting multiple sclerosis. Results of a longitudinal magnetic resonance spectroscopy study. Brain 1998;121:1469–1477.

147. Parry A, Corkill R, Blamire AM, et al. Beta-Interferon treatment does not always slow the progression of axonal injury in multiple sclerosis. J Neurol 2003;250:171–178.

4

Cognitive Dysfunction in Multiple Sclerosis

Darcy Cox, PsyD and Laura Julian, PhD

INTRODUCTION

Cognitive dysfunction is one of the more common symptoms of multiple sclerosis (MS), with an estimated point prevalence of 30 to 60%. The lifetime prevalence may be closer to 50 to 75%, as cognitive symptoms tend to progress with disease progression. Unfortunately, cognitive dysfunction can also be one of the more disabling symptoms of MS *(1–3)*. This chapter reviews the prevalence, diagnosis, possible etiologies, assessment, and treatment of cognitive disorders in MS.

DIAGNOSIS, CHARACTERIZATION, AND PREVALENCE

Cognitive dysfunction is diagnosed when patients experience a change in their cognitive functioning that produces functional impairment. The *Diagnostic and Statistical Manual of Psychiatric Disorders*, the primary diagnostic system used in American psychiatry, lists two cognitive disorders caused directly by MS: Dementia due to Multiple Sclerosis and Cognitive Disorder Not Otherwise Specified (NOS) due to Multiple Sclerosis *(4)*.

Dementia resulting from MS is characterized by memory impairment and impairment in at least one other cognitive domain, which may manifest as aphasia, apraxia, agnosia, or disturbed executive functioning. This impairment must produce significant decline in social and occupational functioning. Frequently, this level of impairment precludes participation in most basic daily activities, including driving, shopping independently, and managing household finances, and may require that the patient be conserved.

Cognitive disorder NOS as a result of MS is a much milder condition, which may include memory dysfunction, and although producing some disturbance in social and/or occupational functioning, does not result in the broad functional impairments seen in dementia resulting from MS. Patients with cognitive disorder NOS resulting from MS may complain of difficulty with memory, attention, multitasking, wordfinding, and problems with organization and scheduling. These

From: *Current Clinical Neurology: Multiple Sclerosis*
Edited by: M. J. Olek © Humana Press Inc., Totowa, NJ

complaints tend to be persistent, but they can wax and wane with fatigue and disease activity. These symptoms may reach a level where they result in occupational disability or unemployment, particularly in patients with intellectually challenging occupations. However, many patients with cognitive disorder NOS resulting from MS are able to continue working with some accommodations. Symptoms of cognitive disorder NOS resulting from MS can produce discord and difficulties in the patient's social and recreational functioning, but this discord is frequently a result of others in the patient's life attributing the patient's symptoms to willful ignoring rather than acknowledging the presence of cognitive change. Patients themselves may misattribute cognitive symptoms to depression, stress, aging, or "losing their minds."

Historically, researchers considered MS to be a subcortical dementia, consisting of recall failure with intact encoding and storage, impaired conceptualization reasoning, slowed information processing, and personality disturbance in the context of normal or near-normal intellectual and language functioning (5,6). However, this characterization does not adequately describe the presentation of many patients with MS and does not address recent imaging and immunological work that demonstrates that MS is truly a whole-brain disease rather than a disease affecting the white-matter tracts alone.

Numerous studies illustrate the depth and breadth of cognitive impairments that can be seen in MS. Thorton and Raz (7) and Zakzanis (8) in their meta-analyses found that impairments in all domains of memory, including problems with encoding and storage, were common in MS. Problems with processing speed, attention, and concentration may be among the most common problems (9–12). Wordfinding deficits and problems with fluency are often seen, particularly with timed generative naming or listing tasks (8,13,14). Difficulties with visual-spatial learning and memory, visuoperceptive organization, and visual-spatial construction tasks are found (8,15), and difficulties with executive functioning, including problems reasoning, sequencing, problem-solving, and shifting sets, can be seen (8,16,17). Executive dysfunction may be more common in primary-progressive MS (PPMS) than in relapsing-remitting MS (RRMS) or secondary-progressive (SPMS) (8). Cognitive symptoms can occur at any point in the disease course and have been confirmed in patients who are in the early stage of the disease, when their diagnosis remains probable rather than definite (18,19). These symptoms, even when individually fairly mild, have a negative cumulative effect on the patient's social and occupational functioning and level of independence. The seminal studies documenting this effect were by Rao, who found difficulties with memory and speed of processing to be the most common cognitive symptoms in MS (2). Patients who have these cognitive impairments are significantly more likely to be unemployed, report social difficulties, and need more personal assistance than patients who are not cognitively impaired, regardless of their level of physical disability (3,20). More recent data developed by the National Multiple Sclerosis Society found that 30 to 40% of Americans living with MS work full- or part-time outside the home, compared to 64% of Americans in the general population *(21)*. These data, although suggesting that many patients with MS are able to continue working in some capacity, do not address several important issues. Many people with MS are able to continue working but only by accepting accommodations, including reductions in hours, reductions in pay, and changing positions to easier or less personally fulfilling roles.

ETIOLOGY: IMAGING FINDINGS

Numerous factors contribute to cognitive dysfunction in patients with MS. Of these, neuropathological changes in the white matter are best understood, although promising lines of research are developing our understanding of the roles of neuro-pathology in the gray matter, changes in neurochemistry, and neuroimmunology.

Techniques for imaging the in vivo brain have greatly expanded our understanding of cognitive dysfunction in MS. Although earlier research focused on white-matter pathology in MS, newer imaging techniques are allowing exploration of gray-matter pathology, axonal damage, and the subsequent atrophy seen in these patients. All these factors play a role in the cognitive dysfunction seen in patients with MS. Imaging studies find modest correlations between T1 and T2 lesion load, proton density (PD)-magnetic resonance imaging (MRI) lesion load, various measures of brain atrophy, various magnetic transfer ratio (MTR) histogram parameters, and cognitive dysfunction. Newer imaging techniques, such as spectroscopy and diffusion tensor imaging, are also likely to provide interesting insights about the causes of cognitive dysfunction in patients with MS.

LONGITUDINAL STUDIES OF CONVENTIONAL IMAGING

The earliest MRI measures found to correlate with cognition in MS were T2 and T1 lesion burden. There is a well-established moderate correlation between these conventional imaging parameters and cognitive dysfunction *(14,17,22–24)*. Although total T2 and T1 lesion burden acts as an adequate predictor of cognitive dysfunction, these measures alone do not account for all the variance in cognitive functioning. Several other factors are crucial, including disease duration, atrophy, axonal degeneration, and other changes in the normal-appearing white matter (NAWM).

Some studies have examined the relationships between cognitive dysfunction and lesion burden longitudinally. Sperling and colleagues *(25)* found that T2 lesion burden in the frontal and parietal white matter correlated with performance on measures of attention, processing speed, and verbal learning in their group of patients with RRMS and SPMS who were cognitively stable for a 4-year period. Hohol and colleagues *(24)* found significant correlations between total T2 lesion volume and ventricular enlargement and nonverbal memory, attention, and processing speed in their mixed group (RRMS, SPMS, and PPMS) of patients who were cognitively stable for 1 year and who demonstrated a statistically significant increase in ventricle size. Neither of these samples demonstrated a statistically significant increase in lesion load, although both groups evidenced this trend. These studies suggest that the rate of change in both lesion volume and cognitive dysfunction is fairly slow, while establishing the significant effect of cortical atrophy. However, in both studies, some patients were receiving interferon (IFN)-β or glatiramer acetate while enrolled, and some were not. Thus, it is possible that the relative stability in both cognitive and MRI measures of these groups reflect the benefits of treatment with immunomodulating agents.

A study providing 10-year follow-up data on the cognitive performance of early RRMS patients further supports the idea that cognitive progression is fairly slow for most patients, regardless of treatment *(20)*. Even though no imaging data were available for these subjects, Amato and colleagues found significant increases in the number of patients considered to be mildly cognitively impaired 4 years after baseline assessment and the number of patients considered to be moderately cognitively impaired 10 years after the initial assessment. Of their 45 patients sample, only 7 received IFN medications, so this data may provide a more accurate view of the natural history of cognitive dysfunction in MS.

NONCONVENTIONAL IMAGING

Although most studies have examined the relationship between T1 and T2 lesion volumes and neuropsychological test scores, there have also been promising studies correlating MTR histograms with neuropsychological functioning *(14,18,26)*. Rovaris and colleagues, in two separate studies, found significant correlations between MTR mean histograms and the measures of verbal fluency, verbal learning and memory, and processing speed and cognitive flexibility. They also found that the average height of the MTR histogram and the peak location of this histogram accounts for 68% of the variance in cognitive functioning in their sample *(27,28)*. In their sample of patients with RRMS and CPMS, Van Buchem and colleagues *(26)* found correlations between MTR histograms and numerous neuropsychological measures, including processing speed, memory, and conceptual processing. Zinadinov and colleagues *(18)* found significant relationships between MTR histogram parameters and cognitive dysfunction quite early in the disease course, further supporting the finding that cognitive symptoms are often seen in the initial presentation.

Studies have attempted to correlate protein magnetic resonance spectroscopy HMRS metabolite ratios and neuropsychological functioning. In their examination of the relationship between spectroscopy and neuropsychological functioning, Foong and colleagues *(29)* found no significant correlations between NAA/Cr ratios and neuropsychological measures. They split their sample into thirds, and the third with the lowest NAA/Cr ratio differed significantly from the other groups on spatial working memory test scores. The use of spectroscopy to develop a better understanding of cognitive dysfunction in MS is likely to lead to additional interesting findings. Krupp and colleagues found significant relationships between verbal learning and memory and problem solving and *N*-acetylaspartate (NAA) concentrations in the left periventricular regions *(30–33)*.

ATROPHY

Atrophy plays a significant role in the development of cognitive difficulties in MS, perhaps particularly in patients with frontal syndromes and more severe behavioral difficulties. Atrophy can begin early in the disease course. Zivadinov and colleagues found evidence of atrophy in the first 5 years after diagnosis in RRMS patients with low levels of physical disability. Following these patients for 5 years, they found that decreased brain parenchymal volume during this time predicts cognitive dysfunction and that patients who experienced greater levels of physical disability also demonstrated more atrophy *(34)*. Frontal atrophy, supratentorial atrophy, and atrophy of the corpus callosum correlate with numerous cognitive problems, including problems with learning and memory, reasoning and attention, as well measures of global cognitive impairment and dementia *(34–36)*. These findings suggest that frontal atrophy may predispose MS patients to mood and behavioral disturbance *(37)*.

FUNCTIONAL IMAGING

Functional MRI is also likely to provide valuable information about how cognitive dysfunction in MS develops. Staffen and colleagues found different activation patterns between controls and patients with MS performing a visual analog of the Paced Auditory Serial Addition Test (PASAT) *(38)*. This line of work is particularly exciting because it may help us better understand both the neuropathology that causes cognitive dysfunction in MS and neuroprotective processes in the brain that contribute to cognitive reserve in these patients.

In summary, cognitive dysfunction is an early symptom of the disease for many patients and tends to be the result of several pathological changes in the brain, including discrete lesions, atrophy, and changes in the NAWM and likely in the gray matter as well.

OTHER FACTORS IMPLICATED IN COGNITIVE DYSFUNCTION

Depression

In addition to neuropathology, several other factors are implicated in disturbed cognitive functioning in patients with MS. Depression is another common symptom of MS, and it frequently has a negative effect on cognition (particularly memory), attention, and concentration. Depression, lack of social support, and cognitive impairment correlate with each other, independent of level of physical disability *(39)*. Depression is also clearly correlated with the use of less effective coping styles, such as emotion-focused coping *(40)*. These relationships are likely to be complex and interactive. The ability of severe clinical depression to reduce performance on neuropsychological measures is well established in healthy controls and in patients with known risk factors for cognitive dysfunction, such as traumatic brain injury (TBI). In patients with MS, Arnett and colleagues found that 25% of the variance in measures of depression is predicted by difficulties with attention/working memory and that these difficulties are particularly apparent on timed tasks of reasoning and problem solving *(41)*. This suggests that cognitive dysfunction may lead to impaired problem solving and poor coping in real-world situations, where people frequently must make flexible and instantaneous coping choices.

A cognitive domain that is especially vulnerable to depression in MS includes working memory and other aspects of executive functioning. Using the working memory system conceptualized by Baddeley and Hitch *(42)*, deficits have been observed in the domains of central executive functioning. Furthermore, patients with MS who are depressed perform poorly when measures of central executive function include a speeded component. Using a capacity-demanding reading-span task and a less demanding word-span task, Arnett et al. *(43)* demonstrated significantly worse performance by patients with MS who were depressed when compared to patients with MS who were not depressed. Although differences in working memory have been noted in patients with MS regardless of depressive status, Arnett and colleagues have demonstrated that depression accounts for a significant proportion of the variance in central executive processes of working memory in MS. These findings are consistent with those of other researchers *(44)* and suggest that depression may exacerbate and/or contribute to existing deficits in central executive processing.

In another investigation, Arnett and colleagues *(41)* also demonstrated decreased functioning in planning abilities among patients with MS who were depressed compared to non-patients with MS who were not depressed using the Tower of London task. In addition to planning abilities, deficits were noted among other measures conceptualized as speeded central executive tasks, namely, the Symbol Digit Modalities Test (SDMT), the PASAT, a reading-span test, and the Visual Elevator subtest of the Test of Everyday Attention. In summary, among other cognitive domains, speeded attentional processing and nonspeeded central executive functioning are specifically susceptible to depression in MS *(41,45,46)*.

Pain

Pain is another frequent symptom of MS that has a well-established negative effect on cognitive functioning. People with MS can experience pain related to spasticity, paroxysmal symptoms, and headache, as well as neuropathic pain. The experience of MS-related pain can range from mild to fairly severe and may or may not be easily treated through medication, physical therapy, or other relief strategies. Pain produces both a direct and an indirect effect on cognitive functioning. People experiencing chronic or acute pain demonstrate decreased attention, processing speed, and difficulties with encoding. Indirectly, pain can produce changes in mood, including depression, and medications used to treat pain frequently have adverse effects on cognitive functioning. In MS, spasticity and muscle tension are often treated with benzodiazepines, which have a direct negative effect on cognition. Antiepileptic medicines frequently used to manage neuropathy also can produce changes in cognitive functioning, particularly difficulties with attention and processing speed.

Fatigue

However, the most common clinical symptom of MS is fatigue, and people with MS can experience worsening of cognitive symptoms both as a direct result of physical fatigue and as a result of cognitive fatigue. Cognitive fatigue is defined as a decline in cognitive performance during a brief time period, such as a neuropsychological testing session or part of the patient's workday. This decline occurs even though the patient is not participating in any physically fatiguing activities. Krupp and colleagues found that patients with MS demonstrated clear declines in performance on measures of verbal memory and executive functioning for a 4-hour session, whereas medically healthy controls demonstrated improvement in memory and executive functioning during the same time period, likely because of practice effects *(32)*. As such, it is particularly important for patients with MS to adequately pace themselves to keep fatigue to a minimum.

ASSESSMENT OF COGNITIVE DYSFUNCTION IN MULTIPLE SCLEROSIS

Clinical Neuropsychological Assessment

Complete and accurate assessment of cognitive dysfunction in patients with MS is important, particularly in those patients who do not have dementia but who, nonetheless, may be experiencing social and occupational difficulties as a result of MS-related cognitive dysfunction. There are several issues related to the assessment of patients with MS. The "gold standard" for assessment is a full neuropsychological battery administered and interpreted by a clinical neuropsychologist. There are several strengths associated with this approach, including an in-depth understanding of the neurological and neuropathological causes of the difficulties the patient is experiencing and the ability to compare the patient against normative standards for the population as a whole, other similar patients with MS, and against the patient's premorbid functioning. Neuropsychologists are able to work with the patient and his or her family or caretakers to develop an individualized plan to understand, manage, and, when possible, remedy the difficulties the patient is experiencing. Neuropsychologists can determine what types of compensatory and rehabilitative approaches will be most helpful for the patient. In addition, neuropsychologists can continue to follow the patient while assessing progression of difficulties and effectiveness of strategies to manage and remediate them.

However, there are numerous potential problems associated with neuropsychological assessment. A full battery usually takes between 6 and 8 hours to administer. This can lead to several difficulties, including problems related to the patient's fatigue, issues with cost and reimbursement, and issues of accessibility, given the limited number of neuropsychologists in many geographic areas. Therefore, numerous other options must be considered.

Recently, a group of prominent MS neuropsychologists have recommended a minimal neuropsychological battery for use with patients with MS. This battery, well-described elsewhere, specifies the need to assess a number of areas of cognitive functioning, including attention, processing speed, mood, verbal and visual learning and memory, language, and verbal and visual-spatial reasoning and judgment *(47)*. Although these measures are still administered by a neuropsychologist or trained psychometrician, most patients should take between 90 and 120 minutes to complete them. This is an excellent option for screening patients, or tracking known progression of deficits in patients who have undergone a more throughout assessment in the past. The downside of this approach is that it still requires a neuropsychologist or trained psychometrician, and issues related to access may still pose barriers for the patient.

One solution under consideration for this access problem is the use of a brief screening questionnaire in the neurologist's office. The MS Neuropsychological Questionnaire, a 15-item measure designed by Benedict and colleagues, can be administered to both patients and significant others in any clinic setting *(48)*. Interestingly, the patient report form of this questionnaire correlates significantly with depression, rather than cognitive functioning. However, the significant-other version has good sensitivity and specificity to cognitive dysfunction in the patient.

Assessment in Research and Clinical Trial Settings

Several outcome measures, are used in randomized controlled clinical trials to assess cognitive functioning as a secondary outcome. Of these, the most commonly used is the Multiple Sclerosis Functional Composite (MSFC). This measure consists of an assessment of lower-limb function/ambulation, the 25-foot walk, a measure of upper-limb function, the nine-hole peg test, and a measure of attention/working memory, the Rao version of the PASAT *(49)*. The MSFC is generally used in conjunction with Expanded Disability Status Scale (EDSS) scores as an outcome measure for clinical trials. It has numerous strengths but also some significant weakness. The PASAT is highly sensitive to MS-related cognitive dysfunction, but it is not specific. Poor performance on the PASAT can be attributed to several factors other than MS cognitive dysfunction, including anxiety, poor math skills, or difficulties in attention and working memory secondary to fatigue, pain, or medication.

TREATMENT

Effect of the Disease Modifying Medications on Cognitive Functioning

Some of the current disease-modifying medications slow the progression of cognitive dysfunction in MS. Intramuscular IFN-β-1a (Avonex) and IFN-β-1b (Betaseron) help preserve cognitive functioning, whereas no effect on cognition is seen for glatiramer acetate (Copaxone) *(50–52)*. IFN-β-1b has a positive effect on visual memory in a small group of patients with RRMS *(51)*. Intramuscular IFN-β-1a has several preservative effects on a much larger group of patients with RRMS *(50)*. Specifically, intramuscular IFN-β-1a helps preserve cognitive functioning during a 2-year period in many key areas, including processing speed, visual-spatial learning and memory, and executive functioning *(50)*. No data on the effects of subcutaneous IFN-β-1a (Rebif) on cognitive functioning are available at this time. The effect of chemotherapy agents commonly used in MS on cognitive functioning has not yet been studied.

Other Approaches to Managing Cognitive Dysfunction in Multiple Sclerosis

In addition to treatments designed to slow the progression of MS itself, several approaches to managing or remediating cognitive symptoms themselves have been suggested.

Symptomatic treatments have been examined in the hope that they would lead to a beneficial effect on cognitive function. No effect on cognition has been seen for pemoline and amantadine or 4-aminopyaride. There have been small, non-randomized, open-label trials of donepezil hydrochloride in patients with MS with cognitive dysfunction and dementia, finding some benefit, but no randomized placebo-controlled trials as yet in this class of medications *(53)*. Clinically, the treatment of depression and pain may also have a significant effect on the patient's experience of cognitive dysfunction.

The research into the application of cognitive rehabilitation techniques has been limited. One study finds no benefit on cognition in a small trial of a cognitive rehabilitation program *(54)*, although this study finds benefit of their program on quality of life for patients. Plohmann and colleagues demonstrated some benefit for a computerized attention training program in patients with MS with mild attentional deficits *(55)*. Canellopoulou and colleagues demonstrated some benefit for memory training in a clinical setting, although these strategies did not independently generalize to the patients' daily lives *(33)*. Further research into the application of cognitive rehabilitation techniques, particularly newer, computer-assisted techniques, is clearly needed.

Currently, because the benefits of medication and rehabilitation are fairly limited, the most common strategies for managing cognitive difficulties associated with MS require the patient to compensate for these difficulties and accommodate them when unable to compensate. There are numerous strategies that patients may find useful for managing specific types of cognitive problems. For patients with memory and organizational difficulties, the use of personal organizers, particularly those with alarms, can be helpful. Compensating for these kinds of difficulties frequently involves a fair amount of assistance from others in the patient's life, including both family members and coworkers. The use of written reminders and directions, telephone logs, and help maintaining a clean and organized home environment can be important. In addition, pacing to manage physical and cognitive fatigue can be helpful. For patients who wish to keep working outside the home, appropriate pacing can be crucial. Several accommodations designed to allow the person with MS adequate opportunities to rest, such as telecommuting and job-sharing, can help keep patients productive in the workforce.

SUMMARY

Cognitive dysfunction is a common symptom of MS, present in as many as three-fourths of patients. It frequently appears early in the disease course. Cognitive dysfunction arises from many of the neuropathological changes seen in the brains of patients with MS, including atrophy, discrete lesions, and changes to NAWM. Cognitive dysfunction is a particularly disabling symptom because of its effects on a patient's social functioning and ability to continue paid employment, as well as the support services that it requires. Cognitive symptoms can vary a great deal from patient to patient and are affected by several other MS symptoms. Depression, fatigue, anxiety, and pain can worsen or mimic cognitive symptoms. Immuno-modulating therapies have some positive effect on cognition, but currently, most patients will receive most benefit from developing individualized plans to manage and compensate for these problems.

ACKNOWLEDGMENT

Dr. Julian is supported by a National Multiple Sclerosis Society Fellowship Grant (FG 1481-A1).

REFERENCES

1. Amato MP, Ponziani G, Siracusa G, Sorbi S. Cognitive dysfunction in early-onset multiple sclerosis: a reappraisal after 10 years. Arch Neurol 2001;58:1602–1606.
2. Rao SM, Leo GJ, Bernardin L, Unverzagt F. Cognitive dysfunction in multiple sclerosis. I. Frequency, patterns, and prediction. Neurology 1991;41:685–691.
3. Rao SM, Leo GJ, Ellington L, Nauertz T, Bernardin L, Unverzagt F. Cognitive dysfunction in multiple sclerosis II. Impact on employment and social functioning. Neurology 1991;41:692–696.
4. American Psychiatric Association. Diagnostic and Statistical Manual of Mental Disorders (4th ed). American Psychiatric Association, Washington, DC, 1994.
5. Rao S. Neuropsychology of multiple sclerosis: a critical review. J Clin Exp Neuropsychol 1986;8:503–542.
6. Beatty WW, Goodkin DE, Monson N, Beatty P. Cognitive disturbances in patients with relapsing remitting multiple sclerosis. Arch Neurol 1989;46:1113–1119.
7. Thornton AE, Raz N. Memory impairment in multiple sclerosis: a quantitative review. Neuropsychology 1997;11:357–366.
8. Zakzanis K. Distinct neurocognitive profiles in multiple sclerosis subtypes. Arch Clin Neuropsychol 2000;15:115–136.
9. Kujala P, Portin R, Ruutianen J, Memory deficits and early cognitive deterioration in MS. Acta Neurologica Scand 1996;93:329–335.
10. Kail R. Speed of information processing in patients with Multiple Sclerosis. J Clin Exper Neuropsychol 1998;20:1–9.
11. Grant I, McDonald WI, Trimble M. Neuropsychological impairment in early multiple sclerosis. In: Jensen K, et al. eds. Mental Disorders and Cognitive Deficits in Multiple Sclerosis John Libbey, London, 1989, pp. 17–26.
12. Brassington JC, Marsh NV. Neuropsychological aspects of multiple sclerosis. Neuropsychol Rev 1998;8:43–77.
13. Basso MR, Beason-Hazan S, Lynn J, Rammochan K, Bornstein RA. Screening for cognitive dysfunction in multiple sclerosis. Arch Neurol 1996;53:980–984.
14. Rovaris M, Fillippi M, Falautano M, et al. Relation between MR abnormalities and patterns of cognitive impairment in multiple sclerosis. Neurology 1998;50:1601–1608.

15. DeLuca J, Barbieri-Berger S, Johnson SK. The nature of memory impairments in multiple sclerosis: acquisition versus retrieval. J Clin Exp Neuropsychol 1994;16:183–189.
16. Beatty W, Monson N. Picture and motor sequencing in Multiple Sclerosis. J Clin Exp Neuropsychol 1994;16:165–172.
17. Foong J, et al. Executive function in multiple sclerosis: the role of frontal lobe pathology. Brain 1997;120:15–26.
18. Zivadinov R, De Masi R, NaSuelli D, et al. MRI techniques and cognitive impairment in the early phase of relapsing-remitting multiple sclerosis. Neuroradiology 2001;43:272–278.
19. Achiron A, Barak Y. Cognitive impairment in probable multiple sclerosis. J Neurol Neurosurg Psychiatry, 2003;74:443–446.
20. Amato M, Ponziani G, Siracusa G, Sorbi S. Cognitive dysfunction in early-onset multiple sclerosis: a reappraisal after 10 years. Arch Neurol 2001;58:1602–1606.
21. LaRocca, N.G., Personal Communication. 2001.
22. Camp S, Stevenson V, Thompson A, et al. Cognitive function in primary progressive and transitional progressive multiple sclerosis: a controlled study with MRI correlates. Brain 1999;122:1341–1348.
23. Comi G, Fillipi M, Marinelli V, et al. Brain MRI correlates of cognitive impairment in primary and secondary progressive multiple sclerosis. J Neurol Sci, 1995;132:222–227.
24. Hohol MJ, Guttman CRG, Orav J, et al. Serial neuropsychological assessment and magnetic resonance imaging analysis in multiple sclerosis. Arch Neurol 1997;54:1018–1025.
25. Sperling RA, Guttman CR, Hohol MJ, et al. Regional magnetic resonance imaging lesion burden and cognitive functioning in multiple sclerosis: a longitudinal study. Arch Neurol 2001;58:115–121.
26. van Buchem MA, McGowan JC, Gossmann RI. Magnetization transfer histogram methodology: its clinical and neuropsychological correlates. Neurology 1999;53(S3):S23–S28.
27. Rovaris M, Filippi M, Minicucci L, et al. Cortical/subcortical disease burden and cognitive impairment in patients with multiple sclerosis. AJNR Am J Neuroradiol 2000;21:402–408.
28. Rovaris M, Filippi M. MRI correlates of cognitive dysfunction in multiple sclerosis patients. J Neurovirol 2000;6(Suppl 2):S172–S175.
29. Foong J, Rozewicz L, Bavieca, Thompson AJ, Miller DH, Ron MA, et al. Correlates of executive function in multiple sclerosis: the use of magnetic resonance spectroscopy as an index of focal pathology. J Neuropsychiat Clin Neurosci 1999;11:54–50.
30. Krupp LB, Alvarez LA, LaRocca NG, Scheinberg LC, et al. Fatigue in multiple sclerosis. Arch Neurol 1988;45:435–437.
31. Krupp LB, Sliwinski M, Masur DM, Friedberg F, Coyle PK, et al. Cognitive functioning and depression in patients with chronic fatigue syndrome and multiple sclerosis. Arch Neurol 1994;51:705–710.
32. Krupp LB, Elkins LE. Fatigue and declines in cognitive functioning in multiple sclerosis. Neurology 2000;55:934–939.
33. Canellopoulou M, Richardson JTE. The role of executive function in imagery mnemonics: evidence from multiple sclerosis. Neuropsychologia 1998;36:1181–1188.
34. Zivadinov R, Sepcic J, Nasuelli D, et al. A longitudinal study of brain atrophy and cognitive disturbances in the early phase of relapsing-remitting multiple sclerosis. J Neurol Neurosurg Psychiatry 2001;70:773–780.
35. Edwards S, Liu C, Blumhardt L. Cognitive correlates of supratentorial atrophy on MRI in multiple sclerosis. Acta Neurologica Scand 2001;104:214–223.
36. Benedict R, Bakshi R, Simon JH, Priore R, Miller C, Munschauer F, et al. Frontal cortex atrophy predicts cognitive impairment in multiple sclerosis. J Neuropsychiatry Clin Neurosci 2002;14:44–51.
37. Huber SJ, Rammohan KW, Bornstein RA, Christy JA, et al. Depressive symptoms are not influenced by severity of multiple sclerosis. Neuropsychiatry Neuropsychol Behav Neurol 1993;6:177–180.
38. Staffen W, Mair A, Zauner H, et al. Cognitive function and fMRI in patients with multiple sclerosis: evidence for compensatory cortical activation during an attention task. Brain 2002;125:1275–1282.

39. Gilchrist AC, Creed FH. Depression, cognitive impairment and social stress in multiple sclerosis. J Psychosomat Med 1994;38:193–201.
40. Mohr DC, Goodkin DE, Gatto N, Van Der Wende J, et al. Depression, coping, and level of neurological impairment in multiple sclerosis. Mult Scler 1997;3:254–258.
41. Arnett PA, Higgenson CI, Randolph JJ. Depression in multiple sclerosis: relationship to planning ability. J Intl Neuropsychol Soc 2001;7:665–674.
42. Baddeley AD, Hitch GJ. Working memory. In: The Psychology of Learning and Motivation, Bower GH, ed. Academic Press, San Diego, 1974, pp. 47–90.
43. Arnett PA, Higginson CI, Voss ND, et al. Depressed mood in multiple sclerosis: relationship to capacity-demanding memory and attentional functioning. Neuropsychology 1999;13:434–446.
44. Thornton AE, Raz N. Memory impairment in multiple sclerosis: a quantitative review. Neuropsychology, 1997;11:357–366.
45. Arnett PA, Higginson CI, Voss WD, Bender WI, Wurst JM, Tippin JM. Depression in multiple sclerosis: relationship to working memory capacity. Neuropsychology 1999;13:546–556.
46. Arnett PA, Higginson CT, Voss WD, et al. Depressed mood in multiple sclerosis: relationship to capacity-demanding memory and attentional functioning. Neuropsychology 1999;13:434–446.
47. Benedict R, Fischer JS, Archibald CJ, et al. Minimal neuropsychological assessment of MS patients: a consensus approach. Clin Neuropsychologist 2002;16:381–397.
48. Benedict R, et al. Screening for multiple sclerosis cognitive impairment using a self-administered 15-item questionnaire. Mult Scler 2003;9:95–101.
49. Rao SM. Neuropsychology Screening Battery for Multiple Sclerosis [unpublished manuscript]. Medical College of Wisconsin, Milwaukee, WI.
50. Fischer JS, Priore RL, Jacobs LD, et al., Neuropsychological effects of interferon beta-1a in relapsing multiple sclerosis. Multiple Sclerosis Collaborative Research Group. Ann Neurol 2000;48:885–892.
51. Pliskin NH, Hamer DP, Goldstein DS, et al. Improved delayed visual reproduction test performance in multiple sclerosis patients receiving interferon beta-1b. Neurology 1996;47:1463–1468.
52. Weinstein A, Schwid SI, Schiffer RB, McDermott MP, Giang DW, Goodman AD. Neuropsychologic status in multiple sclerosis after treatment with glatiramer. Arch Neurol 1999;56:319–324.
53. Greene Y, Tariot P, Wishart H, et al. 12-week, open trial of donepezil hydrochloride in patients with multiple sclerosis and associated cognitive impairments. J Clin Psychopharmacol 2000;20:350–356.
54. Jønsson A, Korfitzen EM, Heltberg A, Ravnborg MH, Byskov-Ottosen E. Effects of neuropsychological treatment in patients with multiple sclerosis. Acta Neurologica Scand 1993;88:394–400.
55. Plohmann AM, Kappos L, Ammann W, et al. Computer assisted retraining of attentional impairments in patients with multiple sclerosis. J Neurol Neurosurg Psychiatry 1998;64:455–462.

5

Multiple Sclerosis, Genetics, and Autoimmunity

Michael Demetriou, PhD, MD

INTRODUCTION

Multiple sclerosis (MS) afflicts approximately 250,000 to 350,000 individuals in the United States and is the most common autoimmune disease involving the nervous system. Multifocal immune-mediated destruction of the myelin sheath and secondary axonal damage in the central nervous system (CNS) results in variable neurological dysfunction, most commonly altered vision, incoordination, gait ataxia, paralysis, and sensory disturbances *(1)*. Relapsing-remitting MS (RRMS), where patients have attacks of neurological dysfunction lasting days to weeks followed by complete to near complete recovery, accounts for approximately 85% of patients with MS. After approximately 10 years, the majority of patients with RRMS have entered secondary-progressive MS (SPMS), where there is gradual accumulation of neurological dysfunction without recovery. This may represent a neurodegenerative phase of the disease that results from axon transfection and neuronal loss *(2,3)*. Primary-progressive MS (PPMS), accounting for approximately 15% of patients with MS, is similar to SPMS, except that these patients do not have a preceding relapsing-remitting phase.

Although the cause of MS is unknown, both environmental and genetic factors are believed to interact to induce the development of disease *(4,5)*. The strongest evidence for a genetic role in susceptibility to MS comes from a study of Canadian twins *(6,7)*. This work demonstrated that the risk of MS within a family increases directly proportional to the amount of shared genetic information, reaching a concordance rate of approximately 30% in monozygotic twins, compared to approximately 3 to 5% for first-degree relatives and 0.1% for the general population. Whole genome screens in patients and similar studies in mice have identified several loci associated with MS and its animal model experimental autoimmune encephalomyelitis (EAE) *(8–12)*. However, except for the class II major histocompatibility complex (MHC) alleles HLA-DR and HLA-DQ, specific candidate genes having a

From: *Current Clinical Neurology: Multiple Sclerosis*
Edited by: M. J. Olek © Humana Press Inc., Totowa, NJ

strong association with MS have yet to be identified. A heterozygous point mutation in PTPRC, the gene encoding the tyrosine phosphatase CD45, was associated with MS, but this was not confirmed in subsequent studies *(13–15)* and is of uncertain significance.

The dominant theory for the pathogenesis of MS centers on the formation of abnormal T-helper cells that are autoreactive against myelin antigens. These T-cells cross the blood–brain barrier (BBB) via adhesion molecules, such as very late antigen-4 (VLA-4), and are stimulated by myelin antigens presented by local antigen presenting cells and differentiate predominantly into T-helper type 1 (T_H1) cells that secrete proinflammatory cytokines, such as interferon-γ (IFN-γ) and tumor necrosis factor-α (TNF-α). This, coupled with activation of B-cells, cytotoxic T-cells, and macrophages, results in inflammatory demyelination and associated neurological symptoms *(1,2,4,5)*. Although each step in this model is important, the formation of abnormal myelin-specific T-cells is the first key event, without which disease cannot develop. This is best demonstrated by two key experiments in mice. First, myelin-specific T-cell clones isolated from mice with EAE, unlike B-cells, can adoptively transfer disease to naïve mice *(16,17)*. Second, transgenic mice, where the only lymphocytes present in the mouse are transgenic T-cell clones specific for myelin basic protein (MBP) (i.e., Rag1$^{-/-}$ mice with a MBP-specific T-cell antigen receptor [TCR] transgene) *(18)*, uniformly develop spontaneous EAE. Combined, these studies indicate that abnormal myelin-specific T-cells are necessary and sufficient to induce and sustain EAE in the absence of any other lymphocyte, including B-cells. Although B-cells may worsen disease severity, they are not required to initiate or sustain disease.

T-cells directed against myelin antigens can be detected in the blood of normal individuals at a frequency similar to that of patients with MS *(19,20)*. This is not surprising because the major myelin proteins are expressed in the thymus during T-cell maturation *(21)*, and T-cells only exit the thymus into the periphery if bind with low affinity to self-peptide/MHC complexes *(22)*. Once in the periphery, T-cells continue to require low-affinity stimulation by self-peptide/MHC for survival. Despite this, self-tolerance is maintained in normal individuals and autoimmune disease does not develop. Therefore, the simple presence of myelin-specific T-cells is not abnormal; rather, a qualitative change in these T-cells is likely required to induce disease. As such, the discovery of genes and associated molecular mechanisms that regulate T-cell function and self-tolerance should provide prime candidates for MS susceptibility genes and new targets for disease therapy.

THE ADAPTIVE AND INNATE IMMUNE SYSTEMS

The immune system can be divided into two broad categories: the innate immune system and the adaptive immune system. The former consists predominantly of phagocytic cells (e.g., macrophages and polymorphonuclear cells), whereas the latter are lymphocytes (e.g., T-cells and B-cells). The defining distinction between these two arms of the immune system is the unique ability of lymphocytes to generate a huge repertoire of high-affinity antigen receptors and the maintenance of the encounter with antigen as immunological memory. Although innate immune system cells also have cell surface antigen receptors, termed toll-like receptors (TLRs), these receptors are invariant and only recognize conserved pathogen-associated molecular patterns (PAMPs), such as lipopolysaccharide, peptidoglycan, CpG DNA motifs, dsRNA, and bacterial flagellen *(23)*. In contrast, adaptive immune system cells have marked variation in their antigen receptors, with each cell's antigen receptor recognizing a degenerate number of antigenic determinants with varying affinity. Recognition of antigen by these receptors leads to clonal expansion of that cell, providing both immunological specificity and memory.

The adaptive system is divided into humoral and cellular immune responses, which are mediated by B-cells and T-cells, respectively. Antigen recognition by B-cell antigen receptors (i.e., membrane-bound immunoglobulin [Ig]M) induces B-cell proliferation and differentiation into antibody-secreting plasma cells, which, in turn, secrete high-affinity antibodies. These antibodies help clear extracellular infectious agents by promoting complement fixation and targeting pathogens for phagocytosis via interaction with Fc receptors on phagocytic cells. In contrast to B-cells, T-cells cannot recognize soluble antigen, but rather require a peptide antigen to be bound to and presented by an MHC. T-cells are divided into two main subtypes: $CD4^+$ T-helper cells, which require MHC class II, and $CD8^+$ cytotoxic T-cells, which require MHC class I. T-helper-cells activate the innate immune system and B-cells via cytokine release, while cytotoxic T-cells kill virally infected cells. Although cytotoxic T-cells, B-cells, and innate immune system cells contribute to inflammatory demyelination, it is the T-helper cell that is key to the initiation and pathogenesis of autoimmune demyelination and is the focus of this chapter.

T-CELLS, SELF-TOLERANCE, AND AUTOIMMUNITY

For many years it was believed that the adaptive immune system evolved to recognize the difference between self and nonself, but we now know that this model is incorrect. In fact, the adaptive immune system not only normally recognizes self-antigens but also requires them for normal homeostasis. Rather, the defining characteristic of interactions with self vs nonself is that lymphocytes are tolerant of self-antigen and nontolerant to foreign antigen. Although lymphocyte antigen receptors bind and recognize self-antigen, this does not normally induce lymphocyte activation and proliferation. Autoimmune disease, including MS, develops when this tolerance to self-antigen is lost. Multiple mechanisms have been proposed for the maintenance of T-cell tolerance to self-antigen *(24)*, several of which are discussed.

T-cells develop in the thymus from stem cells that originated in the bone marrow. Once in the thymus, T-cell receptor (TCR) genes in individual cells undergo gene rearrangement, leading to a large repertoire of TCR specificities. Once this TCR gene rearrangement has occurred, immature T-cells or thymocytes undergo one of three fates: positive selection (5%), negative selection (5%), or death by neglect (90%). Negative selection occurs when a newly rearranged TCR binds to self-antigen/MHC with high affinity, inducing cell death by apoptosis (i.e., programmed cell death). The elimination of T-cells with high affinity to self-antigen in this manner represents an important mechanism for the maintenance of self-tolerance. In contrast, if TCR does not bind self-antigen/MHC at all, then the cells also die by apoptosis. This is termed death by neglect and occurs in approximately 90% of thymocytes. Low-affinity interactions of TCR with self-peptide/MHC provide a survival signal to the developing thymocytes, and only these cells mature, leave the thymus, and enter the periphery. Thus, all mature T-cells are positively selected to bind self-antigen/MHC with low affinity, which explains why normal individuals have myelin-reactive T-cells.

Once in the periphery, naïve T-cells continue to engage self-antigen/MHC. Although these interactions promote T-cell survival *(25–27)*, they normally do not induce significant T-cell proliferation *(28)*. An exception to this occurs in the presence of lymphopenia, when self-peptide-MHC interactions induce a strong proliferative response *(29)*, albeit less vigorous than stimulation with foreign antigen. This has been termed homeostatic proliferation because it is believed to be a mechanism to quickly repopulate an individual to near-normal numbers of T-cells.

Why do these physiological self-peptide-MHC interactions not induce T-cell activation, breakdown of self-tolerance, and the development of autoimmunity? Activation of naive T-cells normally requires not only the recognition of peptide/MHC by the TCR but also other cosignaling events. The combination of these two signals initiates a signaling cascade that results in actin cytoskeleton reorganization and the formation of a specialized contact area between the T-cell and the APC termed the immune synapse *(30–33)*. The formation and integrity of the immune synapse is essential for the activation and proliferation of T-cells *(34,35)*. Although several "cosignals" have been described, the most important is the interaction of the T-cell surface receptor CD28 with its ligands B7-1 and B7-2, which are present on the surface of activated APCs *(36,37)*. Costimulation by CD28 recruits protein kinase-enriched lipid rafts to the immune synapse *(32,33)*, thereby enhancing TCR-mediated signaling and lowering T-cell activation thresholds. TCR signaling in the absence of CD28-B71/2 costimulation not only results in reduced T-cell proliferation but also induces a state of anergy or nonresponsiveness to subsequent stimulation via TCR and CD28 *(38)*. The absence of CD28 in mice leads to T-cell hypoproliferation in response to antigen receptor stimulation *(39)* and resistance to the induction of EAE *(40)* and other autoimmune diseases, indicating that anergy plays an important role in the maintenance of self-tolerance.

Resting APCs, such as dendritic cells and macrophages, express minimal levels of the CD28 receptor B7-1 and no B7-2, thus providing only limited costimulatory signals to T-cells. Recognition of nonself microbial products by dendritic cell and macrophage pattern recognition receptors, such as TLRs, leads to a marked upregulation of the CD28 costimulatory receptors B7-1/B7-2, as well as the secretion of inflammatory cytokines, such as TNF-α and interleukin (IL)-1. This significantly enhances their ability to activate naïve T-cells (23). Because self-antigens do not bind TLRs and do not activate APCs, the innate immune system, via TLR signaling and associated upregulation of costimulatory molecules, plays a key role in communicating to the adaptive immune system whether the antigen it presents is self or nonself (41). The inability of self-antigen to upregulate costimulatory signals in APCs prevents the normal physiological interactions of TCR with self-peptide/MHC from inducing T-cell activation and represents another important mechanism for the maintenance of self-tolerance.

Although T-cell anergy is initiated by TCR signaling in the absence of CD28 costimulation, it also requires the subsequent expression of the CD28 homolog cytotoxic T-lymphocyte-associated antigen-4 (CTLA-4) to maintain it. CTLA-4 is upregulated after T-cell activation (42) and engagement of CTLA-4 with B7-1 and B7-2 transduces a negative signal that inhibits T-cell proliferation. Mice that are deficient in CTLA-4 develop a lethal inflammatory/autoimmune disease characterized by severe inflammatory infiltrates in multiple organs (43). Antibody blockade of CTLA-4 interaction with B7-1 and B7-2 in vivo exacerbates EAE severity (44). In humans, a functional role for CTLA-4 in the prevention of autoimmunity has recently been established by the association of Grave's disease, autoimmune hypothyroidism, and type 1 diabetes with polymorphisms in CTLA-4 that significantly reduce its expression (45). A study of the same polymorphisms in patients with MS has yet to be reported. Other polymorphisms in CTLA-4 have been assessed in patients with MS by multiple groups, for the most part with contradictory results (46–52).

PD-1 and ICOS are two additional members of the CD28/CTLA-4 costimulatory family that, like CTLA-4, are upregulated after T-cell activation and negatively regulate autoimmune disease susceptibility (53). However, they have distinct receptors and do not interact with B7-1 or B7-2. PD-1 is similar to CTLA-4 in that it inhibits T-cell activation, and mice that are deficient in this gene spontaneously develop autoimmune disease (53). In contrast, ICOS regulates T-cell differentiation without significantly altering the initial activation thresholds of naïve T-cells. Deficiency or blockade of ICOS in mice promotes EAE, possibly by inhibiting differentiation of naïve T-cells into autoimmune suppressing T_H2 cells (53). T_H2 cells secrete immunosuppressive cytokines, such as IL-4, IL-5, IL-10, and IL-13, which inhibit proinflammatory T_H1 cells and suppress autoimmunity.

Although CD28 costimulation markedly lowers T-cell activation thresholds, it is not absolutely required to induce full T-cell stimulation. It has been estimated that clustering of approximately 8000 TCRs is sufficient to activate T-cells, a number that is reduced by approximately fivefold by CD28 coreceptor stimulation (54). Thus, one potential mechanism for the abnormal activation of T-cells by self-peptide would be a gene mutation that directly enhances TCR clustering, thereby allowing T-cell activation in the absence of CD28 cosignals. Indeed, two mouse genes, Mgat5 and cbl-b, display this precise phenotype. Deficiency in either gene results in enhanced ligand-induced TCR clustering, CD28 independent T-cell activation, increased susceptibility to EAE, and the development of spontaneous autoimmune disease. Although mutations in these two genes produce the same phenotype, the molecular mechanisms involved are distinct. Mgat5 is an enzyme in the Asn (N)-linked protein glycosylation pathway that modifies cell surface receptors (e.g., TCR) with a high-affinity ligand for a family of carbohydrate-binding proteins termed galectins. Multivalent interactions of galectins with Mgat5-modified glycoproteins sequester the TCR complex within a cell surface galectin-glycoprotein lattice that restricts ligand-induced TCR recruitment to the immune synapse. The absence of Mgat5 glycans disrupts this lattice, thereby enhancing agonist-induced TCR clustering, downstream signaling, T-cell activation, and, in mice, spontaneous autoimmunity. In contrast, cbl-b is an E3 ubiquitin ligase that negatively regulates the guanine nucleotide exchange factor Vav by targeting phosphatidylinositol 3 (PI3)-kinase for ubiquitination. This inhibits actin cytoskeleton reorganization and associated TCR receptor clustering at the immune synapse *(55–57)*. The key point is that in the absence of either Mgat5 or cbl-b, TCR clustering is enhanced, leading to antigen-induced T-cell hyperproliferation and spontaneous autoimmunity in mice. Although mutations in Mgat5 and cbl-b have not been reported in humans, they represent prime candidate susceptibility genes for autoimmune diseases, such as MS.

Taken together these data strongly indicate that multiple genes involved in the T-cell costimulatory pathway can independently regulate the same endpoint: T-cell hyperproliferation and autoimmune disease. Therefore, it is likely that dysregulation of T-cell costimulatory pathways play a key role in the loss of immune tolerance in MS and represent prime targets for therapeutic intervention.

MOLECULAR MIMICRY, IMMUNE TOLERANCE, AND MULTIPLE SCLEROSIS

The previous discussion centered on molecular mechanisms in the regulation of immune tolerance. Because they are not specific for a particular antigen, they can be applied to the pathogenesis of multiple autoimmune diseases. However, they do not address why one individual develops MS and another develops type 1 diabetes. Although the answer to this question is unknown, it is likely differences in environmental risk factors, or more precisely exposure to different pathogens. It is well established that numerous human pathogens contain peptide sequences that are molecular mimics of endogenous self-antigens *(58,59)*. For example, the myelin antigen MBP shares homology with multiple microbes, including measles, hepatitis B, influenza, adenovirus, herpes simples virus (HSV), Epstein-Barr virus (EBV), PPV, and pseudomonas *(60)*. In addition, TCR binds peptide/MHC with very low-affinity (K_D approximately $10^{-5}M$), resulting in a highly degenerate specificity for peptide/MHC. Thus, in a genetically susceptible individual who has the appropriate MHC haplotype and dysfunction in one or more of the pathways described, infection with one of these pathogens may lead to cross-activation of myelin-reactive T-cells and the development of MS. This model is supported by the fact that relapses in MS are frequently triggered by viral infections, that pathogen peptides with homologies at specific MHC and TCR contact sites are able to stimulate MBP-specific T-cell clones from patients with MS *(60)*, and that clinical and pathological EAE can be induced by immunization with peptide from a microbe that has homology to a myelin antigen *(61–64)*. However, the strongest evidence for this model is work with a transgenic mouse that expresses a MBP-specific TCR *(65)*. When these mice were housed under pathogen-free conditions, they displayed no phenotype. However, when they were housed in a nonsterile animal colony with mouse pathogens, such as mouse hepatitis virus, pinworm, and trichomonas-type flagellates, approximately 14–44% of the mice spontaneously developed clinical and pathological EAE. This indicates that exposure to pathogens and associated activation of the MBP-specific T-cells were required to trigger spontaneous EAE and provides a model to define how genetic susceptibility and environmental factors can interact to induce autoimmune demyelination. Because humans do not live in sterile environments, a similar experiment in humans is not possible. Instead, we must rely on these types of animal experiments to provide the best evidence for molecular mimicry in the pathogenesis of MS.

SUMMARY

The best available evidence, both from human studies and animal models, such as EAE, strongly indicate that MS is initiated and sustained by T-cells. Other leukocytes, such as B-cells, may regulate severity of disease but are insufficient to cause disease. Complex interactions between an individual's genetic background and his or her environment are required for disease to develop. Although we do not yet know the precise genetic and environmental factors required, mutations in genes that regulate T-cell activation thresholds and/or costimulatory pathways in combination with exposure to pathogens with cross-reactivity to myelin antigens currently represents the best model for the pathogenesis of MS. Confirmation of this model and the determination of these factors should eventually lead to better preventative and treatment strategies for this disabling disease.

REFERENCES

1. Noseworthy JH, Lucchinetti C, Rodriguez M, Weinshenker BG. Multiple sclerosis. Progress in determining the causes and treatment of multiple sclerosis. N Engl J Med 2000;343:938–952.
2. Steinman L. Multiple sclerosis: a two-stage disease. Nat Immunol 2001;2:762–764.
3. Lucchinetti C, Bruck W, Noseworthy J. Multiple sclerosis: recent developments in neuropathology, pathogenesis, magnetic resonance imaging studies and treatment. Curr Opin Neurol 2001;14:259–269.
4. Noseworthy JH. Progress in determining the causes and treatment of multiple sclerosis. Nature 1999;399:A40–A47.
5. Steinman L. Multiple sclerosis: a coordinated immunological attack against myelin in the central nervous system. Cell 1996;85:299–302.
6. Ebers GC, Sadovnick AD, Risch NJ. A genetic basis for familial aggregation in multiple sclerosis. Canadian Collaborative Study Group. Nature 1995;377:150–151.

7. Ebers GC, Bulman DE, Sadovnick AD, et al. A population-based study of multiple sclerosis in twins. N Engl J Med 1986;315:1638–1642.

8. Ebers GC, Kukay K, Bulman DE, et al. A full genome search in multiple sclerosis. Nat Genet 1996;13:472–476.

9. Haines JL, Ter-Minassian M, Bazyk A, Feakes R, et al. A complete genomic screen for multiple sclerosis underscores a role for the major histocompatability complex. The Multiple Sclerosis Genetics Group. Nat Genet 1996;13:469–471.

10. Sawcer S, Jones HB, et al. A genome screen in multiple sclerosis reveals susceptibility loci on chromosome 6p21 and 17q22. Nat Genet 1996;13:464–468.

11. Becker KG, Simon RH, Bailey-Wilson JE, et al. Clustering of non-major histocompatibility complex susceptibility candidate loci in human autoimmune diseases. Proc Natl Acad Sci U S A 1998;95:9979–9984.

12. Butterfield RJ, Sudweeks JD, Blankenhorn EP, et al. New genetic loci that control susceptibility and symptoms of experimental allergic encephalomyelitis in inbred mice. J Immunol 1998;161:1860–1867.

13. Vorechovsky I, Kralovicova J, Tchilian E, et al. Does 77C→G in PTPRC modify autoimmune disorders linked to the major histocompatibility locus? Nat Genet 2001;29:22–23.

14. Barcellos LF, et al. PTPRC (CD45) is not associated with the development of multiple sclerosis in U.S. patients. Nat Genet 2001;29:23–24.

15. Jacobsen M, et al. A point mutation in PTPRC is associated with the development of multiple sclerosis. Nat Genet 2000;26:495–499 (2000).

16. Ben Nun A, Cohen IR. Experimental autoimmune encephalomyelitis (EAE) mediated by T cell lines: process of selection of lines and characterization of the cells. J Immunol 1982;129: 303–308.

17. Zamvil S, et al. T-cell clones specific for myelin basic protein induce chronic relapsing paralysis and demyelination. Nature 1985;317:355–358.

18. Lafaille JJ, Nagashima K, Katsuki M, Tonegawa S. High incidence of spontaneous autoimmune encephalomyelitis in immunodeficient anti-myelin basic protein T cell receptor transgenic mice. Cell 1994;78:399–408.

19. Burns J, Rosenzweig A, Zweiman B, Lisak RP. Isolation of myelin basic protein-reactive T-cell lines from normal human blood. Cell Immunol 1983;81:435–440.

20. Jingwu Z, Medaer R, Hashim GA, Chin Y, van der Berg-Loonen E, Raus JC. Myelin basic protein-specific T lymphocytes in multiple sclerosis and controls: precursor frequency, fine specificity, and cytotoxicity. Ann Neurol 1992;32:330–338.

21. Pribyl TM, Campagnoni C, Kampf K, Handley VW, Campagnoni AT. The major myelin protein genes are expressed in the human thymus. J Neurosci Res 1996;45:812–819.

22. Abbas AK, Janeway CA, Jr. Immunology: improving on nature in the twenty-first century. Cell 2000;100:129–138.

23. Barton GM, Medzhitov R. Control of adaptive immune responses by Toll-like receptors. Curr Opin Immunol 2002;14:380–383.

24. Walker LS, Abbas AK. The enemy within: keeping self-reactive T cells at bay in the periphery. Nat Rev Immunol 2002;2:11–19.

25. Takeda S, Rodewald HR, Arakawa H, Bluethmann H, Shimizu T. MHC class II molecules are not required for survival of newly generated CD4+ T cells, but affect their long-term life span. Immunity 1996;5:217–228.

26. Tanchot C, Lemonnier FA, Perarnau B, Freitas AA, Rocha B. Differential requirements for survival and proliferation of CD8 naive or memory T cells. Science 1997;276:2057–2062.

27. Brocker T. Survival of mature CD4 T lymphocytes is dependent on major histocompatibility complex class II-expressing dendritic cells. J Exp Med 1997;186:1223–1232.

28. Tough DF, Sprent J. Turnover of naive- and memory-phenotype T cells. J Exp Med 1994;179:1127–1135.

29. Jameson SC. Maintaining the norm: T-cell homeostasis. Nat Rev Immunol 2002;2:547–556.

30. Monks CR, Freiberg BA, Kupfer H, Sciaky N, Kupfer A. Three-dimensional segregation of supramolecular activation clusters in T cells. Nature 1998;395:82–86.

31. Grakoui A, Bromley SK, Sumen C, et al. The immunological synapse: a molecular machine controlling T cell activation. Science 1999;285:221–227.

32. Wulfing C, Davis MM. A receptor/cytoskeletal movement triggered by costimulation during T cell activation. Science 1998;282:2266–2269.

33. Viola A, Schroeder S, Sakakibara Y, Lanzavecchia A. T lymphocyte costimulation mediated by reorganization of membrane microdomains. Science 1999;283:680–682.

34. Dustin ML, Chan AC. Signaling takes shape in the immune system. Cell 2000;103:283–294.

35. Bromley SK, et al. The immunological synapse. Annu Rev Immunol 2001;19:375–396.

36. Lenschow DJ, Walunas TL, Bluestone JA. CD28/B7 system of T cell costimulation. Annu Rev Immunol 1996;14:233–258.

37. Chambers CA. The expanding world of co-stimulation: the two-signal model revisited. Trends Immunol 2001;22:217–223.

38. Harding FA, McArthur JG, Gross JA, Raulet DH, Allison JP. CD28-mediated signalling co-stimulates murine T cells and prevents induction of anergy in T-cell clones. Nature 1992;356:607–609.

39. Shahinian A, Pfeffer K, Lee KP, et al. Differential T cell costimulatory requirements in CD28-deficient mice. Science 1993;261:609–612.

40. Oliveira-dos-Santos AJ, Ho A, Tada Y, et al. CD28 costimulation is crucial for the development of spontaneous autoimmune encephalomyelitis. J Immunol 1999;162:4490–4495.

41. Janeway CA, Jr. The immune system evolved to discriminate infectious nonself from noninfectious self. Immunol Today 1992;13:11–16.

42. Alegre ML, Frauwirth KA, Thompson CB. T-cell regulation by CD28 and CTLA-4. Nat Rev Immunol 2001;1:220–228.

43. Waterhouse P, Penninger JM, Timms E, et al. Lymphoproliferative disorders with early lethality in mice deficient in Ctla-4. Science 1995;270:985–988.

44. Hurwitz AA, Sullivan TJ, Krummel MF, Sobel RA, Allison JP. Specific blockade of CTLA-4/B7 interactions results in exacerbated clinical and histologic disease in an actively-induced model of experimental allergic encephalomyelitis. J Neuroimmunol 1997;73:57–62.

45. Ueda H, et al. Association of the T-cell regulatory gene CTLA4 with susceptibility to autoimmune disease. Nature 2003;423:506–511.

46. Fukazawa T, Yanagawa T, Kikuchi S, et al. CTLA-4 gene polymorphism may modulate disease in Japanese multiple sclerosis patients. J Neurol Sci 1999;171:49–55.

47. Harbo HF, Celius EG, Vartdal F, Spurkland A. CTLA4 promoter and exon 1 dimorphisms in multiple sclerosis. Tissue Antigens 1999;53:106–110.

48. Ligers A, Xu C, Saarinen S, Hillert J, Olerup O. The CTLA-4 gene is associated with multiple sclerosis. J Neuroimmunol 1999;97:182–190.

49. Rasmussen HB, Kelly MA, Francis DA, Clausen J. CTLA4 in multiple sclerosis. Lack of genetic association in a European Caucasian population but evidence of interaction with HLA-DR2 among Shanghai Chinese. J Neurol Sci 2001;184:143–147.

50. Dyment DA, Steckley JL, Willer CJ, et al. No evidence to support CTLA-4 as a susceptibility gene in MS families: the Canadian Collaborative Study. J Neuroimmunol 2002;123:193–198.

51. Kantarci OH, Hebrink DD, Achenbach SJ, et al. CTLA4 is associated with susceptibility to multiple sclerosis. J Neuroimmunol 2003;134:133–141.

52. Alizadeh M, Babron MC, Birebent B, et al. Genetic interaction of CTLA-4 with HLA-DR15 in multiple sclerosis patients. Ann Neurol 2003;54:119–122.

53. Sharpe AH, Freeman GJ. The B7-CD28 superfamily. Nat Rev Immunol 2002;2:116–126.

54. Viola A, Lanzavecchia A. T cell activation determined by T cell receptor number and tunable thresholds. Science 1996;273:104–106.

55. Chiang YJ, Kole HK, Brown K, et al. Cbl-b regulates the CD28 dependence of T-cell activation. Nature 2000;403:216–220.

56. Bachmaier K, Krawczyk C, Kozieradzki I, et al. Negative regulation of lymphocyte activation and autoimmunity by the molecular adaptor Cbl-b. Nature 2000;403:211–216.
57. Fang D, Wang HY, Fang N, Altman Y, Elly C, Liu YC. Cbl-b, a RING-type E3 ubiquitin ligase, targets phosphatidylinositol 3- kinase for ubiquitination in T cells. J Biol Chem 2001;276: 4872–4878.
58. Albert LJ, Inman RD. Molecular mimicry and autoimmunity. N Engl J Med 1999;341:2068–2074.
59. Benoist C, Mathis D. Autoimmunity provoked by infection: how good is the case for T cell epitope mimicry? Nat Immunol 2001;2:797–801.
60. Wucherpfennig KW, Strominger JL. Molecular mimicry in T cell-mediated autoimmunity: viral peptides activate human T cell clones specific for myelin basic protein. Cell 1995;80:695–705.
61. Fujinami RS, Oldstone M.B. Amino acid homology between the encephalitogenic site of myelin basic protein and virus: mechanism for autoimmunity. Science 1985;230:1043–1045.
62. Gautam AM, Liblau R, Chelvanayagam G, Steinman L, Boston T. A viral peptide with limited homology to a self peptide can induce clinical signs of experimental autoimmune encephalomyelitis. J Immunol 1998;161:60–64.
63. Mokhtarian F, Zhang Z, Shi Y, Gonzales E, Sobel RA. Molecular mimicry between a viral peptide and a myelin oligodendrocyte glycoprotein peptide induces autoimmune demyelinating disease in mice. J Neuroimmunol 1999;95:43–54.
64. Grogan JL, Kramer A, Nogai A, et al. Cross-reactivity of myelin basic protein-specific T cells with multiple microbial peptides: experimental autoimmune encephalomyelitis induction in TCR transgenic mice.J Immunol 1999;163:3764–3770.
65. Goverman J, Woods A, Larson L, Weiner LP, Hood L, Zaller DM. Transgenic mice that express a myelin basic protein-specific T cell receptor develop spontaneous autoimmunity. Cell 1993;72:551–560.

6

B-Cell Immunity in Multiple Sclerosis

Yufen Qin, MD and Pierre Duquette, MD

INTRODUCTION

Multiple sclerosis (MS) is the most common chronic neurological disorder in young Caucasian adults *(1–3),* but after more than a century of active research, its etiology remains unknown. It is a peculiar disease, because it is restricted to the central nervous system (CNS), is not associated with any other neurological or systemic disorder, and has no animal counterpart. In the typical form, MS evolves through relapses and remissions, although, in the majority of patients, a secondary progressive phase ensues *(4–7).* Its classic pathological hallmark is the plaque, which, in the acute form of the disease, shows perivascular infiltration and contains macrophages filled with myelin debris *(8–16).* This classic view is challenged by magnetic resonance imaging (MRI) and pathological studies, which reveal substantial early axonal damage.

MS was formerly described as a strictly demyelinating disease but is now known to affect both axons and myelin *(17–19).* Several MRI studies have shown signs of preplaque anomalies, the pathological nature of which is controversial. MS is considered to have an inflammatory and a degenerative component, although whether the degenerative component is secondary to inflammation or is caused by primary axonal damage, remains unclear.

The prevailing etiological hypothesis for MS is that it is a multifactorial disorder, affecting individuals predisposed by a combination of several susceptibility genes and environmental factors (which are mainly infectious in nature) *(20–30).* Plaque formation is attributed to immune mechanisms, triggered by an autoimmune attack directed against antigens in the myelin membrane. Experimental authoimmune encephalomyelitis (EAE) is an animal model induced in mammals by injection with either whole-brain tissue or specific myelin proteins, such as myelin basic protein (MBP) *(31–33),* myelin oligodendrocyte glycoprotein (MOG) *(34–38),* myelin-associated glycoprotein (MAG) *(39,40),* or proteolipid protein (PLP) *(41,42).* The disease can be transmitted from an affected to a naïve animal by

From: *Current Clinical Neurology: Multiple Sclerosis*
Edited by: M. J. Olek © Humana Press Inc., Totowa, NJ

T-cell transfer, which has led to the identification, in humans, of T-cell clones specific for these myelin proteins *(43–46)*. These T-cell clones, which can be isolated from normal individuals and patients with MS, are believed to be central to the initiation of the immune process that culminates in plaque formation. Consequently, MS has been seen mainly as a T-cell disease, and therapeutic strategies are based on this concept *(47,48)*.

Recent publications have challenged this view and focused on the possible involvement of B-cells in the immune pathogenesis of MS. This chapter reviews the biology of B-cells in relation to their implication in MS. Findings from various groups, including the author's own, are summarized and their implications discussed.

IMMUNOGLOBULIN IN CEREBROSPINAL FLUID

MS is considered to be a cell-mediated autoimmune disease, and involvement of the humoral immune system is indicated by the presence of oligoclonal immunoglobulin (Ig) proteins (oligoclonal bands) (OCBs) in the CSF of the majority of patients. These proteins are produced by B-cells in the CNS *(49–53)*.

Intrathecal Ig synthesis, reflected by an increased IgG ratio and presence of OCBs, is a general feature of chronic brain inflammation and is of diagnostic use in MS. Naturally produced intrathecal OCBs are restricted to the IgG1 and IgG3 subclasses in most patients *(54,55)*. Much lower amounts of IgM and IgA are sometimes present *(56)*, and local production of IgM is often detected in the CSF of patients with early MS *(57,58)*. A significant relationship between IgA and a progressive disease course *(59)* and the presence of OCBs has been reported, the latter in approximately 90 to 95% of patients with clinically definite MS (CDMS). Presence of OCBs is important in the diagnosis of early MS, particularly in those patients with normal brain magnetic resonance imaging (MRI) scans *(60,61)*; it has been suggested that they appear early in the course of MS. The frequency of OCBs in patients with optic neuritis (ON), one of the earliest manifestations of MS, is between 34 and 72%, depending on the detection technique used *(62–64)*.

Several approaches have been used to identify the antigens recognized by these IgG antibodies (Abs). Intrathecal Ig bands recognize several myelin proteins (MBP, PLP, MOG, and MAG) *(65–70)* and viruses (measles, rubella, varicella zoster, and herpes simplex) *(71,72)*. Heterogeneity of antigen specificity of intrathecal IgG has been observed, but only a small proportion of total Ig may be MS-related. Attempts to absorb non-MS-specific Ig with viral or endogenous antigens have proved unsuccessful *(73)*. These early findings raised the question of whether OCBs resulted after an MS-related antigen-driven B-cell response or an MS-unrelated B-cell response. Different groups have shown more recently that an antigen-driven adaptive immune response occurs in the CNS. By examining B-cell Ig genes, it was found that MS lesions and CSF contain B-cells with characteristics of an antigen-driven adaptive immune response, including T–B-cell interaction, somatic hypermutation, immune memory development, and B-cell clonal selection and expansion *(74–80)*.

INNATE AND ADAPTIVE IMMUNITY

Immune responses have both an innate and an adaptive component. The defense mechanisms involved in innate immunity consist of phagocytes (neutrophils and macrophages), natural killer (NK) cells, natural IgM-secreting natural autoreactive B-cells, and plasma proteins (including complement system proteins). NK cells produce interferon (IFN)-γ, a macrophage-activating cytokine. Natural autoreactive B-cells, which react with one or more self-antigens independent of T-cell help, account for most of the B-cell repertoire in the fetus and healthy adult individuals. These B-cells have no memory and are usually encoded by unmutated germline variable region genes. Macrophages secrete cytokines that stimulate inflammation and immune responses, whereas the complement system lyses and opsonizes microbes for phagocytosis. The adaptive immune component involves specificity for distinct macromolecules, and an ability to remember and respond more vigorously to repeated exposures to the same molecule. Adaptive immune responses are initiated by the interaction of a foreign antigen with mature T- and B-lymphocytes that express diverse, clonally expressed antigen receptors. T-cells mature in the thymus, where they express antigen receptors and coreceptors (CD4 or CD8), the latter recognizing peptides displayed by the body's own major histocompatibility complex (MHC) molecules. Immature B-cells mature in bone marrow where they express antigen receptors (IgM and IgD) and become functionally competent. Immature T- and B-cells expressing high-affinity receptors for self-antigens, which are present in the generative lymphoid organs, are eliminated; this process is referred to as negative deletion, or central tolerance to self-antigens.

LYMPHOID TISSUES

All adaptive immune responses are initiated in the peripheral lymphoid tissues, namely the lymph nodes, spleen, and mucosa. Mature naïve T- and B-cells leave the generative lymphoid organs (thymus and bone marrow) and circulate through the peripheral lymphoid tissues, where foreign antigens are filtered out and concentrated. The net result of adaptive immune responses is generation of effector and memory cells. Effector CD4 and CD8 T-cells secrete cytokines that activate B-cells, macrophages, granulocytes, and vascular endothelial cells. Plasma and memory B-cells secrete antibodies into the circulation, and both the cells and the antibody bind to antigen in the tissues.

HUMORAL IMMUNITY

The majority of humoral immunity results from an antigen-driven T-cell-dependent B-cell reaction in lymphoid tissue. Adaptive humoral immune responses against lymph-borne proteins are initiated in the lymph nodes. Circulating mature naïve T- and B-cells migrate through venule walls and take up temporary residence in lymphoid tissue. T- and B-cells are sequestered in particular areas: the follicles are B-cell-rich areas (B-cell-zones); primary follicles contain mainly mature, naïve B-cells; and T-cells are located between the follicles (in T-cell zones). Antigen-activated follicular B-cells migrate toward the interface between the follicles and T-cell zones, where they present antigen to helper T-cells specific for that antigen *(81,82)*. B-cells are activated by T-cell generated lymphokines to enter the cell cycle and undergo mitosis to generate a clone of cells with identical B-cell receptors. These form germinal centers (GCs) in the follicles, called secondary follicles. GCs are the sites of B-cell proliferation, B-cell Ig V gene mutation, B-cell clone selection, and memory B-cell generation. Selection of antigen receptors is based on antigen affinity *(83–85)*. B-cells with the highest affinity receptor are selected to survive and differentiate into antibody-secreting plasma cells *(86–88)*. GCs play a critical role in the generation of high-affinity humoral immune responses via Ig gene somatic hypermutation.

IG GENE SOMATIC HYPERMUTATION

Unlike T-cells, B-cells are subject to antigen-dependent mutations and selection processes in the secondary lymphoid tissues, designed to increase the affinity and functional efficiency of the memory Ig repertoire *(83,89)*. Like T-lineage repertoire selection in the thymus, B-lineage repertoire selection is closely regulated and functionally linked with a specialized microenvironment—the GC *(85,90–94)*.

Both Ig gene somatic hypermutation and B-cell clonal expansion play critical roles in the generation of high-affinity humoral immune responses. B-cell surface Ig is composed of heavy and light chains encoded by the variable (V), diversity (D), and joining (J) genes in the case of the heavy chains (V_H, D_H, and J_H) and by the V_L and J_L genes in the case of the light chains *(95–98)*. Each V_H or V_L segment contains three regions of especially high variability (hypervariable regions) corresponding to the protein loops that contact the antigen and are known as complementarity determining regions (CDRs) *(99)*. The genes V_H and V_L code for CDR1 and CDR2, respectively, whereas CDR3 is encoded by a combination of the V_H, D_H, J_H, V_L, and J_L genes. The regions between CDRs are the framework regions, and they are responsible for maintaining the structure. Each B-cell expresses a particular pair of heavy and light V regions, representing the molecular basis of the clonal selection theory, which postulates that each B-cell and its progeny are predestined to have a single antibody specificity *(100)*.

In T-cell-dependent antibody responses, antigen-specific B-cells undergo rapid and extensive clonal expansion in GCs. During this process, somatic point mutations are introduced into the Ig gene of the proliferating B-cells. Mutations are concentrated in the hypervariable region that forms the antigen binding site *(85,86,101)*. Some of these may generate a binding site with increased affinity for its antigen, leading to antibodies of improved binding affinity after further antigen selection. Therefore, repeated antigenic challenge leads to "affinity maturation" of the response, resulting in production of antibodies with high affinity for the antigen. B-cells with the highest affinity are selected to survive and differentiate into memory and antibody-secreting B-cells. Rechallenge with a persistent antigen results in massive proliferation of clonal memory B-cells into high-affinity antibody-secreting plasma cells. These cells dominate the humoral immune response after vaccination and in autoimmunity and B-cell malignancy.

Somatically mutated B-cell Ig V genes are considered to be the hallmark of antigen-driven humoral immunity.

IMMUNE MEMORY AND B-CELL CLONAL EXPANSION

Studies have shown that clonal expansion is based on immune memory and results in an enhanced response on restimulation with the same antigen. Memory is generated by an increased affinity of B-cell clones for antigen, resulting from somatic mutation of the Ig V gene. The B-cells undergo a Darwinian positive selection process based on their affinity for antigen held on follicular dendritic cells in GCs. High-affinity mutants survive, whereas low-affinity mutants cannot bind antigen and die by apoptosis *(102,103)*. Positively selected B-cells differentiate to short-lived plasma cells, which secrete antibody, and to long-lived memory plasma cells that persist in the lymph nodes, spleen, and bone marrow *(90,104–106)*. Long-lived memory cells are clones that maintain the established phase of the T-cell-dependent antibody response. Under persistent antigen stimulation, memory B-cell clones proliferate and dominate a specific B-cell mediated humoral immune response throughout the organism's lifetime. Such antigen stimulation might be necessary to maintain antigen-specific serum antibody in inflammatory tissue at high levels for long periods. Therefore, B-cell clones require antigen for their maintenance *(106–108)* and in the absence of antigen are lost from the adoptive host *(107)*. The role of antigen in memory maintenance and clonal expansion is important, and antigen persistence might be a key factor in (auto)immune diseases.

THE ROLE OF B-CELLS IN MULTIPLE SCLEROSIS

For the last two decades, T-cell-mediated immunity has dominated studies of MS pathogenesis. This emphasis on T-cells mainly resulted from detection of activated T-cells in MS lesions and analogies with the animal model EAE. T-cells can transfer EAE between animals with particular MHC class II alleles and are believed to break down the blood–brain barrier (BBB) in early MS and predominate within acute lesions. The type 1 helper T-cell (Th1), cytokines, interleukin IL-2, IFN-γ, and tumor necrosis factor-α, are involved in the inflammatory reaction in active MS lesions *(109,110)*. The α-chemokines, IFN-inducible protein 10, and monokine induced by IFN-γ (Mig), which attract Th1 cells, are mainly secreted by macrophages and reactive astrocytes within actively demyelinating MS lesions *(111)*. Overexpression of type 5 Chemokine C-motif Receptor and type 3 Chemokine XC-motif Receptor, the receptors for these chemokines, is seen in lesion-derived T-cells and peripheral T-cells in patients with MS *(112–114)*. Recently, there has been considerable progress in this field *(74–77)* using investigations based mainly on molecular studies of the Ig V_H genes expressed by B-cells in CSF or lesions in patients with MS. These studies have shown that B-cell immunity, including antigen-driven B-cell somatic hypermutation, T–B-cell interaction, memory B-cell and plasma cell development in GCs, tissue-specific migration, and B-cell clonal expansion in the CNS, are actively involved in MS development. They occur during the early stages of MS and continue through later disease stages. Increased intrathecal oligoclonal Ig synthesis, the most common abnormality detected in patients with CDMS, suggests ongoing B-cell proliferation in the CNS. The specific binding of antibodies to their antigen in brain tissue could cause tissue damage by activation of innate immunity, including complement and phagocytes.

B-CELL CLONAL EXPANSION: COMMON AND CONSISTENT FEATURE OF MULTIPLE SCLEROSIS

The advent of the polymerase chain reaction (PCR) and sequencing techniques and knowledge of characteristics of the GC differentiation pathway have enabled adaptive humoral immune responses to be studied during MS pathogenesis. Real-time PCR and sequence analysis of Ig V_H genes demonstrated a dominant B-cell clonal expansion in CSF of 10 out of 12 patients with MS and 3 out of 15 patients with other neurological diseases *(74)*. The nucleotide sequences of V_H genes in clonally expanded CSF B-cells from patients with MS shows preferential usage of the V_H IV family. Numerous somatic mutations were seen, mainly in the CDRs with a high replacement-to-silent ratio, distributed in a way suggestive of migration into the CNS after positive selection of B-cells in the GCs through their antigen receptor. Another report also showed preferential use and somatic hypermutation of the V_H IV family genes in lesion biopsies from two patients with acute MS *(75)*. These results were confirmed by observations of B-cell clonal expansion in frozen plaque sections from 10 patients with MS and increased use of VH1-69, VH4-34, and VH4-39 in these lesions *(76)*. Accumulation of oligoclonal B-cells was seen in 10 out of 10 patients with MS, but only 3 out of 10 patients with other neurological disorders. The V(D)J genes used by B-cells in the CSF were much less represented in peripheral blood lymphocytes, indicating tissue-specific clonal B-cell localization *(77)*. Recently, the authors have shown B-cell clonal expansion in 11 out of 12 patients with chronic progressive MS (unpublished data). These findings indicate that most patients with MS with early or chronic disease have predominant B-cell clonal expansion and confirm the significance of intrathecal B-cell clonal expansion in the clinical and pathobiological aspects of MS. Analysis of CSF B-cell clonality provides an objective assessment of an autoimmune process in MS evolution.

B-CELL CLONAL EXPANSION IN EARLY MULTIPLE SCLEROSIS

Several studies demonstrate that permanent tissue damage occurs in early MS *(11,115–117)*. The ability to recognize an autoimmune reaction in the CNS during the early disease stages is important in establishing a diagnosis, and early therapy may prevent or delay early tissue damage. Analysis of Ig V_H genes in CSF B-cells means that a wider range of patients with different clinical courses can be studied.

It is particularly suitable for patients in the early stages of disease, who have a first attack suggestive of MS (clinically isolated syndrome [CIS]). Progress in imaging techniques and laboratory tests have improved MS diagnosis, but MS-like lesions or OCBs are seen in only 50–70% of patients with CIS *(118–122)*. The presence of both lesions and OCBs is highly predictive of CDMS *(60,120,123–125)*, and the predictive value of OCBs for CDMS development is important in patients with CIS with normal brain MRI scans *(61,126,127)*. However, a special diagnostic problem is presented by patients with CIS with recurrent myelitis in one locus but no other signs of demyelination on MRI imaging *(128)* and by patients with normal MRI results and no OCBs *(129,130)*.

The authors' ongoing studies examine the clinical diagnostic value of B-cell clonal expansion in predicting the development of MS after CIS. Of 20 patients with CIS suggestive of MS examined, 8 had 3 or more high-signal lesions (2 of whom had no CSF OCBs [group 1]), 4 had 1 high-signal lesion in the spinal cord (2 of these had no OCBs [group 2]), and 8 had normal MRI and no OCBs (group 3). Nucleotide sequencing of the Ig V_H genes showed that intrathecal B-cell clonal expansion had occurred in all 8 patients in group 1 (including the 2 patients negative for OCBs), in 3 out of 4 patients in group 2 (including 1 with no OCBs), and in 2 out of 8 patients in group 3. CDMS developed within the 5-year follow-up in 10 of the 13 patients who showed intrathecal B-cell clonal expansion: 6 from group 1 (2 with no OCBs), 2 from group 2 (1 with no OCBs), and 2 from group 3 (normal MRI and no OCBs). None of the 7 patients who did not show intrathecal B-cell clonal expansion demonstrated any further neurological manifestations within the 5-year follow-up. These results indicate that clonal B-cell infiltration precedes the appearance of MRI lesions and OCBs.

Early histoimmunostaining studies of MS lesions showed an inflammatory, primarily lymphocytic, infiltration of the vessels and capillaries of the brain parenchyma that did not lead to changes in the myelin sheaths and could not be demonstrated by gadolinium (Gd)-enhanced MRI. This "vasculitis" may allow B-cells to penetrate the CNS, where they produce Igs that are detected as OCBs. These changes have been well demonstrated in normal white matter *(8,131–133)*. Such findings support the hypothesis that clinical symptoms and intrathecal B-cell clonal expansion can occur before CNS dissemination, indicating the importance of B-cell-mediated humoral immunity during the early stages of lesion development. The authors' results confirm and extend those of previous reports and indicate the value of detection of intrathecal B-cell clonal expansion at presentation as a predictive and prognostic indicator in patients presenting with CIS suggestive of MS.

ANTIBODY-MEDIATED INNATE AND ADAPTIVE IMMUNE RESPONSES IN MULTIPLE SCLEROSIS

Antibodies in Demyelinated Lesions of Multiple Sclerosis

Infiltrated B-cell clones are clearly required for development of humoral immunity-induced demyelination. These clones produce monoclonal (auto)antibodies that damage myelin by several mechanisms. They can specifically bind antigen in myelin, then activate the classic complement cascade as a result of binding complement component C1q to the Fc region of the antigen-bound antibody *(134)*. This induces production of the membrane attack complex (MAC), which inserts itself into cell membranes causing lysis and cell death *(135,136)*. The Fc region of the antibody can also bind to Fc receptors on macrophages, neutrophils, and NK cells, causing these innate immune cells to specifically attack myelin by antibody-dependent cell-mediated cytotoxicity.

The role of autoantibodies in demyelination was first noted in the EAE model. Classical EAE, induced in susceptible animal strains (i.e., Lewis rats) by immunization with myelin antigens and Freund's adjuvant, is usually monophasic with acute inflammation in the CNS and no demyelination. However, when anti-MOG antibody is given as a single injection after immunization with MBP, demyelination is induced. During the last 30 years, myelin protein-specific B-cells and antibodies have been extensively studied in MS. High-affinity antibodies to MBP and MOG have been purified from MS lesions *(137)*, and B-cells and antibodies to PLP *(138)*, MAG, and other CNS antigens *(139,140)* are found in the CSF of patients with MS (the antibodies also being found in serum) *(139)*. Genain et al. used immunogold-labeled MOG and MBP to locate antigen-specific plasma cells and antibodies in MS lesions and demonstrated that MOG- and MBP-specific antibodies are present on the surface of plasma cells in the parenchyma, in areas undergoing demyelination, on the myelin networks around scattered axons, and on droplets of myelin debris in the parenchyma *(70)*. These findings strongly support the idea that infiltration of MOG- and MBP-specific plasma cells and the local secretion of autoantibodies play an important role in demyelination and lesion formation. Deposition of antibodies and complement and infiltration of T- and B-cells and macrophages into the perivascular region are coupled with the destruction of the myelin sheath and axons *(141)*—the most common pattern of pathology in the majority of MS lesions.

Complement in Demyelinated Lesions of Mutiple Sclerosis

On binding antigen, an (auto)antibody can activate proinflammatory complement components, such as C1, C3, and C9, and cause tissue damage. Activation of the first part and terminal components of the classic complement cascade can be assessed by measuring activation of the C3 and C9 terminal complement complex, respectively. Deposits of antibody and complement, activated macrophages and microglial cells, and T- and B-cell infiltration are seen in the CSF in MS cases and are considered to be involved in lesion formation *(142–146)*. Full activation of the complement cascade, especially of C9, during MS attacks may be restricted to patients with more advanced disease and is significantly correlated with degree of neurological disability *(147)*. In the brain, oligodendroglial cells may be more sensitive to complement damage *(148)* than microglia and astrocytes *(149)*.

In MS, complement in the peripheral blood may be transported into the CNS as a result of leakage of the BBB. Alternatively, there may be local synthesis of complement by astrocytes, microglia, and infiltrated macrophages, especially in an environment containing high levels of proinflammatory cytokines *(150)*. The most convincing data for a role of complement activation in MS come from histopathologic studies showing presence of IgG and complement protein C1q within the plaque *(151)*, C3 around the demyelinating borders of MS plaques *(152)*, and C3d on macrophages in the most active lesions *(132)*. There is evidence that initial demyelination is caused by binding of Ig to myelin, which results in activation of complement, phagocytes, and resident microglia. However, the antigens involved are unknown; further analysis of the oligoclonal B-cell response may help to identify the primary provoking antigens *(131)*. In MS, the activated lytic complement complex generated by C9 activation is exclusively deposited in areas of active myelin and oligodendrocyte destruction *(153)*.

Antibody-Dependent Cell-Mediated Cytotoxicity

The Fc region of the molecule mediates many effects of antibodies. This region of IgG1 and IgG3 binds Fc receptors on phagocytes (macrophages and neutrophils) and promotes phagocytosis of antibody-bound antigen in different tissues. The consequences of phagocytosis are activation of the enzyme phagocyte oxidase and secretion of hydrolytic enzymes, which induce tissue inflammation and tissue damage. The hyperactive early plaque is usually infiltrated around its central vein with monocytes, lymphocytes, and plasma cells *(154)*. The phagocytic element contributes to myelin breakdown *(155,156)*; phagocytosis was seen in the periplaque white matter of autopsy plaques from two patients with secondary-progressive MS (SPMS). Immunohistochemical staining showed microglia engaging short segments of disrupted myelin bearing C3d deposits *(157,158)*. Phagocytosis of myelin by macrophages, triggering the production of reactive oxygen species (ROS), has been observed in EAE *(157)*. These studies show that antibody can cause demyelination by three main mechanisms:

1. Opsonization and phagocytosis of cells.
2. Complement- and Fc-receptor-mediated inflammation and tissue injury.
3. Interference with normal cellular functions by antibody binding to physiologically important molecules or cellular receptors.

NEW APPROACH TO MULTIPLE SCLEROSIS-RELATED ANTIBODY

The finding that clonal expansion of hypermutated B-cells occurs in lesions and in the CSF during different disease stages could mean that persistent antigen-driven adaptive immunity is responsible for disease progression. MS-related antigens have been investigated extensively using patient CSF and serum antibodies. Antibodies against infectious agents and autoantigens have been identified in the CSF and in the lesions, but the data are not convincing, because most of them might not be MS-related. The clonal expansion of B-cells in CSF and lesions could indicate that MS is driven by persistent restricted antigen(s) and provides the opportunity to study MS-related antigens using in vitro recombinant antibody synthesis techniques developed in the last decade. This approach, which makes it possible to synthesize antibodies using the Ig V_H and V_L genes expressed in a B-cell clone, uses PCR and sequential cloning of gene sequences coding for the Ig V_H and V_L chains in a phage display vector to produce single-chain Fv antibody. Brain cDNA banks and phage display peptide libraries have provided peptide ligands that can be used to identify the antigen recognized by the antibody, using an in vitro selection process called panning. This technique allows the study of antigens recognized by clonally expanded CSF-B-cells. The feasibility of this approach was recently demonstrated in studies using an antibody phage display library, generated from brains of humans with subacute sclerosing panencephalitis (SSPE) or MS, which showed that recombinant antibody prepared from SSPE brain reacted with the nucleocapsid protein of measles virus *(159–161)*. Williamson et al. showed that recombinant antibody, engineered from the Ig genes of B-cells obtained from either active plaques and periplaque regions in MS brain or from the CSF of a patient with MS, bound tightly and specifically to double-stranded DNA *(162)*. These early findings demonstrate that such techniques may have a significant effect on the study of MS-related antigens in the CSF and lesions of MS.

CONCLUSIONS

The outstanding fact of this review is that the presence of B-cell clonal expansion, in CSF and plaques of patients with MS, is indicative of an ongoing antigen-driven response in the CNS. These somatically hypermutated B-cells are found early in the disease, sometimes in the absence of OCBs and MRI lesions, as well as in latter stages. These findings have several possible implications:

- Increased diagnostic sensitivity.
- Prognosis.
- Role in immunopathogenesis.
- Role in primary and secondary progression.
- Effect on therapy.

Evidence that MS is an autoimmune disease remains inconclusive, but one can at least presume that humoral immunity plays a role in lesion formation and perpetuation; alternatively, it could be involved in tissue-repair mechanisms.

The antigen inducing this humoral response remains unknown, and it is important to identify it as either a self- or foreign-protein—a goal that several laboratories are actively pursuing. Given the complexity of MS and what we currently know about CSF IgGs, many antigens could be involved.

The authors believe that the paradigm of MS as a T-cell disease must be revisited, because B-cells are involved during the initial and late diseases. There is mounting evidence that a degenerative process, in addition to and possibly even preceding inflammation, is also implicated, but currently the biological basis of this degeneration, as distinct from inflammation, is obscure. Finally, it is suspected that inflammation as a whole may play a part in tissue reconstitution and B-cell immune responses might be involved in all or part of these processes.

These studies will be pursued and will hopefully unravel further aspects of the perceived complexity of MS.

REFERENCES

1. Page WF, Kurtzke JF, Murphy FM, Norman JE, Jr. Epidemiology of multiple sclerosis in U.S. veterans: V. Ancestry and the risk of multiple sclerosis. Ann Neurol 1993;33:632-639.
2. Poser CM. The epidemiology of multiple sclerosis: a general overview. Ann Neurol 1994;36(Suppl 2):S180–S193.
3. Rothwell PM, Charlton D. High incidence and prevalence of multiple sclerosis in south east Scotland: evidence of a genetic predisposition. J Neurol Neurosurg Psychiatry 1998;64:730–735.
4. Lublin FD, Reingold SC. Defining the clinical course of multiple sclerosis: results of an international survey. National Multiple Sclerosis Society (USA) Advisory Committee on Clinical Trials of New Agents in Multiple Sclerosis. Neurology 1996;46:907–911.
5. Confavreux C, Compston DA, Hommes OR, McDonald WI, Thompson AJ. EDMUS, a European database for multiple sclerosis. J Neurol Neurosurg Psychiatry 1992;55:671–676.
6. Poser CM, Paty DW, Scheinberg L, et al. New diagnostic criteria for multiple sclerosis: guidelines for research protocols. Ann Neurol 1983;13:227–231.
7. Poser CM. Onset symptoms of multiple sclerosis. J Neurol Neurosurg Psychiatry 1995;58:253–254.
8. Adams CW, Poston RN, Buk SJ, Sidhu YS, Vipond H. Inflammatory vasculitis in multiple sclerosis. J Neurol Sci 1985;69:269–283.
9. Tran EH, Hoekstra K, van Rooijen N, Dijkstra CD, Owens T. Immune invasion of the central nervous system parenchyma and experimental allergic encephalomyelitis, but not leukocyte extravasation from blood, are prevented in macrophage-depleted mice. J Immunol 1998;161: 3767–3775.
10. Lassmann H, Raine CS, Antel J, Prineas JW. Immunopathology of multiple sclerosis: report on an international meeting held at the Institute of Neurology of the University of Vienna. J Neuroimmunol 1998;86:213–217.
11. Trapp BD, Peterson J, Ransohoff RM, Rudick R, Mork S, Bo L. Axonal transection in the lesions of multiple sclerosis. N Engl J Med 1998;338:278–285.
12. Ffrench-Constant C. Pathogenesis of multiple sclerosis. Lancet 1994;343:271–275.
13. Boyle EA, McGeer PL. Cellular immune response in multiple sclerosis plaques. Am J Pathol 1990;137:575–584.
14. Ozawa K, Suchanek G, Breitschopf H, et al. Patterns of oligodendroglia pathology in multiple sclerosis. Brain 1994;117(Pt 6):1311–1322.
15. Lassmann H. Neuropathology in multiple sclerosis: new concepts. Mult Scler 1998;4:93–98.
16. Waxman SG. Demyelinating diseases—new pathological insights, new therapeutic targets. N Engl J Med 1998;338:323–325.
17. McDonald WI, Compston A, Edan G, et al. Recommended diagnostic criteria for multiple sclerosis: guidelines from the International Panel on the diagnosis of multiple sclerosis. Ann Neurol 2001;50:121–127.
18. Thorpe JW, Kidd D, Moseley IF, et al. Serial gadolinium-enhanced MRI of the brain and spinal cord in early relapsing-remitting multiple sclerosis. Neurology 1996;46:373–378.
19. Poser CM, Kleefield J, O'Reilly GV, Jolesz F. Neuroimaging and the lesion of multiple sclerosis. AJNR Am J Neuroradiol 1987;8:549–552.
20. Ebers GC, Sadovnick AD, Risch NJ. A genetic basis for familial aggregation in multiple sclerosis. Canadian Collaborative Study Group. Nature 1995;377:150–151.
21. Doolittle TH, Myers RH, Lehrich JR, et al. Multiple sclerosis sibling pairs: clustered onset and familial predisposition. Neurology 1990;40:1546–1552.
22. Cowan EP, Pierce ML, McFarland HF, McFarlin DE. HLA-DR and -DQ allelic sequences in multiple sclerosis patients are identical to those found in the general population. Hum Immunol 1991;32:203–210.

23. Ebers GC, Bulman DE, Sadovnick AD, et al. A population-based study of multiple sclerosis in twins. N Engl J Med 1986;315:1638–1642.
24. Pringle CE, McEwan LM, Ebers GC. Laryngeal Uhthoff's phenomenon: a case report. Mult Scler 1995;1:163–164.
25. Haines JL, Ter-Minassian M, Bazyk A, et al. A complete genomic screen for multiple sclerosis underscores a role for the major histocompatability complex. The Multiple Sclerosis Genetics Group. Nat Genet 1996;13:469–471.
26. Hutter CD, Laing P. Multiple sclerosis: sunlight, diet, immunology and etiology. Med Hypotheses 1996;46:67–74.
27. Dean G, McLoughlin H, Brady R, Adelstein AM, Tallett-Williams J. Multiple sclerosis among immigrants in Greater London. Br Med J 1976;1:861–864.
28. Detels R, Visscher BR, Haile RW, Malmgren RM, Dudley JP, Coulson AH. Multiple sclerosis and age at migration. Am J Epidemiol 1978;108:386–393.
29. Gershon AA, Raker R, Steinberg S, Topf-Olstein B, Drusin LM. Antibody to Varicella-Zoster virus in parturient women and their offspring during the first year of life. Pediatrics 1976;58: 692–696.
30. Gray GC, Palinkas LA, Kelley PW. Increasing incidence of varicella hospitalizations in United States Army and Navy personnel: are today's teenagers more susceptible? Should recruits be vaccinated? Pediatrics 1990;86:867–873.
31. Ben-Nun A, Wekerle H, Cohen IR. Vaccination against autoimmune encephalomyelitis with T-lymphocyte line cells reactive against myelin basic protein. Nature 1981;292:60–61.
32. Wekerle H. The viral triggering of autoimmune disease. Nat Med 1998;4:770–771.
33. Mokhtarian F, McFarlin DE, Raine CS. Adoptive transfer of myelin basic protein-sensitized T cells produces chronic relapsing demyelinating disease in mice. Nature 1984;309:356–358.
34. Amor S, Groome N, Linington C, et al. Identification of epitopes of myelin oligodendrocyte glycoprotein for the induction of experimental allergic encephalomyelitis in SJL and Biozzi AB/H mice. J Immunol 1994;153:4349–4356.
35. Schluesener HJ, Sobel RA, Weiner HL.. Demyelinating experimental allergic encephalomyelitis (EAE) in the rat: treatment with a monoclonal antibody against activated T cells. J Neuroimmunol 1988;18:341–351.
36. Schluesener HJ, Lider O, Sobel RA. Induction of hyperacute brain inflammation and demyelination by activated encephalitogenic T cells and a monoclonal antibody specific for a myelin/oligodendrocyte glycoprotein. Autoimmunity 1989;2:265–273.
37. Lassmann H, Brunner C, Bradl M, Linington C. Experimental allergic encephalomyelitis: the balance between encephalitogenic T lymphocytes and demyelinating antibodies determines size and structure of demyelinated lesions. Acta Neuropathol (Berl) 1988;75:566–576.
38. Lyons JA, San M, Happ MP, Cross AH. B cells are critical to induction of experimental allergic encephalomyelitis by protein but not by a short encephalitogenic peptide. Eur J Immunol 1999;29:3432–3439.
39. Itoyama Y, Webster HD. Immunocytochemical study of myelin-associated glycoprotein (MAG) and basic protein (BP) in acute experimental allergic encephalomyelitis (EAE). J Neuroimmunol 1982;3:351–364.
40. Sternberger NH, McFarlin DE, Traugott U, Raine CS.. Myelin basic protein and myelin-associated glycoprotein in chronic, relapsing experimental allergic encephalomyelitis. J Neuroimmunol 1984;6:217–229.
41. Yoshimura T, Kunishita T, Sakai K, Endoh M, Namikawa T, Tabira T. Chronic experimental allergic encephalomyelitis in guinea pigs induced by proteolipid protein. J Neurol Sci 1985;69:47–58.
42. Yamamura T, Namikawa T, Endoh M, Kunishita T, Tabira T.. Passive transfer of experimental allergic encephalomyelitis induced by proteolipid apoprotein. J Neurol Sci 1986;76:269–275.
43. Martin R, Voskuhl R, Flerlage M, McFarlin DE, McFarland HF. Myelin basic protein-specific T-cell responses in identical twins discordant or concordant for multiple sclerosis. Ann Neurol 1993;34:524–535.

44. Kerlero de Rosbo N, Milo R, Lees MB, Burger D, Bernard CC, Ben-Nun A. Reactivity to myelin antigens in multiple sclerosis. Peripheral blood lymphocytes respond predominantly to myelin oligodendrocyte glycoprotein. J Clin Invest 1993;92:2602–2608.

45. Sun JB, Olsson T, Wang WZ, et al. Autoreactive T and B cells responding to myelin proteolipid protein in multiple sclerosis and controls. Eur J Immunol 1991;21:1461–1468.

46. Trotter JL, Wegescheide CL, Garvey WF, Tourtellotte WW.. Studies of myelin proteins in multiple sclerosis brain tissue. Neurochem Res 1984;9:147–152.

47. Bansil S, Cook SD, Rohowsky-Kochan C. Multiple sclerosis: immune mechanism and update on current therapies. Ann Neurol 1995;37(Suppl 1):S87–S101.

48. Maffione AB, Tato E, Losito S, et al. In vivo effects of recombinant-interferon-beta1b treatment on polymorphonuclear cell and monocyte functions and on T-cell-mediated antibacterial activity in patients with relapsing-remitting multiple sclerosis. Immunopharmacol Immunotoxicol 2000;22:1–18.

49. Tourtellotte W. On cerebrospinal fluid immunoglobulin-G (IgG) quotients in multiple sclerosis and other diseases. A review and a new formula to estimate the amount of IgG synthesized per day by the central nervous system. J Neurol Sci 1970;10:279–304.

50. Tourtellotte WW, Murthy K, Brandes D, et al. Schemes to eradicate the multiple sclerosis central nervous system immune reaction. Neurology 1976;26:59–61.

51. Tibbling G, Link H, Ohman S. Principles of albumin and IgG analyses in neurological disorders. I. Establishment of reference values. Scand J Clin Lab Invest 1977;37:385–390.

52. Lefvert AK, Link H. IgG production within the central nervous system: a critical review of proposed formulae. Ann Neurol 1985;17:13–20.

53. Esiri MM. Immunoglobulin-containing cells in multiple-sclerosis plaques. Lancet 1977;2:478.

54. Grimaldi LM, Maimone D, Reggio A, Raffaele R.. IgG1,3 and 4 oligoclonal bands in multiple sclerosis and other neurological diseases. Ital J Neurol Sci 1986;7:507–513.

55. Sesboue R, Daveau M, Degos JD, et al. IgG (Gm) allotypes and multiple sclerosis in a French population: phenotype distribution and quantitative abnormalities in CSF with respect to sex, disease severity, and presence of intrathecal antibodies. Clin Immunol Immunopathol 1985;37:143–153.

56. Giles PD, Wroe SJ.. Cerebrospinal fluid oligoclonal IgM in multiple sclerosis: analytical problems and clinical limitations. Ann Clin Biochem 1990;27(Pt 3):199–207.

57. Lolli F, Siracusa G, Amato MP, et al. Intrathecal synthesis of free immunoglobulin light chains and IgM in initial multiple sclerosis. Acta Neurol Scand 1991;83:239–243.

58. Sharief MK, Thompson EJ. The predictive value of intrathecal immunoglobulin synthesis and magnetic resonance imaging in acute isolated syndromes for subsequent development of multiple sclerosis. Ann Neurol 1991;29:147–151.

59. Egg R, Reindl M, Deisenhammer F, Linington C, Berger T. Anti-MOG and anti-MBP antibody subclasses in multiple sclerosis. Mult Scler 2001;7:285–289.

60. Rolak LA, Beck RW, Paty DW, Tourtellotte WW, Whitaker JN, Rudick RA. Cerebrospinal fluid in acute optic neuritis: experience of the optic neuritis treatment trial. Neurology 1996;46:368–372.

61. Cole SR, Beck RW, Moke PS, Kaufman DI, Tourtellotte WW. The predictive value of CSF oligoclonal banding for MS 5 years after optic neuritis. Optic Neuritis Study Group. Neurology 1998;51:885–887.

62. Filippini G, Comi GC, Cosi V, et al. Sensitivities and predictive values of paraclinical tests for diagnosing multiple sclerosis. J Neurol 1994;241:132–137.

63. Nikoskelainen E, Frey H, Salmi A.. Prognosis of optic neuritis with special reference to cerebrospinal fluid immunoglobulins and measles virus antibodies. Ann Neurol 1981;9:545–550.

64. Sandberg-Wollheim M, Bynke H, Cronqvist S, Holtas S, Platz P, Ryder LP. A long-term prospective study of optic neuritis: evaluation of risk factors. Ann Neurol 1990;27:386–393.

65. Warren KG, Catz I, Johnson E, Mielke B. Anti-myelin basic protein and anti-proteolipid protein specific forms of multiple sclerosis. Ann Neurol 1994;35:280–289.

66. Olsson T, Zhi WW, Hojeberg B, et al. Autoreactive T lymphocytes in multiple sclerosis deter-
    mined by antigen-induced secretion of interferon-gamma. J Clin Invest 1990;86:981–985.
67. Zhou SR, Maier CC, Mitchell GW, LaGanke CC, Blalock JE, Whitaker JN. A cross-reactive anti-
    myelin basic protein idiotope in cerebrospinal fluid cells in multiple sclerosis. Neurology
    1998;50:411–417.
68. Raine CS, Cannella B, Hauser SL, Genain CP. Demyelination in primate autoimmune encephalo-
    myelitis and acute multiple sclerosis lesions: a case for antigen-specific antibody mediation. Ann
    Neurol 1999;46:144–160.
69. Cross AH, Trotter JL, Lyons JA. B cells and antibodies in CNS demyelinating disease. Journal of
    Neuroimmunology 2001;112:1–14.
70. Genain CP, Cannella B, Hauser SL, Raine CS.. Identification of autoantibodies associated with
    myelin damage in multiple sclerosis. Nat Med 1999;5:170–175.
71. Horikawa Y, Tsubaki T, Nakajima M. Rubella antibody in multiple sclerosis. Lancet 1973;1:996–997.
72. Catalano LW, Jr. Herpesvirus hominis antibody in multiple sclerosis and amyotrophic lateral
    sclerosis. Neurology 1972;22:473–478.
73. Oger J, Roos R, Antel JP. Immunology of multiple sclerosis. Neurol Clin 1983;1:655–679.
74. Qin YF, Duquette P, Zhang YP, Talbot P, Poole R, Antel J.. Clonal expansion and somatic
    hypermutation of V-H genes of B cells from cerebrospinal fluid in multiple sclerosis. Journal of
    Clinical Investigation 1998;102:1045–1050.
75. Owens GP, Kraus H, Burgoon MP, Smith-Jensen T, Devlin ME, Gilden DH. Restricted use of
    V(H)4 germline segments in an acute multiple sclerosis brain. Ann Neurol 1998;43:236–243.
76. Baranzini SE, Jeong MC, Butunoi C, Murray RS, Bernard CCA, Oksenberg JR. B cell repertoire
    diversity and clonal expansion in multiple sclerosis brain lesions. J Immunol 1999;163:
    5133–5144.
77. Colombo M, Dono M, Gazzola P, et al. Accumulation of clonally related B lymphocytes in the
    cerebrospinal fluid of multiple sclerosis patients. J Immunol 2000;164:2782–2789.
78. Cross AH. MS: the return of the B cell. Neurology 2000;54:1214–1215.
79. Correale J, de Los Milagros Bassani Molinas M.. Oligoclonal bands and antibody responses in
    Multiple Sclerosis. J Neurol 2002;249:375–389.
80. Archelos JJ, Storch MK, Hartung HP. The role of B cells and autoantibodies in multiple sclerosis.
    Ann Neurol 2000;47:694–706.
81. Jacob J, Kassir R, Kelsoe G. In situ studies of the primary immune response to (4-hydroxy-3-
    nitrophenyl)acetyl. I. The architecture and dynamics of responding cell populations. J Exp Med
    1991;173:1165–1175.
82. Liu YJ, Zhang J, Lane PJ, Chan EY, MacLennan IC. Sites of specific B cell activation in primary
    and secondary responses to T cell-dependent and T cell-independent antigens. Eur J Immunol
    1991;21:2951–2962.
83. Vitetta ES, Berton MT, Burger C, Kepron M, Lee WT, Yin XM. Memory B and T cells. Annu
    Rev Immunol 1991;9:193–217.
84. MacLennan IC, Liu YJ, Johnson GD. Maturation and dispersal of B-cell clones during T cell-
    dependent antibody responses. Immunol Rev 1992;126:143–161.
85. Nossal GJ. The molecular and cellular basis of affinity maturation in the antibody response. Cell
    1992;68:1–2.
86. Siekevitz M, Kocks C, Rajewsky K, Dildrop R. Analysis of somatic mutation and class switching
    in naive and memory B cells generating adoptive primary and secondary responses. Cell
    1987;48:757–770.
87. Shlomchik MJ, Marshak-Rothstein A, Wolfowicz CB, Rothstein TL, Weigert MG. The role of
    clonal selection and somatic mutation in autoimmunity. Nature 1987;328:805–811.
88. Levy NS, Malipiero UV, Lebecque SG, Gearhart PJ. Early onset of somatic mutation in immuno-
    globulin VH genes during the primary immune response. J Exp Med 1989;169:2007–2019.
89. Cochet M, Pannetier C, Regnault A, Darche S, Leclerc C, Kourilsky P. Molecular detection
    and in vivo analysis of the specific T cell response to a protein antigen. Eur J Immunol 1992;22:
    2639–2647.

90. MacLennan IC, Gray D. Antigen-driven selection of virgin and memory B cells. Immunol Rev 1986;91:61–85.
91. Tsiagbe VK, Inghirami G, Thorbecke GJ.. The physiology of germinal centers. Crit Rev Immunol 1996;16:381–421.
92. Berek C, Jarvis JM, Milstein C. Activation of memory and virgin B cell clones in hyperimmune animals. Eur J Immunol 1987;17:1121–1129.
93. Jacob J, Kelsoe G. In situ studies of the primary immune response to (4-hydroxy-3-nitrophenyl)acetyl. II. A common clonal origin for periarteriolar lymphoid sheath-associated foci and germinal centers. J Exp Med 1992;176:679–687.
94. Liu YJ, Johnson GD, Gordon J, MacLennan IC. Germinal centres in T-cell-dependent antibody responses. Immunol Today 1992;13:17–21.
95. Schroeder HW, Jr, Hillson JL, Perlmutter RM. Structure and evolution of mammalian VH families. Int Immunol 1990;2:41–50.
96. Kirkham PM, Mortari F, Newton JA, Schroeder HW, Jr. Immunoglobulin VH clan and family identity predicts variable domain structure and may influence antigen binding. Embo J 1992;11:603–609.
97. Kroemer G, Helmberg A, Bernot A, Auffray C, Kofler R. Evolutionary relationship between human and mouse immunoglobulin kappa light chain variable region genes. Immunogenetics 1991;33:42–49.
98. Frippiat JP, Williams SC, Tomlinson IM, et al. Organization of the human immunoglobulin lambda light-chain locus on chromosome 22q11.2. Hum Mol Genet 1995;4:983–991.
99. Roberts S, Cheetham JC, Rees AR. Generation of an antibody with enhanced affinity and specificity for its antigen by protein engineering. Nature 1987;328:731–734.
100. Burnet FM. A modification of Jerne's theory of antibody production using the concept of clonal selection. CA Cancer J Clin 1976;26:119–121.
101. Griffiths GM, Berek C, Kaartinen M, Milstein C. Somatic mutation and the maturation of immune response to 2-phenyl oxazolone. Nature 1984;312:271–275.
102. Liu YJ, Joshua DE, Williams GT, Smith CA, Gordon J, MacLennan IC. Mechanism of antigen-driven selection in germinal centres. Nature 1989;342:929–931.
103. Hollowood K, Macartney JC. Reduced apoptotic cell death in follicular lymphoma. J Pathol 1991;163:337–342.
104. Bachmann MF, Kundig TM, Odermatt B, Hengartner H, Zinkernagel RM. Free recirculation of memory B cells versus antigen-dependent differentiation to antibody-forming cells. J Immunol 1994;153:3386–3397.
105. Kraal G, Weissman IL, Butcher EC. Memory B cells express a phenotype consistent with migratory competence after secondary but not short-term primary immunization. Cell Immunol 1988;115:78–87.
106. Slifka MK, Antia R, Whitmire JK, Ahmed R.. Humoral immunity due to long-lived plasma cells. Immunity 1998;8:363–372.
107. Gray D, Skarvall H. B-cell memory is short-lived in the absence of antigen. Nature 1988;336:70–73.
108. Gray D, Matzinger P. T cell memory is short-lived in the absence of antigen. J Exp Med 1991;174:969–974.
109. Cannella B, Raine CS. The adhesion molecule and cytokine profile of multiple sclerosis lesions. Ann Neurol 1995;37:424–435.
110. Navikas V, Link H.. Review: cytokines and the pathogenesis of multiple sclerosis. J Neurosci Res 1996;45:322–333.
111. Simpson JE, Newcombe J, Cuzner ML, Woodroofe MN. Expression of the interferon-gamma-inducible chemokines IP-10 and Mig and their receptor, CXCR3, in multiple sclerosis lesions. Neuropathol Appl Neurobiol 2000;26:133–142.
112. Balashov KE, Rottman JB, Weiner HL, Hancock WW. CCR5(+) and CXCR3(+) T cells are increased in multiple sclerosis and their ligands MIP-1alpha and IP-10 are expressed in demyelinating brain lesions. Proc Natl Acad Sci U S A 1999;96:6873–6878.
113. Sorensen TL, Tani M, Jensen J, et al. Expression of specific chemokines and chemokine receptors in the central nervous system of multiple sclerosis patients. J Clin Invest 1999;103:807–815.

114. Strunk T, Bubel S, Mascher B, Schlenke P, Kirchner H, Wandinger KP. Increased numbers of CCR5+ interferon-gamma- and tumor necrosis factor-alpha-secreting T lymphocytes in multiple sclerosis patients. Ann Neurol 2000;47:269–273.
115. Bruck W, Porada P, Poser S, et al. Monocyte/macrophage differentiation in early multiple sclerosis lesions. Ann Neurol 1995;38:788–796.
116. Ferguson B, Matyszak MK, Esiri MM, Perry VH.. Axonal damage in acute multiple sclerosis lesions. Brain 1997;120(Pt 3):393–399.
117. Ganter P, Prince C, Esiri MM.. Spinal cord axonal loss in multiple sclerosis: a post-mortem study. Neuropathol Appl Neurobiol 1999;25:459–467.
118. Morrissey SP, Miller DH, Kendall BE, et al. The significance of brain magnetic resonance imaging abnormalities at presentation with clinically isolated syndromes suggestive of multiple sclerosis. A 5-year follow-up study. Brain 1993;116(Pt 1):135–146.
119. Beck RW, Cleary PA, Trobe JD, et al. The effect of corticosteroids for acute optic neuritis on the subsequent development of multiple sclerosis. The Optic Neuritis Study Group. N Engl J Med 1993;329:1764–1769.
120. Frederiksen JL, Larsson HB, Olesen J. Correlation of magnetic resonance imaging and CSF findings in patients with acute monosymptomatic optic neuritis. Acta Neurol Scand 1992;86:317–322.
121. Soderstrom M.. The clinical and paraclinical profile of optic neuritis: a prospective study. Ital J Neurol Sci 1995;16:167–176.
122. Hawkes CH, Thompson EJ, Keir G, et al. Iso-electric focusing of aqueous humour IgG in multiple sclerosis. J Neurol 1994;241:436–438.
123. Optic Neuritis Study Group. The 5-year risk of MS after optic neuritis. Experience of the optic neuritis treatment trial. Neurology 1997;49:1404–1413.
124. Paolino E, Fainardi E, Ruppi P, et al. A prospective study on the predictive value of CSF oligoclonal bands and MRI in acute isolated neurological syndromes for subsequent progression to multiple sclerosis. J Neurol Neurosurg Psychiatry 1996;60:572–575.
125. Bosch X. Imaging the brain. N Engl J Med 1998;339:407; discussion 408–409.
126. Soderstrom M, Ya-Ping J, Hillert J, Link H.. Optic neuritis: prognosis for multiple sclerosis from MRI, CSF, and HLA findings. Neurology 1998;50:708–714.
127. Plante-Bordeneuve V, Lalu T, Misrahi M, et al. Genotypic-phenotypic variations in a series of 65 patients with familial amyloid polyneuropathy. Neurology 1998;51:708–714.
128. Bashir K, Whitaker JN. Importance of paraclinical and CSF studies in the diagnosis of MS in patients presenting with partial cervical transverse myelopathy and negative cranial MRI. Mult Scler 2000;6:312–316.
129. Stendahl-Brodin L, Link H. Relation between benign course of multiple sclerosis and low-grade humoral immune response in cerebrospinal fluid. J Neurol Neurosurg Psychiatry 1980;43:102–105.
130. Zeman AZ, Kidd D, McLean BN, et al. A study of oligoclonal band negative multiple sclerosis. J Neurol Neurosurg Psychiatry 1996;60:27–30.
131. Gay FW, Drye TJ, Dick GWA, Esiri MM. The application of multifactorial cluster analysis in the staging of plaques in early multiple sclerosis—identification and characterization of the primary demyelinating lesion. Brain 1997;120:1461–1483.
132. Gay D, Esiri M.. Blood–brain barrier damage in acute multiple sclerosis plaques. An immunocytological study. Brain 1991;114(Pt 1B):557–572.
133. Pozzilli C, Bernardi S, Mansi L, et al. Quantitative assessment of blood–brain barrier permeability in multiple sclerosis using 68-Ga-EDTA and positron emission tomography. J Neurol Neurosurg Psychiatry 1988;51:1058–1062.
134. Loos M. Biosynthesis of the collagen-like C1q molecule and its receptor functions for Fc and polyanionic molecules on macrophages. Curr Top Microbiol Immunol 1983;102:1–56.
135. Esser AF. Big MAC attack: complement proteins cause leaky patches. Immunol Today 1991;12:316–318; discussion 321.

136. Bhakdi S, Tranum-Jensen J. Complement lysis: a hole is a hole. Immunol Today 1991;12:318–320; discussion 321.
137. Wucherpfennig KW, Catz I, Hausmann S, Strominger JL, Steinman L, Warren KG. Recognition of the immunodominant myelin basic protein peptide by autoantibodies and HLA-DR2-restricted T cell clones from multiple sclerosis patients. Identity of key contact residues in the B-cell and T-cell epitopes. J Clin Invest 1997;100:1114–1122.
138. Sun JP, Olsson T, Wang WZ, et al. Autoreactive T-Cell and B-Cell Responding to Myelin Proteolipid Protein in Multiple-Sclerosis and Controls. Eur J Immunol 1991;21:1461–1468.
139. Cruz M, Olsson T, Ernerudh J, Hojeberg B, Link H. Immunoblot detection of oligoclonal antimyelin basic protein IgG antibodies in cerebrospinal fluid in multiple sclerosis. Neurology 1987;37:1515–1519.
140. Olsson T, Baig S, Hojeberg B, Link H.. Antimyelin basic protein and antimyelin antibody-producing cells in multiple sclerosis. Ann Neurol 1990;27:132–136.
141. Lucchinetti C, Bruck W, Parisi J, Scheithauer B, Rodriguez M, Lassmann H. Heterogeneity of multiple sclerosis lesions: implications for the pathogenesis of demyelination. Ann Neurol 2000;47:707–717.
142. Compston DA, Morgan BP, Campbell AK, et al. Immunocytochemical localization of the terminal complement complex in multiple sclerosis. Neuropathol Appl Neurobiol 1989;15:307–316.
143. Scolding NJ, Morgan BP, Houston WA, Linington C, Campbell AK, Compston DA. Vesicular removal by oligodendrocytes of membrane attack complexes formed by activated complement. Nature 1989;339:620–622.
144. Link H. Complement factors in multiple sclerosis. Acta Neurol Scand 1972;48:521–528.
145. Patterson V. C9 in multiple sclerosis. Lancet 1984;2:458.
146. Morgan BP, Campbell AK, Compston DA.. Terminal component of complement (C9) in cerebrospinal fluid of patients with multiple sclerosis. Lancet 1984;2:251–254.
147. Sellebjerg F, Jaliashvili I, Christiansen M, Garred P.. Intrathecal activation of the complement system and disability in multiple sclerosis. J Neurol Sci 1998;157:168–174.
148. Wren DR, Noble M. Oligodendrocytes and oligodendrocyte/type-2 astrocyte progenitor cells of adult rats are specifically susceptible to the lytic effects of complement in absence of antibody. Proc Natl Acad Sci U S A 1989;86:9025–9029.
149. Davoust N, Nataf S, Holers VM, Barnum SR. Expression of the murine complement regulatory protein crry by glial cells and neurons. Glia 1999;27:162–170.
150. Morgan BP, Gasque P. Expression of complement in the brain: role in health and disease. Immunol Today 1996;17:461–466.
151. Woyciechowska JL, Brzosko WJ. Immunofluorescence study of brain plaques from two patients with multiple sclerosis. Neurology 1977;27:620–622.
152. Lumsden CE. The immunogenesis of the multiple sclerosis plaque. Brain Res 1971;28:365–390.
153. Storch MK, Piddlesden S, Haltia M, Iivanainen M, Morgan P, Lassmann H. Multiple sclerosis: in situ evidence for antibody- and complement-mediated demyelination. Ann Neurol 1998;43:465–471.
154. Nyland H, Matre R, Mork S. Fc receptors of microglial lipophages in multiple sclerosis. N Engl J Med 1980;302:120–121.
155. Adams CW. The onset and progression of the lesion in multiple sclerosis. J Neurol Sci 1975;25:165–182.
156. Arstila AU, Riekkinen P, Rinne UK, Laitinen L. Studies on the pathogenesis of multiple sclerosis. Participation of lysosomes on demyelination in the central nervous system white matter outside plaques. Eur Neurol 1973;9:1–20.
157. Prineas JW, Kwon EE, Cho ES, et al. Immunopathology of secondary-progressive multiple sclerosis. Ann Neurol 2001;50:646–657.
158. Prineas JW, Graham JS. Multiple sclerosis: capping of surface immunoglobulin G on macrophages engaged in myelin breakdown. Ann Neurol 1981;10:149–158.

159. Gilden DH, Burgoon MP, Kleinschmidt-DeMasters BK, et al. Molecular immunologic strategies to identify antigens and b-cell responses unique to multiple sclerosis. Arch Neurol 2001;58:43–48.
160. Owens GP, Williamson RA, Burgoon MP, et al. Cloning the antibody response in humans with chronic inflammatory disease: immunopanning of subacute sclerosing panencephalitis (SSPE) brain sections with antibody phage libraries prepared from SSPE brain enriches for antibody recognizing measles virus antigens in situ. J Virol 2000;74:1533–1537.
161. Burgoon MP, Williamson RA, Owens GP, et al. Cloning the antibody response in humans with inflammatory CNS disease: isolation of measles virus-specific antibodies from phage display libraries of a subacute sclerosing panencephalitis brain. J Neuroimmunol 1999;94:204–211.
162. Williamson RA, Burgoon MP, Owens GP, et al. Anti-DNA antibodies are a major component of the intrathecal B cell response in multiple sclerosis. Proc Nat Acad Sci U S A 2001;98:1793–1798.
163. Stadelmann C, Kerschensteiner M, Misgeld T, et al. BDNF and gp145trkB in multiple sclerosis brain lesions: neuroprotective interactions between immune and neuronal cells?. Brain 2002;125(Pt 1):75–85.

7

Multiple Sclerosis

A Case for Early Treatment

Alex C. Tselis, PhD, MD and Omar A. Khan, MD

INTRODUCTION

Multiple sclerosis (MS) has emerged as a treatable disorder with several disease-modifying therapies (DMTs) now licensed in the United States for MS treatment. These are interferon (IFN)-β-1a (two formulations, Avonex and Rebif), IFN-β-1b (Betaseron), glatiramer acetate (GA) (Copaxone), and mitoxantrone (Novantrone). Although all five DMTs were tested in phase III randomized controlled trials (RCTs) and shown to be superior to placebo, no therapy has ever been shown to halt disease progression *(1–5)*. Because MS is a chronic, unpredictable disease and clinically variable from patient to patient, treatment choices for patients with MS can pose a dilemma, despite the plethora of information. Nonetheless, the use of DMTs in definite relapsing-remitting MS (RRMS) is well established.

More recently, clinicians and scientists have focused on the early treatment of MS, which presents a new challenge in MS therapeutics. Several lines of evidence suggest that early treatment should be considered. Despite positive outcomes in treatment trials of clinically isolated syndromes (CIS) in patients considered at high risk of developing definite MS, many debate whether early treatment of patients with CIS affects long-term disability. The lack of data demonstrating an effect of DMT on long-term disability in patients with CIS, combined with the economic consequences of these medications, argue in favor of a conservative approach in this population. This argument is further strengthened by the well-established efficacy of IFN-β and GA in RRMS; it is also well recognized that existing DMTs are only partially effective.

On the other hand, a growing body of evidence suggests that treatment with a DMT in patients presenting with CIS is beneficial and may delay the development of clinically definite MS (CDMS). The authors examine data supporting early treatment of MS and also consider the revised diagnostic criteria for MS *(6)*, which enables clinicians to make the diagnosis and initiate treatment early.

From: *Current Clinical Neurology: Multiple Sclerosis*
Edited by: M. J. Olek © Humana Press Inc., Totowa, NJ

A picture of MS pathogenesis is emerging, based in part on the data discussed in this chapter, in which the initial stages of the disease are dominated by inflammatory demyelination, leading to concomitant axonal damage. As the disease progresses, the inflammatory component declines significantly, but a degenerative process is triggered with axonal transection and degeneration proceeding independently (and probably irreversibly) of inflammation. The disease thus evolves into a neurodegenerative process and is less responsive to treatment by immunomodulatory medications, which are primarily directed against the inflammatory component of the disease *(7)*.

APPLICATION OF THE NEW MULTIPLE SCLEROSIS DIAGNOSTIC CRITERIA: SUPPORTING EARLY DIAGNOSIS AND TREATMENT

The diagnosis of MS depends on the demonstration of the presence of at least two separately located lesions (spatial dissemination) in the white matter of the central nervous system (CNS) occurring at two separate times (temporal dissemination), in the absence of any better explanation for these lesions. Formal criteria for the diagnosis were first proposed in 1965 and reflected the understanding of the disease and diagnostic technology available at that time *(8)*. As new diagnostic methods evolved (e.g., measurements of oligoclonal banding and immunoglobulin [Ig] G index in cerebrospinal fluid [CSF], evoked potential tests), new diagnostic criteria were published to incorporate these methods in the diagnosis of MS *(9)*. With the advent of magnetic resonance imaging (MRI) scanning in patients with MS, the diagnostic criteria for MS had to be modified to consider this new method *(6)*.

The importance of MRI for the diagnosis of MS became apparent when patients with CIS who had brain MRIs were followed long-term. In one study of 89 patients with CIS, 57 (64%) had abnormal and 32 (36%) had normal MRIs. After a 5-year follow-up, 72% of patients with an initially abnormal scan had developed CDMS, using the Poser criteria, whereas only 2 of 32 patients (6%) with normal MRIs had CDMS *(10)*. The presence of oligoclonal bands (OCBs) in the CSF was also a risk factor for the development of CDMS, but it was not as strong as that of an abnormal MRI. Further follow-up of 81 of these patients, over 10 years, confirmed and strengthened these results. The risk of progressing to CDMS was 83% (45 out of 54 patients) in those with an abnormal initial MRI and 11% (3 out of 27 patients) in those without *(11)*.

In an important follow-up study by the same group *(12)*, 71 patients with CIS were followed out to an average of 14 years. Those with initially abnormal brain MRIs were at high risk (88%) of developing CDMS, with a median time of 2 years. Of those who developed MS, the degree of disability at 14 years, as measured by the Expanded Disability Status Scale (EDSS) *(13)*, correlated with the increase in lesion volume from onset to 5 years but not the increase in lesion volume from 5 to 14 years. This suggests that disease activity early in the course of MS, within the first 5 years, may have significant prognostic implication. A higher level of early disease activity, as measured by the degree of accumulation of new lesions, may be more damaging to the brain than a similar accumulation of lesions later in the course of the disease.

An international panel on MS diagnosis has published new diagnostic criteria for MS, popularly referred to as the McDonald criteria *(6)*. These new diagnostic criteria have largely replaced the previous MS diagnostic criteria published by Poser and colleagues 20 years ago *(9)*, although the new recommendations have retained the requirement of disease dissemination in time and space. However, the new criteria incorporate paraclinical tools, primarily MRI, to facilitate the diagnosis of MS for patients presenting with CIS suggestive of MS. In addition to a second clinical attack in a different location in the CNS, the McDonald criteria also allow the presence of new lesions on T2 or gadolinium (Gd)-enhanced T1 images 6 or 3 months after onset, respectively, to confirm dissemination in time and space.

Tintore and colleagues *(14)* examined the usefulness of the McDonald criteria in 139 patients with CIS. All patients underwent a brain MRI within 3 months of their attack and again 12 months later. After 12 months, 11% had developed CDMS according to the Poser criteria, compared to 37% with the McDonald criteria. Of the 37%, 80% experienced a second attack within a mean follow-up of 49 months. The new criteria showed a sensitivity of 74% and a specificity of 86% in predicting conversion to CDMS. Dalton and associates *(15)* reported similar findings in 80 patients presenting with CIS. Another study *(12)* demonstrated that 80% of patients presenting with CIS and MRI lesions go on to develop CDMS. Filippi and colleagues *(16)* also found that the presence of multiple T2-weighted lesions on brain MRI scans in patients are highly predictive of progression to clinically definite MS.

The McDonald criteria allow for diagnosis of MS to be made before the patient experiences a second clinical attack, with significant practical implications. Most importantly, we can now identify patients after their first clinical attack by use of MRI methods and predict the likelihood that they will develop CDMS with a reasonably high degree of sensitivity and specificity. This raises the issue of initiating treatment early in these so-called "high-risk" patients, as discussed in this chapter. Further advances in the early diagnosis of MS will sharpen the urgency of making these therapeutic decisions. For example, in a recent study, 103 patients with CIS were evaluated for the presence of anti-myelin basic protein (MBP) and anti-myelin oligodendrocyte glycoprotein (MOG) antibodies *(17)*. Of the 39 patients with no such antibodies, only 9 (23%) had a relapse, in a mean time of 45 months, whereas 21 of 22 (95%) with antibodies to both MBP and MOG relapsed in an average of 7.5 months. The rest of the patients had only anti-MOG antibodies, and 35 of 42 (83%) of them had relapses in 14.6 months. This interesting pilot study implies that serologic tests may be developed to detect MS at early stages of the disease *(18)*.

EVIDENCE BASED ON HISTOPATHOLOGICAL DATA

Irreversible axonal damage in MS has been recognized for more than a century *(19)*. However, only recently has it been eloquently shown with modern histopatho-

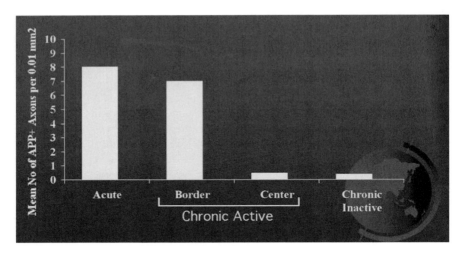

Fig. 1. Axonal transection in acute MS lesions as measured by the area density of amyloid precursor protein (APP)-positive axons.

logical techniques. Two studies revived the concept of axonal damage as a consequence of inflammation occurring during episodes of acute inflammation that may occur even in the early stages of the disease course in MS *(20,21)*. Ferguson and colleagues *(20)* studied 18 MS brains and examined 19 lesions of varying ages. Lesions were evaluated for the presence of amyloid precursor protein (APP), a sensitive marker of axonal damage. They found a high number of APP-positive axons in acute lesions and the edges of chronic active lesions (Fig. 1). Trapp and colleagues *(21)* studied 47 lesions from 11 patients with MS and a disease duration ranging from 2 weeks to 26 years. Using immunohistochemistry and confocal microscopy, they found transected axons to be a consistent feature throughout active lesions, with an average density of 11,236 per mm^3 (Fig. 2).

The presence of axonal transection in patients with a short disease duration implies that axonal transection occurs in MS lesions at an early stage of the disease. These two studies in particular led MS experts to reconsider their approach to treating MS, especially because of the availability of effective and relatively safe DMT. With compelling histopathological data demonstrating irreversible axonal damage early on in MS, the early initiation of antiinflammatory DMT renders itself to be a logical therapeutic approach.

EVIDENCE BASED ON MAGNETIC RESONANCE IMAGING DATA

There has been considerable work examining the severity and extent of brain tissue damage in MS using MRI. Most studies have focused well-established cohorts of patients with MS with considerable disease activity or disability.

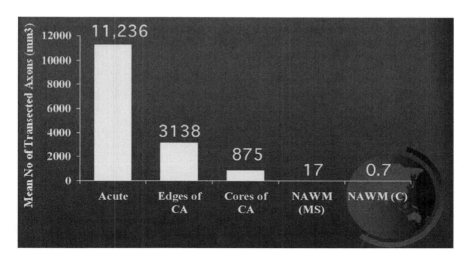

Fig. 2. Axonal transection as measured by confocal microscopy of axonal retraction balls, detected by immunohistochemical staining.

However, more recently much interest has been placed on disease pathology in early MS. MRI studies in MS have shown demyelination and axonal injury in patients with relatively mild disease of short duration. Newer techniques for measuring MS pathology with MRI, including MR spectroscopy and magnetization transfer ratio, have also identified destructive tissue pathology in the early stages of RRMS *(22–25)*.

Rudick and colleagues *(22)* examined brain parenchymal fraction (BPF) in patients with RRMS who had minimal disability and short disease duration and compared them with healthy controls *(22)*. The BPF is the fraction of intracranial volume occupied by brain parenchyma only (i.e., brain parenchyma volume divided by whole-brain volume). They found that, on average, the patients with MS had a BPF that was 2 to 3 standard deviations below the level seen in healthy controls. Chard et al. *(26)* studied brain atrophy in patients in the stage of MS having minimal disability, with a mean EDSS of 1.0 and mean disease duration of 1.8 years. Three-dimensional fast-spoiled gradient recall images were obtained and segmented into gray and white matter, in addition to measuring whole-brain volumes. Patients with MS were compared to 27 normal matched controls. Significant brain atrophy affecting both gray and white matter was seen in the MS patients, suggesting that destructive disease pathology may occur even at an early stage of the disease.

Magnetic resonance spectroscopy (MRS) enables the study of in vivo tissue metabolites that represent axonal integrity. *N*-acetylaspartate (NAA) has been widely evaluated as a marker of neuronal and axonal viability in MR spectroscopic studies. These studies have consistently shown decreased NAA levels and NAA to creatine (Cr) ratios (NAA/Cr) in MS lesions, as well as in the normal-appearing white matter (NAWM) of patients with MS *(27–30)*. In a study by De Stefano and

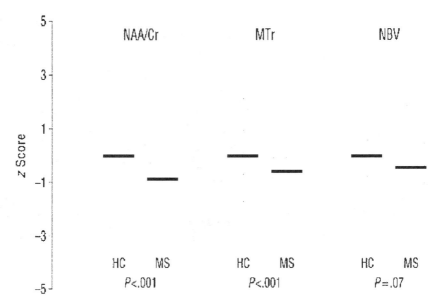

Fig. 3. Comparison of *N*-acetyl-aspartate to creatinine ratio (NAA/Cr), magnetization transfer ratio (MTr), and normalized brain volume (NBV) between healthy controls (HC) and patients with MS. NAA/Cr and MTr values are significantly reduced in patients with MS.

colleagues *(25)*, 60 patients with RRMS, a median disease duration of 2.7 years, and an EDSS score of <2 underwent combined MRIs/MRSs, including magnetization transfer ratios (MTR) and brain volume measurements. They compared these values with those of healthy controls. The patients with MS demonstrated significantly lower NAA/Cr ratios and reduced MTR levels. Brain volume was also decreased (Fig. 3). Subanalysis of patients with a disease duration of <3 years ($n = 36$) and a T2 lesion load <2 cm^3 ($n = 26$) showed lower NAA/Cr, MTR values, and brain volumes than those of healthy controls. This study provided strong evidence of a destructive tissue process as shown by MRS, MTR, and measurements of brain volume in early and patients with minimally affected RRMS. The demographics of the patients in the De Stefano study have been compared to those in the pivotal trials demonstrating efficacy of DMT (Table 1). It is evident that patients with established RRMS participating in phase III trials had greater disability (mean EDSS) and disease duration than the cohort studied by De Stefano. Thus, it would be logical to assume that treatment of MS at an early stage should confer greater advantage to the patient than waiting for the disease to exhibit clinical evidence of disease activity (i.e., occurrence of relapses).

Whole-brain atrophy as measured by BPF, as well as atrophy of the corpus callosum, has previously been observed in relatively milder stages of RRMS *(22)*. Ranjeva and colleagues *(31)* studied the corpus callosum volume in patients with

Table 1
Baseline Demographics:
Phase III Pivotal Trials vs DeStefano Study

Phase III trials	Age	Disease duration	EDSS
Betaseron®	35.2	4.7	3.0
Avonex®	36.7	6.6	2.4
Copaxone®	34.6	7.3	2.7
Rebif®*	35.6	6.4	2.5
Stefano study	35.0	2.7	0–2

CIS suggestive of MS. Forty-six patients with CIS and 24 matched healthy controls underwent various techniques employing MRI, including MRS, MTR, and mean diffusivity (MD) to measure corpus callosum volume and tissue pathology. Decreased MTR and increased MD were consistently seen in patients with CIS, whereas no atrophy was observed, with no statistically significant difference in normalized brain volume between patients with MS and healthy controls. This pattern was seen even in the absence of lesions visible on conventional MRI. These findings suggested that diffuse structural and metabolic changes indicative of myelin pathology occur in the corpus callosum at the earliest stage of MS, even before any atrophy can be detected.

EVIDENCE BASED ON CLINICAL TRIALS IN CLINICALLY ISOLATED SYNDROMES AND MULTIPLE SCLEROSIS

Studies of treatment at the earliest clinical manifestations of MS are of special interest in understanding the stagewise response of the disease to DMTs (Table 2). In particular, the earliest clinical manifestations of MS present with the CIS of optic neuritis (ON), transverse myelopathy, and brainstem demyelinating lesions (typically, internuclear ophthalmoplegia). As discussed, patients with CIS with multiple (though silent) lesions on the MRI are at high risk of developing CSMS within the next few years. The MRI data have been so compelling as to force the incorporation of MRI criteria in the diagnostic criteria for MS, as discussed *(6)*.

Two double-blind, placebo-controlled trials of patients presenting with the first CNS demyelinating event and abnormal MRI scans have shown a benefit of initiating DMT *(32,33)*. In the multi-center Controlled High-Risk Subjects Avonex Multiple Sclerosis Prevention Study (CHAMPS), 383 patients were randomized to receive 30 μg intramusclular (IM) IFN-β-1a weekly vs placebo for 3 years. The primary endpoint was conversion to CDMS, as defined by the occurrence of a second attack. The study was halted at the time of an interim analysis, before its scheduled 3-year duration, when it was shown that treatment with IFN-β-1a significantly delayed time to second attack compared with placebo. The probability of developing CDMS was 50% in the placebo group vs 35% in the IFN-β group ($p = 0.002$). The Food and Drug Administration (FDA) has now approved the use of IFN-β-1a

Table 2
Summary of DMT Pivotal Trials in CIS, RRMS, and SPMS

Agent	Study (ref.)	Primary outcome	Primary outcome achieved		
			CIS	RRMS	SPMS
Interferon (IFN)-β-1a (Avonex)	Controlled High-Risk Subjects Avonex MS Prevention Study (CHAMPS) *(32)*	Second demyelinating event, defining clinically define multiple sclerosis (CDMS)	Yes		
IFN-β-1a (Rebif)	Early Treatment of MS (ETOMS) *(33)*	Second demyelinating event, defining CDMS	Yes		
Glatiramer acetate (Copaxone)	*(4)*	Proportion of patients relapse-free		Yes	
IFN-β-1b (Betaseron)	*(1)*	Rate of MS relapses		Yes	
IFN-β-1a (Avonex)	*(2)*	Accumulation of deficit, defined by Expanded Disability Status Scale (EDSS)		Yes	
Glatiramer acetate (Copaxone)	*(4)*	Rate of MS relapses		Yes	
IFN-β-1a (Rebif)	Pregnancy in Multiple Sclerosis Study (PRIMS) *(3)*	Rate of MS relapses		Yes	
Glatiramer acetate (Copaxone)		Time to confirmed progression			No
IFN-β-1a (Rebif)	SPECTRIMS *(40)*	Progression of deficit defined by EDSS			No
IFN-β-1b (Betaseron)	European Study Group secondary-progressive MS (SPMS) Study *(42)*	Progression of deficit defined by EDSS			Yes
IFN-β-1b (Betaseron)	North American Study Group SPMS Study *(39)*	Progression of deficit defined by EDSS			No
IFN-β-1a (Avonex)	IMPACT *(41)*	Progression of deficit defined by Multiple Sclerosis Functional Composite (MSFC), a composite index			Yes (No effect on EDSS)

given at a dose of 30 µg IM weekly after the first demyelinating episode in patients with CIS suggestive of MS. The Early Treatment of MS (ETOMS) study used an identical primary endpoint in study patients with a first demyelinating event. Investigators randomized 309 patients to receive 22 µg SC IFN-β-1a weekly or placebo for 2 years. Compared with placebo, treatment with IFN-β-1a resulted in fewer patients converting to CDMS (34% vs 45%) ($p = 0.047$).

In one of the earlier trials of GA, 50 patients with RRMS were randomized to either GA 20 mg SC daily for 2 years or placebo, with a primary endpoint of proportion of patients who were exacerbation-free during the course of the trial *(34)*. The results were that 56% of patients in the active treatment arm were exacerbation-free, whereas only 26% of the placebo group had no exacerbations ($p = 0.045$). Interestingly, in a posthoc analysis comparing patients with mild disease (EDSS = 0–2) to those with more severe disease (EDSS = 3–6), there was a much greater reduction in relapse count in the milder patients than the more disabled ones. These results suggest that pharmacologic intervention early in the course of the disease may be more efficacious in the prevention of accumulation of deficit than such intervention later in the disease course, when there is already fixed deficit or after the onset of secondary progression.

Can the initiation of DMT be delayed with no loss of benefit to a patient with CDMS? A reasonable way to test this would be to continue a trial in which patients in a placebo arm are rerandomized to an active treatment arm and followed carefully. Two such studies have been done.

In the first study, a continuation of the PRISMS trial, in which patients with RRMS were randomized to 1 of 3 arms, placebo, 22 µg and 44 µg of IFN-β-1a SC 3 times a week (tiw), patients in the placebo arm were rerandomized, at 2 years, to one of the active IFN-β-1a arms, and followed for another 2 years *(35)*. At the 4-year time point, the high-dose 44 µg tiw group statistically had significantly less progression of disability (defined as an increase of EDSS by at least one step, sustained for at least 3 months) than either of the crossover groups, along with the lower dose 22 µg tiw group. There was also less accumulation of MRI burden of disease during the 4 years of the study in the high-dose 44 µg tiw group than the lower dose group or either of the crossover groups *(35)*.

In the second study, with the longest follow up among all MS treatment trials conducted to date, 251 patients with RRMS were randomized to GA or placebo. At the end of the randomized phase, 209 (83%) of the patients continued onto open-label GA and were followed for up to 10 years after the initial randomization. A total of 128 patients completed 10 total years on the study. Of these, 64 were originally randomized to GA and 69 to placebo, before the open-label phase. Most of the patients originally on GA had stable or improved EDSS scores, although the average EDSS increased by 0.9 points to 3.67. However, the relevant finding was that fewer patients in the GA-at-randomization group ($n = 50$) had progression during the entire study period than those in the placebo-at-randomization group ($n = 72$) ($p = 0.015$) *(36)*.

These studies highlight two significant findings. First, DMT early in the course of disease, at the first clinical attack, significantly delays the occurrence of a second attack, which would satisfy the criteria for CDMS. Second, early treatment results in significantly less progression in the disease than late treatment, and late treatment does not restore lost function *(37)*.

DMT IN SECONDARY PROGRESSIVE MULTIPLE SCLEROSIS

Although the efficacy of DMT in RRMS is firmly established *(1,3,4,32)*, results of studies examining the efficacy of DMT for patients with secondary-progressive MS (SPMS) have either been negative or shown only modest benefit at best *(38–42)* (Table 2).

In one of the first studies of GA, 106 patients with "chronic progressive MS," a mixture of patients with SPMS and primary-progressive MS (PPMS), were recruited at two centers (Albert Einstein College of Medicine, Bronx, NY, and Baylor College of Medicine, Houston, TX) and randomized to GA 20 mg SC every day for 2 years or placebo *(38)*. The primary outcome was time to progression (defined by a 1.0-step increase in EDSS for baseline EDSS > 5 and a 1.5-step increase in EDSS for baseline EDSS <5) sustained for 3 months. There was no difference in outcome between the 2 groups for the 2 years.

In the SPECTRIMS study, 618 patients with SPMS were randomized to 1 of 3 arms: placebo, IFN-β-1a 22 or 44 µg subcutaneously tiw for 3 years. The primary outcome was time to confirmed progression of disability (defined by an increase in EDSS by one point if baseline EDSS <5.5 and by 0.5 point if baseline EDSS >5.5, sustained for 3 months). The primary outcome was not different between the patients in the three arms, although there was a hint of efficacy in a posthoc subgroup analysis favoring patients with prestudy relapses compared to patients without *(40)*.

In the North American Study Group on Interferon β-1b in Secondary Progressive MS study, 939 patients with SPMS were randomized to placebo or IFN-β-1b 5 MIU or 8 MIU/m^2 of body surface area, subcutaneously every other day, for 3 years, with a primary outcome of disease progression defined by a 1.0 point increase in EDSS (or 0.5-point increase if baseline EDSS >6.0). There was no difference on the primary outcome variable between the arms of the study *(39)*.

However, another study of IFN-β-1b showed a positive effect on SPMS, again using the conventional measure of disability, the EDSS, as a primary endpoint. In the European Study Group SPMS study, 718 patients with SPMS with baseline EDSS between 3.0 and 6.5 were randomized to placebo or IFN-β-1b 8 MIU SC every other day for 2 years, with a primary outcome of a 1.0-point increase in EDSS sustained for 3 months (or a 0.5-point increase for baseline EDSS of 6.0 or 6.5). The study found that the drug delayed progression by 9 to 12 months ($p = 0.0008$) during a study period of 2 to 3 years *(42)*. Although the study design and patient populations were similar to the North American SPMS study, there were differences. Subjects in the European SPMS study had more recent relapses than subjects in the North American SPMS study *(43)*. It is interesting that a posthoc analysis of the subjects in the SPECTRIMS trial also showed a hint of efficacy in those SPMS patients with prestudy relapses (*see* above).

CAMPATH-1H, a strong lymphocyte-depleting monoclonal antibody directed against CD52, was used to reduce MRI activity of disease in patients with SPMS. In this study, 25 patients with SPMS, baseline EDSS 4.0–6.0, were infused with CAMPATH-1H and followed clinically and with serial MRIs. Despite a profound decrease in the number and volume of Gd-enhancing lesions on MRI, disability progression continued in 50% of the patients. These patients also had increasing brain atrophy. The atrophy correlated with a decrease in the NAA signal on MRS, indicating that the atrophy most likely resulted from axonal degeneration *(44,45)*.

The effect of CAMPATH-1H may be quite different when used in an earlier stage of disease. In an open-label preliminary study of 22 patients with RRMS, there was a substantial decrease in relapse rate and virtual cessation of accumulation of disability *(46)*. Although these results were preliminary and in a small, selected group of patients, this may be an example of the dichotomy of the response of MS to therapy, depending on the stage of the disease, with earlier disease (RRMS) showing better response than later disease (SPMS).

Some studies found benefit in SPMS only by using sensitive outcomes. For example, the IMPACT study recruited 436 patients with SPMS and randomized them to either placebo or IFN-β-1a 60 μg IM once a week for 2 years. In this study, the primary outcome was change in the MS functional composite (MSFC), which consisted of a combination of measures of ambulation (timed gait), cognition (paced auditory serial addition test), and upper extremity function (nine-hole peg test), from baseline to 24 months. There was a modest but statistically significant effect on the composite score, largely driven by the "nine-hole peg test," but there was no effect on ambulatory ability (timed gait component of the MSFC) or EDSS *(41)*.

CONCLUSIONS

Recognizing the partial efficacy of available DMT in RRMS and modest benefit in SPMS, initiating therapy in patients considered at high risk of developing MS appears reasonable. Given the evidence discussed, one may argue that delaying DMT in this group of patients offers no advantage to the patient and may even be detrimental. However, longer follow-up in patients presenting with CIS and abnormal brain MRI scans is needed to unequivocally settle the issue of early treatment in MS.

REFERENCES

1. IFN-beta Study Group. Interferon beta-1b is effective in relapsing-remitting multiple sclerosis. I. Clinical results of a multicenter, randomized, placebo-controlled trial. Neurology, 1993;43: 655–661.
2. Jacobs L, Cookfair DL, Ruddick RA, et al. Intramuscular interferon beta-1a for disease progression in relapsing multiple sclerosis. Ann Neurol 1996;39:285–294.
3. The PRISMS Study Group. Randomized, double-blind, placebo-controlled study of interferon beta-1a in relapsing-remitting multiple sclerosis. Lancet, 1998;352:1498–1504.

4. Johnson K, Brooks BR, Cohen JA, et al. Copolymer 1 reduces relapse rate and improves disability in remitting-relapsing multiple sclerosis: results of a phase III multicenter, double-blind, placebo-controlled trial. Neurology 1995;45:1268–1276.

5. Hartung H, Gonsette R, Konig N, et al. Mitoxantrone in progressive multiple sclerosis: a placebo-controlled, double-blind, randomized multicentre trial. Lancet 2002;360:2018–2025.

6. McDonald W, Compston A, Edan G, et al. Recommended diagnostic criteria for multiple sclerosis: guidelines from the International Panel on the Diagnosis of Multiple Sclerosis. Ann Neurol 2001;50:121–127.

7. Trapp B, Ransohoff RM, Fischer E, et al. Neurodegeneration in multiple sclerosis: relationship to disability. Neuroscientist 1999;5:48–57.

8. Schumacher G, Beebe G, Kibler RF, et al. Problems of experimental trials of therapy in multiple sclerosis: report by the panel on the evaluation of experimental trials of therapy in multiple sclerosis. Ann N Y Acad Sci 1965;122:552–568.

9. Poser C, et al. New diagnostic criteria for multiple sclerosis: guidelines for research protocols. Ann Neurol 1983;13:227–231.

10. Morrisey S, Miller DH, Kendall BE, et al. The significance of brain magnetic resonance imaging abnormalities at presentation with clinically isolated syndromes suggestive of multiple sclerosis. A 5-year followup study. Brain 1993;116:135–146.

11. O'Riordan J, Thompson AJ, Kingsley DP, et al. The prognostic value of brain MRI in clinically isolated syndromes of the CNS. A 10-year followup. Brain 1998;121:495–503.

12. Brex P, Ciccarelli O, O'Riordan JI, Sailer M, Thompson AJ, Miller DH. A longitudinal study of abnormalities on MRI and disability from multiple sclerosis. N Engl J Med 2002;346:158–164.

13. Kurtzke J. Rating neurologic impairment in multiple sclerosis: an expanded disability status scale (EDSS). Neurology 1983;33:1444–1452.

14. Tintore M, et al. New diagnostic criteria for multiple sclerosis: application in first demyelinating episode. Neurology 2003;60:27–30.

15. Dalton C, et al. Application of the new McDonald criteria to patients with clinically isolated syndromes suggestive of multiple sclerosis. Ann Neurol 2002;52:47–53.

16. Filippi M, Horsfield MA, Morrissey SP, et al. Quantitative brain MRI lesion load predicts the course of clinically isolated syndromes suggestive of multiple sclerosis. Neurology 1994;44: 635–641.

17. Berger T, et al. Antimyelin antibodies as a predictor of clinically definite multiple sclerosis after a first demyelinating event. N Engl J Med 2003;349:139–145.

18. Antel J, Bar-Or A. Do myelin-directed antibodies predict multiple sclerosis? N Engl J Med 2003;349:107–109.

19. Charcot M. Histologie de la sclerose en plaques. Gazette Hospitaux 1868;141:554–558.

20. Ferguson B, Matyszak MK, Esiri MM, Perry VH. Axonal damage in acute multiple sclerosis lesions. Brain 1997;120:393–399.

21. Trapp B, Peterson J, Ransohoff RM, Rudick R, Mork S, Bo L. Axonal transection in the lesions of multiple sclerosis. N Engl J Med 1998;338:278–285.

22. Rudick R, Fisher E, Lee JC, Simon J. Use of the brain parenchymal fraction to measure whole brain atrophy in relapsing-remitting MS. Neurology 1999;53:1698–1704.

23. Arnold D, Shoubridge EA, Villemure JG, Feindel W. Proton magnetic resonance spectroscopy of human brain in vivo in the evaluation of multiple sclerosis: assessment of the load of the disease. Magn Reson Med 1990;14:154–159.

24. Sarchielli P, Presciutti O, Peiliccioli GP, et al. Absolute quantification of brain metabolites by proton magnetic resonance spectroscopy in normal-appearing white matter of multiple sclerosis patients. Brain 1999;122:513–521.

25. De Stefano N, Narayanan S, Francis SJ, et al. Diffuse axonal and tissue injury in patients with multiple sclerosis with low cerebral lesion load and no disability. Arch Neurol 2002;59:26. Chard D, et al. Brain atrophy in clinically early relapsing-remitting multiple sclerosis. Brain 2002;125:327–337.

27. De Stefano N, Matthews PM, Antel JP, Preul M, Francis G, Arnold DL. Chemical pathology of acute demyelinating lesions and its correlation with disability. Ann Neurol 1995;38:901–909.

28. Narayana P, Doyle TJ, Lai D, Wolinsky JS. Serial proton magnetic resonance spectroscopic imaging, contrast-enhanced magnetic resonance imaging, and quantitative lesion volumetry in multiple sclerosis. Ann Neurol 1998;43:56–71.

29. De Stefano N, Matthews PM, Fu L, et al. Axonal damage correlates with disability in patients with relapsing-remitting multiple sclerosis: results of a longitudinal magnetic resonance spectroscopy study. Brain 1998;121:1469–1477.

30. Matthews P, DeStefano N, Narayanan S, et al. Putting magnetic resonance spectroscopy studies in context: axonal damage and disability in multiple sclerosis. Semin Neurol 1998;18:327–336.

31. Ranjeva J, Pelletier J, Confort-Gouny S, et al. MRI/MRS of corpus callosum in patients with clinically isolated syndrome suggestive of multiple sclerosis. Mult Scler 2003;9:554–565.

32. Jacobs L, Beck RW, Simon JH, et al. Intramuscular interferon beta-1a therapy initiated during a first demyelinating event in multiple sclerosis. N Engl J Med 2000;343:898–904.

33. Comi G, Fillippi M, Barkhof F, et al. Effect of early interferon treatment on conversion to definite multiple sclerosis: a randomised study. Lancet 2001;357:1576–1582.

34. Bornstein M, Miller A, Slagle S, et al. A pilot trial of Cop-1 in exacerbating-remitting multiple sclerosis. N Engl J Med 1987;317:408–414.

35. The PRISMS4 Study Group, PRISMS4: Long-term efficacy of interferon beta-1a in relapsing MS. Neurology 2001; 56:1628–1636.

36. Ford C, et al. Sustained efficacy and tolerability of Copaxone (glatiramer acetate) in relapsing-remitting multiple sclerosis patients treated for over 10 years. Mult Scler 2003;9(Suppl 2):S120.

37. Schwid S, Bever CJ. The cost of delaying treatment in multiple sclerosis. What is lost is not regained. Neurology 2001;56:1620.

38. Bornstein M, Miller A, Slagle S, et al. A placebo-controlled, double-blind, randomized, two-center, pilot trial of Cop1 in chronic progressive multiple sclerosis. Neurology 1991;41:533–539.

39. Goodkin D, et al. North American Study Group on Interferon beta-1b in Secondary Progressive MS: clinical and MRI results of a 3-year randomized controlled trial. Neurology 2000;54:2352.

40. Secondary Progressive Efficacy Trial of Recombinant Interferon Beta-1b in MS (SPECTRIMS) Study Group. Randomized controlled trial of interferon beta-1a in secondary progressive MS. Neurology 2001;56:1496–1504.

41. Cohen J, Cutter G, Fischer J, et al. Benefit of interferon beta-1a on MSFC progression in secondary progressive MS. Neurology 2002;59:679–687.

42. European Study Group on Interferon beta-1b in Secondary Progressive MS. Placebo-controlled, multicentre, randomised trial of interferon beta-1b in treatment of secondary progressive multiple sclerosis. Lancet 1998;352:1491–1497.

43. McFarland H. Comparative analysis of the outcome of two phase III studies of interferon beta-1b. Neurology 2000;54:2352.

44. Coles A,Wing MG, Molyneux P, et al. Monoclonal antibody treatment exposes three mechanisms underlying the clinical course of multiple sclerosis. Ann Neurol 1999;46:296–304.

45. Paolillo A, Coles AJ, Molyneux PD, et al. Quantitative MRI in patients with secondary progressive MS treated with monoclonal antibody CAMPATH-1H. Neurology 1999;53:751–757.

46. Coles A, Deans J, Compston A. Campath-1H treatment of multiple sclerosis. Neurology 2003;60:A168–A169.

47. NMSS. National Multiple Sclerosis Society Compendium: Early Treatment Part I. Consensus Statement NMSS. Disease Management Consensus Statement. 1998.

8

Pregnancy and Multiple Sclerosis

Christina Caon, MSN, RN

INTRODUCTION

Numerous autoimmune diseases affect women during their reproductive years, including multiple sclerosis (MS), rheumatoid arthritis, systemic lupus erythematosus, myasthenia gravis, and Sjögren's syndrome *(1–3)*. Most autoimmune diseases become clinically silent or are pushed into so-called "remission" during pregnancy *(4)*. Pregnancy poses a challenge for the immune system because the fetus is essentially an allograft harboring antigens from the father. In response, pregnancy induces immune deviation in the mother, protective to the fetus, and, at the same time, alters autoimmune responses to the benefit of the pregnant woman. Studies examining disease course support the protective effect of pregnancy in the context of autoimmune diseases.

IMMUNOLOGICAL PROFILE OF MULTIPLE SCLEROSIS DURING PREGNANCY

MS is widely believed to be a T-cell-mediated autoimmune disease directed against myelin antigens in the central nervous system (CNS) *(5)*. Although the precise cause and antigens have not been identified, several are candidates in MS. It is also believed that other factors, including genetic susceptibility, exposure to infectious agents, and environmental factors, may interact and render a person susceptible to developing the disease.

Given the autoimmune nature of MS and its predominant occurrence in young women, investigators have started to examine the effect of pregnancy on the immunological profile. T-helper (Th) lymphocytes are classified into Th1 (proinflammatory) and Th2 (antiinflammatory) cell types based on the type of cytokines they secrete *(2)*. Th1 cytokines include interleukin (IL)-1, -2, and -12; tumor necrosis factor (TNF)-α, and interferon (IFN)-γ, whereas Th2 cytokines include IL-4, -5, -6, and -10 *(6)*. This highly simplified view of Th1 and Th2 responses is the focus of several therapeutic strategies in autoimmune diseases, including MS. Currently

From: *Current Clinical Neurology: Multiple Sclerosis*
Edited by: M. J. Olek © Humana Press Inc., Totowa, NJ

available therapies in MS and numerous therapies that are under investigation are targeted at inducing Th2 responses, diminishing Th1 responses, or both *(7)*.

Studies have shown that the immunological profile in MS undergoes numerous distinct changes during pregnancy. Specifically, pregnancy creates a state of natural immunomodulation paralleling the therapeutic effect of currently available disease-modifying therapies (DMT). A protective effect of pregnancy in experimental autoimmune encephalomyelitis (EAE), a commonly studied animal model of MS, has been repeatedly demonstrated. Induction of EAE is diminished in pregnant guinea pigs, rabbits, and Lewis rats *(8–10)*. More specifically, late pregnancy suppresses disease activity in EAE. In one study, serum obtained from mice during late pregnancy decreased proliferative responses and diminished inflammatory Th1 cytokine production *(11)*. Others have shown an altered state of cytokine imbalance favoring Th2 responses during pregnancy *(12,13)*. In pregnancy, humoral immune responses are increased, whereas cellular-immune responses are decreased. Minimizing a strong cellular response against fetal antigens during pregnancy is critical in maintaining pregnancy. Administration of Th1 cytokines causes abortion in normal pregnant mice *(14)*. Moreover, a recent study showed that production of IL-12 and TNF-α was significantly reduced during late pregnancy *(15)*.

Several lines of evidence suggest that estrogens are important immunoregulators and that their relatively high levels during pregnancy promote the development of an antiinflammatory Th2 response *(16)*. After the first 4 weeks of pregnancy, virtually all estrogen production is driven from fetal trophoblast *(17)*. In late pregnancy, there is a disproportionate amount of estriol produced. This has been the focus of intense research as one of the factors conferring a protective effect of pregnancy in autoimmune diseases. In one study, estriol was compared to progesterone and placebo pellets in mice induced with EAE *(18)*. Estriol-treated mice showed reduced severity of EAE compared to no effect with progesterone. This led to a study in human nonpregnant patients with MS treated with 8 mg of orally administered estriol daily for 6 months *(19)*. Pretreatment observation for each patient was used as the control period. During estriol treatment, patients showed reduced relapse frequency, as well as brain magnetic resonance imaging (MRI) lesions. Blood obtained from patients receiving 8 mg of daily estriol showed a distinct deviation toward a Th2 response. Endometrial biopsies showed no evidence of hyperplasia or abnormal menstrual bleeding, suggesting the safety of this therapeutic approach in MS. These preliminary observations warrant a large multicenter, placebo-controlled study to further explore the therapeutic effect of oral estriol in relapsing-remitting MS (RRMS).

Progesterone and prolactin have also been studied as potential immunoregulators during pregnancy. In the presence of progesterone, lymphocytes from pregnant women produce a protein factor capable of inhibiting Th1 cytokine production and stimulating a Th2 shift *(20)*. In contrast, prolactin induces humoral- and cell-mediated immune responses, and its increased secretion during lactation (postpartum) may potentially render women with MS to a higher relapse rate *(21)*.

DISEASE COURSE DURING PREGNANCY

That young women of child-bearing potential are at highest risk for the development of MS has drawn much interest and debate. These patients with MS are often faced with difficult decisions regarding pregnancy and parenthood. Numerous studies have examined the clinical course of MS during pregnancy (Table 1). However, there is a lack of large well-designed studies examining the effect of pregnancy on MS. Furthermore, pregnancy studies in MS are likely to be biased because women with high disease activity and frequent relapses are expected to avoid pregnancy. Until 1990, virtually all studies reported were retrospective. Nevertheless, the majority of studies reported the relapse rate to decrease during pregnancy and increase during the postpartum period. In 1990, the first prospective study by Birk et al. *(22)* was reported, which confirmed previously published retrospective observations. The authors studied eight women and followed them for up to 6 months after delivery. The annualized relapse rate during pregnancy decreased to 0.17 and increased to 1.74 during the 6-month postpartum period with an 18-fold increase in the relapse rate in the first 3 months after delivery. Autoreactive T-lymphocytes were significantly decreased in pregnant women with MS compared to nonpregnant women with MS. Although the study was small, the authors noted no complications as a result of epidural anesthesia or breast-feeding. Sadovnick and colleagues *(23)* observed the relapse rate in 53 women with MS during pregnancy and up to 6 months after delivery. The relapse rate during pregnancy was compared to the prepregnancy annual relapse rate (self-control), as well as the annual relapse rate in 64 matched controls. Results of this study showed that the number of observed relapses during pregnancy was not significantly different when compared to the prepregnancy rate (self-controls). When compared to matched controls, the relapse rate was significantly lower ($p < 0.02$) only during the third trimester. After delivery there was an increase in the relapse rate; however, this was not significant when compared to either the self- or matched controls. The authors concluded that neither pregnancy (entire gestation period) nor the 6-month period after delivery increased the risk of relapses. The results were conflicting with other published reports, suggesting that pregnancy is associated with a decrease and puerperium with an increase in the relapse rate. Study methodology raised questions if the study was truly prospective and data missing from case controls may have affected the outcomes reported in this study *(24)*. In a longitudinal prospective study conducted by Roullet et al. *(25)*, 125 women with RRMS were followed for a mean duration of 10.3 years. During this time, 33 women became pregnant and 32 full-term pregnancies were observed. Women had been followed for at least 1 year at the clinic before pregnancy. Patients were used as their own controls and also compared to nonpregnant controls. Compared to prepregnancy baseline, there was no increase in the relapse rate during the entire pregnancy or any individual trimester. In contrast, when compared to control patients with MS, the relapse rate was lower during pregnancy (0.86 vs 0.54, $p = 0.07$). During the first 3 months after delivery, the relapse rate increased compared to baseline (1.62 vs 0.51, $p = 0.05$). During the next 3

Table 1
Summary of Studies Examining the Relapse Rate of Patients With Multiple Sclerosis During Pregnancy

Published study	Type of study	Number of live births (N)	Control group	Relapse rate prepregnancy	Relapse rate during pregnancy	Relapse rate 6 months postpartum
Confavreux et al., 1998	P	227	Nonpregnant self	0.70	0.43	1.05
Worthington et al., 1994	P	15	Nonpregnant self	0.57	0.48	1.1
Sadovnick et al., 1994	P	58	Nonpregnant self	0.63	0.57	0.93
		42	Matched controls	0.82	0.57	0.95
Roullet et al, 1993	P	32	Nonpregnant self	0.51	0.79	1.06
Bernardi et al, 1991	R-questionnaire	66	Nonpregnant self	0.65	0.1	0.79
Birk et al., 1990	P	8	Anticipated relapse rate	0.66	0.17	1.74
Frith & McLeod, 1988	R-interview	85	Nonpregnant self	0.53	0.3	0.99

Abbr: P, prospective; R, retrospective.

months, the relapse rate returned to the baseline level (0.46 vs 0.51). The authors also noted that relapses were generally mild or moderate during pregnancy in contrast to the postpartum period when relapses were more severe. Neurologic disability did not increase during follow-up after pregnancy. Another prospective observation reported the effect of pregnancy on the relapse rate in 52 patients with RRMS who had 66 pregnancies during an 8-year period *(26)*. Compared to baseline, the relapse rate during pregnancy decreased significantly (0.65 vs 0.10, $p < 0.01$). Interestingly, a rebound effect was observed in this study. There were no relapses observed during the last trimester of pregnancy in contrast to the puerperium where a relapse rate of 0.79 was observed.

Worthington et al. *(27)* also examined the relationship between pregnancy and MS in a prospective fashion. They compared the relapse rate in 15 women who became pregnant to 22 matched controls for up to 3 years after pregnancy. The relapse rate showed a decrease from 0.57 before pregnancy to 0.48 during pregnancy. During the postpartum period, there was a significant increase in the number of relapses in the first 6 months ($p < 0.02$), with 75% of the relapses occurring in the first 3 months after delivery. However, at the end of the 3-year follow-up period after pregnancy, the annual relapse rate was 0.50 and similar to prepregnancy relapse rate (0.50 vs 0.57, $p = NS$). Relapses occurring during the 6 months postpartum were more severe than those during or before pregnancy. However, compared to matched controls, there was no significant difference between the relapse rates (0.50 vs 0.48), the severity of relapses, or in neurologic disability at 3 years after pregnancy.

The Pregnancy in Multiple Sclerosis Study (PRIMS) was the most comprehensive study to date examining the effect of pregnancy on MS disease activity *(28)*. The PRIMS study was a multicenter prospective study in which 254 women from 12 centers in Europe participated. A total of 269 pregnancies were observed, and participants were followed for up to 12 months after delivery. Full data on pregnancy and delivery were available for 256 pregnancies in 241 women. The relapse rate during each trimester of pregnancy and 1 year after delivery were compared to the baseline relapse rate during the year before pregnancy (self-control). Compared to the baseline relapse rate of 0.7, there was a slight decrease in the relapse rate during the first and second trimesters (0.5 and 0.6, $p = 0.03$ and $p = 0.17$, respectively). However, in the third trimester, the relapse rate was reduced to 0.2 (0.2 vs 0.7, $p < 0.001$). The relapse rate during the first 3 months after delivery increased significantly to 1.2 (1.2 vs 0.7, $p < 0.001$) and returned to prepregnancy baseline level 12 months after delivery (0.6 vs 0.7, $p = 0.59$). Forty-two women received epidural analgesia during labor, which was not associated with an increased risk of a relapse during puerperium. Women who breast-fed ($n = 122$) had a significantly lower relapse rate compared to women who did not ($p = 0.02$). Neurologic disability assessed at 36 weeks of pregnancy and at 3, 6, and 12 months after delivery showed mild worsening. The use of epidural analgesia or breast-feeding did not correlate with increased disability. This study confirmed previously published observations on the effect of pregnancy on MS and provided clinicians and patients with reassuring information. Women with MS who are contemplating pregnancy may be informed that conception, gestation, epidural analgesia, and breast-feeding are not likely to alter the natural history of the disease.

A unique study in which serial brain MRI scans were performed in pregnant women with MS showed that MRI activity, including new and enlarging lesions, decreased during pregnancy *(29)*. Two patients participating in a monthly brain MRI protocol became pregnant and were imaged during and after pregnancy. Both patients demonstrated a significant decrease in the number of lesions during pregnancy, with no active lesions seen during the third trimester. During postpartum, both patients exhibited several new lesions. Although the study had only two patients, serial brain MRI scans supported the clinical evidence from other prospective studies showing the protective effect of pregnancy on MS, particularly during the third trimester.

In conclusion, most observations, both prospective and retrospective, indicate a reduction in the relapse rate during pregnancy, particularly during the third trimester. This is followed by an increased risk of a relapse during the postpartum period, especially in the first 3 months after delivery. Overall, pregnancy does not seem to affect the long-term course of MS.

DISEASE MANAGEMENT DURING PREGNANCY

Management of Pregnancy

Prepregnancy Counseling

Three important aspects of prepregnancy counseling for patients with MS need consideration. First, couples contemplating pregnancy may need counseling regarding the effect of pregnancy on MS and vice versa. Second, potential parents often face the anxiety of "transmitting the disease" to the newborn and are eager to learn about the chances of the baby developing MS. It is important to note that there are no prenatal tests or amniotic fluid tests for MS. There is a well-defined genetic predisposition, and the incidence of familial MS is estimated to be 10% to 15% *(30)*. In general, if one parent has MS, the lifetime risk of a child developing MS is between 3 and 5%, compared with the general population of 0.5% *(31)*. However, there are no well-defined modes of transmission associated with MS (i.e., autosomal dominant or recessive). The third aspect of preconception counseling involves fertility and the ability to conceive. MS has no known physiologic effect on fertility, and retrospective studies have shown that MS does not increase the risk of ectopic pregnancies *(32)*, spontaneous abortions *(33)*, or stillbirths when compared to the general population. However, sexual dysfunction may occur in 50 to 90% of patients *(34)*. Psychological stress associated with sexual dysfunction may be challenging to treat if it impairs the ability to conceive. Sexual dysfunction can occur in males or females with MS and includes difficulties such as erectile dysfunction, vaginal dryness, bladder and bowel incontinence, or positional difficulties. In one study, more than 70% of the patients reported improved relationship with their partner after discussing sexuality related issues with the healthcare professional *(35)*. If the issues surrounding sexual dysfunction have been addressed and the couple continues to have difficulties conceiving, fertility may have to be assessed by fertility disorder specialists. Although no large well-designed studies have been conducted to examine the effect of fertility-enhancing medications on disease activity in MS, one study did report an increased relapse rate in three women who used clomiphene citrate, a commonly used fertility-enhancing drug *(36)*. Finally, patients who were previously treated with immunosuppressive agents for MS may have prolonged periods of amenorrhea and infertility *(37)*. Although patients who receive intense immunosuppressive and chemotherapy agents have clinically aggressive disease and are more likely to avoid pregnancy, potential infertility as a result of these interventions should be carefully discussed.

Obstetrical Care

Prenatal care of patients with MS should not differ from that of women who do not have MS *(38)*. Women with MS may experience aggravation of their bowel and bladder symptoms during pregnancy. This may warrant close monitoring of urinary tract infections. Mueller et al. studied pregnancy-related complications in 198 women with MS and found that they were no more likely to have pregnancy or delivery complications than more than 1500 women without MS observed for 2 years after delivery *(39)*. However, they did note a possible increased risk of maternal anemia. With respect to infants, there was no difference in the incidence of low birth weight, congenital malformations, or higher infant mortality rates in the two groups. Patients with relatively greater neurologic disability at the time of pregnancy or unexpected disease activity during pregnancy may require special care, including a multidisciplinary approach involving the obstetrician and the neurologist. More specifically, preexisting motor deficits and increased fatigue may cause difficulty during labor and require assisted delivery *(38)*. Overall, there is no evidence to suggest that pregnant women with MS should be considered "high-risk pregnancy" simply because of the diagnosis of MS. High risk should be based primarily on obstetrical status or in the event of neurologic worsening.

Delivery and Anesthesia

The method of delivery should be determined by the obstetrician as deemed appropriate. Caesarean section should not be considered as the preferred route of delivery in patients with MS unless clinically indicated *(40)*. Similarly, there is no conclusive evidence contraindicating the use of anesthesia for delivery in patients with MS. The use of epidural anesthesia in patients with MS has been the focus of much debate. Two studies have suggested that spinal anesthesia may increase the risk of relapses *(41,42)*. However, others have not found epidural or other forms of anesthesia to increase the risk of relapses *(28,43,44)*. A modest association between an increase in the relapse rate and the use of bupivacaine regional blockade given at concentrations higher than 0.25% for a prolonged period was reported in one study

(45). However, there was no increased risk observed with epidural anesthesia. These findings were confirmed in the PRIMS study *(28)*. Currently, there is little evidence to support an association between either epidural anesthesia or regional blockade and increased risk of relapses. Larger well-designed studies are needed to provide conclusive information regarding the use of analgesia and anesthesia in MS during labor.

Management of Multiple Sclerosis During Pregnancy (Fig. 1)

The Food and Drug Administration (FDA) designates safety categories to drugs based on risk to fetus and overall safety during pregnancy (Table 2). There are five categories currently assigned by the FDA. These are discussed in descending order of safety.

- Category A: Controlled human studies have shown no fetal risks. This is the safest category.
- Category B: No controlled human studies are available. Animal studies show either no risk or minimal risk to the fetus.
- Category C: No human studies are available. Adverse fetal effects have been shown in animals.
- Category D: Evidence of human risk has been shown, but benefits may outweigh risks.
- Category X: Well-described and proven fetal risks have been shown. Use in pregnancy is contraindicated.

Treatment During Pregnancy

Relapses: Treatment of relapses should depend on a risk–benefit assessment. Relapses characterized by severe motor, cerebellar, or sensory deficits leading to gait ataxia should be considered for treatment because these deficits are more likely to cause injury to the mother and potentially harm the fetus. Intravenous (IV) methylprednisolone (IVMP) (category C) given at a dose of 1 g for 3 to 5 days is an appropriate first-choice treatment *(46)*. Cleft lip and palate have been associated with the use of IVMP during pregnancy, although the overall incidence is low *(47)*. Alternate treatment strategies include plasmapheresis; this is considered to be a safe alternative to IVMP for the treatment of relapses with virtually no risk to the fetus and can be used safely during breast-feeding *(48)*. It poses minimal risk to the mother, mostly related to shifts in fluid volume during pheresis *(49)*. Several investigators have also studied the effect of IV immunoglobulin (IVIg) (category C) as a preventive therapy for relapses in the postpartum period and found IVIg to be effective in preventing relapses during the immediate postpartum period *(50,51)*.

Disease-modifying therapies: Currently, two categories of DMT, β-(IFN) (category C) and glatiramer acetate (GA) (category B) are effective and are available for long-term use in the treatment of RRMS *(52)*. At this time, there is insufficient data to support elective or continuous use of DMT during pregnancy. Some reports have suggested that DMT, particularly glatiramer acetate, may be safe during pregnancy *(53,54)*. β-IFNs (category C) are abortifacient *(55)* and are best avoided during pregnancy. For couples contemplating pregnancy, it is generally

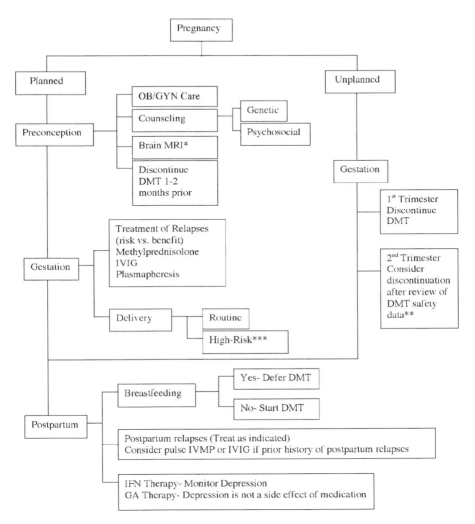

Fig. 1. Flow chart showing the management of multiple sclerosis in pregnancy. *Obtain brain MRI scan prior to conception in patients with clinically active disease. **GA is category B in pregnancy and may be used in some patients. IFNs can be abortifacient and should be discontinued. ***High risk delivery should be determined by obstetrical status. Worsening of neurologic disability may also place a patient at high risk.

recommended that DMT be discontinued at least one to two menstrual cycles before planned conception. It may be helpful to obtain a brain MRI scan before the decision to conceive, especially in patients with a history of clinically active disease. Brain MRI scans with multiple active lesions may predict relapses *(56)*. There-

Table 2
US Food and Drug Administration Categorization
of Medications Used in Multiple Sclerosis

Category B	Category C	Category D
Bupropion	Amitriptyline	Azathioprine
Glatiramer acetate	Avonex	Benzodiazepines
Loperamide	Baclofe	Carbamazepine
Sildenafil	Betaseron	Cyclophosphamide
Oxybutynin	Donepezil	Mitoxantrone
Pemoline	Fluoxetine	Phenytoin
	Gabapentin	
	IVIg	
	Methylprednisolone	
	Nortriptyline Paroxetine	
	Rebif	
	Sertraline	
	Symmetrel	
	Tizanidine	
	Venlafaxine	
	4-aminopyridine	

Notes: Category A: controlled human studies have shown no fetal risks; category B: no controlled human studies are available. Animal studies show either no risk or minimal risk to the fetus; category C: no human studies are available. Adverse fetal effects have been shown in animals; category D: evidence of human risk has been shown but benefits may outweigh risks; category X: well described and proved fetal risks have been shown. Use in pregnancy is contraindicated.

fore, in the presence of disease activity on a brain MRI scan or significant worsening of brain MRI lesions compared to a previous scan, it may be advisable to postpone pregnancy and repeat the brain MRI after a 6-month interval. Even more challenging for the clinician is the issue of unplanned pregnancy or if pregnancy is confirmed after the critical first trimester. Information on the risks and benefits of continuing therapy should be discussed with the patient so that an informed decision can be made. Although discontinuation of DMT in these circumstances is commonly practiced, one may consider elective use of DMT, particularly with Copaxone (category B), after the first trimester, given the safety profile of this agent. However, multicenter MS pregnancy registries may be the only practical method to examine the safety of DMT during pregnancy.

Postpartum Management

Management of MS in the postpartum period can be a challenge, given the responsibility of a newborn, along with the uncertainty about the disease. A multidisciplinary approach involving the neurologist, pediatrician, psychosocial counseling, and, most importantly, family support *(57)* may be needed in some instances. In one study, despite deciding to become pregnant, patients with MS perceived this decision as risky behavior *(58)*.

Depression

Depression is frequently encountered during postpartum *(59)* and is also well-recognized in MS *(60)*. Patients with a history of depression or "pregnancy blues" should be carefully monitored. Despite the joy of having a newborn, providing care to the infant can place enormous strain on the mother, the couple, and their resources. Patients with MS may be more susceptible to such stress and thus require closer monitoring. Up to 30% of patients with MS may be unable to provide adequate care for the infant because of disability *(61)*. This, in turn, may precipitate depression in addition to the higher risk of relapses making the postpartum period challenging and highly stressful necessitating the importance of a good family support system *(62)*. Finally, feeling depressed and stressed may need to be carefully distinguished from a true relapse to avoid unnecessary use of steroids. Antidepressants and counseling should be considered. IFN-β may precipitate or cause depression *(63)*. Its use during the postpartum period is not contraindicated but should be closely monitored.

Breast-Feeding

Breast-feeding is not contraindicated in patients with MS. Pregnant women may be concerned about transmitting the disease to the infant through breast-feeding *(64)*, which is not the case. Furthermore, there is no conclusive evidence to suggest that breast-feeding has a harmful effect on the disease course or precipitates exacerbations. Nelson et al. *(65)* conducted a study where 435 women were interviewed regarding breast-feeding and postpartum relapses. Information was collected on 191 pregnancies, and no significant difference in exacerbation rate was found between women who breast-fed and those who did not. In the PRIMS study, breast-feeding was associated with a lower risk of a relapse during the postpartum period *(28)*. A rare condition affecting vision, known as "lactation optic neuritis" (ON), has been reported in women during the postpartum period *(66)*. This should not deter patients to breast-feed but merely alert them to report symptoms for careful evaluation. Overall, patients who are contemplating breast-feeding may need to be advised regarding the use of medications during breast-feeding. DMT for MS may be secreted in the breast milk and therefore should not be prescribed during breast-feeding. However, history of clinically active disease or occurrence of relapses during postpartum may warrant immediate resumption of DMT. Breast-feeding should be avoided in these cases.

Treatment of Relapse

As discussed, the bulk of data indicate that there is an increase in the relapse rate during the postpartum period. Relapses should be treated with steroids if warranted. Higher doses of IVMP are generally the most efficient and fastest method to treat a relapse, although there is no consensus on the ideal dosing regimen of steroids. The use of an oral prednisone taper after high doses of IVMP makes no difference on neurologic outcome *(67)*. This is useful to know because prolonged use of steroids can lead to weight gain, mood irritability, and worsening of depression. Thus, eliminating unnecessary use of steroids during postpartum may be beneficial to the patient. In cases of caesarean section deliveries, treatment with high doses of IVMP may impair wound healing. Plasmapheresis remains as the only alternative to steroids for the treatment of a relapse, especially in steroid-resistant cases *(68)*. Currently, there is insufficient data to support the routine use of IVIg during postpartum to prevent relapses. Only patients at high risk of relapses during puerperium should be considered as a candidate for IVIg treatment. High risk may be arbitrarily defined as history of relapses after previous pregnancies or relapses during pregnancy. These decisions require careful consideration and should be made on a case-by-case basis until studies are performed that provide more conclusive data.

Resumption of Disease-Modifying Therapies

In general, resumption of treatment with DMT should occur soon after delivery if breast-feeding is not planned. Ideally, patients should resume the same DMT as before pregnancy. Treatment-naïve patients or newly diagnosed patients should be given information on all available DMTs to make an informed choice. Consideration should be given to two aspects regarding the use of DMT after delivery. First, all currently available DMT are injectable medications requiring self-administration by the patient. This may be somewhat trying for many patients during the postpartum period when they are already undergoing significant stress and strain. Thus, compliance with the injections and management of side effects should be given special attention. Second, patients need to be informed that DMT may not show immediate clinical benefits and their effect on reducing the relapse rate is generally observed after several months *(69–72)*. Therefore, one may still experience a relapse during therapy with DMT, especially in the first few months after initiating therapy. The purpose of DMT is to alter the long-term natural history of the disease and minimize ensuing disability. Consequently, the most important message delivered to the patient should emphasize that some form of DMT is better than none, which is a view strongly endorsed by the National Multiple Sclerosis Society (1998).

REFERENCES

1. Cutolo M, Sulli A, Seriolo B, Acardo S, Masi AT. Estrogens, the immune response and auotimmunity. Clin Exp Rheumatol 1995;13:217–226.
2. Geenen V, Perrier de Hauterive, Puit M, et al. Autoimmunity and pregnancy: theory and practice. Acta Clinica Beligica 2002;57:317–324.
3. Zurier RB. Pregnancy in patients with rheumatic diseases. Rheum Dis Clin North Am 1989; 2:193–405.
4. Buyon JP. The effect of pregnancy on autoimmune diseases. J Leukocyte Biol 1998;63:281–287.
5. Martin R, McFarland HF, McFarlin DE. Immunological aspects of demyelinating diseases. Annu Rev Immunol 1992;10:153–187.

6. Sharief K. Cytokines in multiple sclerosis: pro-inflammation or pro-remyelination? Mult Scler 1998;4:169–173.

7. Stuve O, Cree BC, Von Budingen HC, et al. Approved and future pharmacotherapy for multiple sclerosis. Neurology 2002;8:290–301.

8. Abramsky O. Pregnancy and multiple sclerosis. Ann Neurol 1994;36(Suppl):S38–S41.

9. Voskhul RR, Palaszynski K. Sex hormones and experimental autoimmune encephalomyelitis: implications for multiple sclerosis. Neuroscientist 2001;7:258–270.

10. Keith AB. The effect of pregnancy on experimental allergic encephalomyelitis in guinea pigs and rats. J Neuro Sci 1978;38:317.

11. Langer-Gould A, Hideki G, Slansky A, Ruitz PJ, Steinman L. Late pregnancy suppresses relapses in experimental autoimmune encephalomyelitis: evidence for a suppressive pregnancy-related serum factor. J Immunol 2002;169:1084–1091.

12. Wegmann T, Lin H, Guilbert L, Mosmann TR. Bidirectional cytokine interactions in maternal-fetal relationship: Is successful pregnancy a Th2 phenomenon? Immunol Today 1993;14:353.

13. Marzi M, Vigano D, Trabattoni D, et al. Characterization of type 1 and type 2 cytokine production profile in physiologic and pathologic human pregnancy. Clin Exp Immunol 1996;106:127.

14. Haynes MK, Smith JB. Can Th1 like immune response explain the immunopathology of recurrent spontaneous miscarriage? J Reprod Immunol 1997;35:65-71.

15. Elenkov IA, Wilder RL, Bakalov VK, et la. IL-12, TNF-α, hormonal changes during late pregnancy and early postpartum: implications for autoimmune disease activity during these times. J Clin Endocrinol Metab 2001;86:4933–4938.

16. Voskuhl R. Gender issues and multiple sclerosis. Curr Neurol Neurosci Reports 2002;2:277–286.

17. Draca S. Is pregnancy a model how we should control some autoimmune diseases. Autoimmunity 2002;35:307–312.

18. Sicotte NL, Liva SM, Klutch R, et al. Treatment of multiple sclerosis with the pregnancy hormone estriol. Ann Neurol 2002;52:421–428.

19. Kim S, Liva SM, Dalal MA, Verity MA, Voskuhl RR. Estriol ameliorates autoimmune demyelinating disease: implications for multiple sclerosis. Neurology 1999;52:1230–1238.

20. Szekeres-Bartho J, Wegmann TG. A progesterone dependent immunomodulatory protein alters Th1/Th2 balance. J Reproduc Immunol 1996;31:81–95.

21. Hartmann DP, Holaday JW, Bernton EW. Inhibition of lymphocyte proliferation by antibodies to prolactin. FASEB J 1989;3:2194–2202.

22. Birk K, Ford C, Smeltzer S, Ryan D, Miller R, Rudick, RA. The clinical course of multiple sclerosis during pregnancy and the puerperium. Arch Neurol 1990;47:738–742.

23. Sadovnick AD, Eisen K, Hashimoto SA, et al. Pregnancy and multiple sclerosis. Arch Neurol 1994;51:1120–1124.

24. Rudick RA, Sadovnick AD. Pregnancy and multiple sclerosis. Arch Neurol 1995;52:849–850.

25. Roullet E, Verdier-Taillefer MH, Amarenco P, et al. Pregnancy and multiple sclerosis: a longitudinal study of 125 remittent patients. J Neurol Neurosurg Psychiatry 1993;56:1062–1065.

26. Bernardi S, Grasso MG, Bertollini R, Orzi F, Fieschi C. The influence of pregnancy on relapses in multiple sclerosis: a cohort study. Acta Neurol Scand 1991;84:403–406.

27. Worthington J, Jones R, Crawford M, Forti A. Pregnancy and multiple sclerosis—a 3-year prospective study. J Neurol 1994;241:228–233.

28. Confavreux C, Hutchinson M, Hours MM, Cortinovis- Tourniaire P, Moreau T, PRIMS group. Rate of pregnancy-related relapse in multiple sclerosis. N Engl J Med 1998;339:285–291.

29. Van Walderveen MAA, Tas MW, Barkhof F, et al. Magnetic resonance evaluation of disease activity during pregnancy in multiple sclerosis. Neurology 1994;44:327–329.

30. Herrera BM, Ebers GC. Progress in deciphering the genetics of multiple sclerosis. Curr Opin Neurol 2003;16:253–258.

31. Ebers GC, Sadovnick AD. The role of genetic factors in multiple sclerosis susceptibility. J Neuroimmunol 1994;53:1–17.

32. Rubin GL, Peterson HB, Dorfman SF, et al. Ectopic pregnancy in the United States: 1970–1978. JAMA 1983;13:1725–1729.
33. Poland BJ, Miller JR, Harris M, Livingston J. Spontaneous abortion. A study of 1,961 women and their conceptuses. Acta Obstet Gynecol Scand 1981;102:1–32.
34. DasGupta R, Fowler CJ. Sexual and urological dysfunction in multiple sclerosis: better understanding and improved therapies. Curr Opin Neurol 2002;15:271–278.
35. Zorzon M, Zivadinov R, Bosco A, et al. Sexual dysfunction in multiple sclerosis: a case-control study. I. Frequency and comparison of groups. Mult Scler 1999;5:418–427.
36. Moreau T, Gere J, Vernay D, Clavelou P, Giroud M. Clomiphene citrate can increase relapse rate in mulitiple sclerosis. Mult Scler 2002;8(Supp 1):S85.
37. Sanders JE, Hawley J, Levy W, et al. Pregnancies following high-dose cyclophosphamide with or without high-dose busulfan or total-body irradiation and bone marrow transplantation. Blood 1996;84:3045–3052.
38. Davis RK, Maslow AS. Multiple sclerosis in pregnancy: a review. Obs Gyn Surv 1992;47:290–296.
39. Mueller BA, Zhang J, Critchlow CW. Birth outcomes and need for hospitalization after delivery among women with multiple sclerosis. Am J obstet Gynecol 2002;186:446–452.
40. Kaufman KE, Bailit JL, Grobman W. Elective induction: an analysis of economic and health consequences. Am J Obstet Gynecol 2002;187:853–863.
41. Stenuit J, Marchand P. Les sequelles de rachi-anaesthesie. Act Neurol Belg 1968;68:626–635.
42. Bamford C, Sibley W, Laguna J. Anaesthesia in multiple sclerosis. Can J Neurol Sci 1978;5:41–44.
43. Salvador M, Redin J, de Carlos J, Abad L. Esclerosis multiple y analgesia epidural obstetrica. Rev Esp Anestesiol Reanim 1997;44:33–35.
44. Crawford JS, James FM, Nolte H, Van Steenberg A, Shah JL. Regional analgesia for patients with chronic neurological disease and similar conditions. Anaesthesia 1981;36:821.
45. Bader AM, Hunt CO, Datta S, Naulty JS, Ostheimer GW. Anesthesisa for the obstetric patient with multiple sclerosis. J Clin Anesth 1988;1:21–23.
46. Martinez-Caceres EM, Carrau MA, Brieva L, Espejo C, Barbera N, Montalban X. Treatment with methylprednisolone in relapses of multiple sclerosis patients: immunological evidence of immediate and short-term but not long-lasting effects. Clin Exp Immunol 2002;127:165–171.
47. Kusanagi T. Dose-response relations of palatal slit, cleft palate, and fetal mortality in mice treated with a glucocorticoid. Teratology 1983;28:165–168.
48. Khatri BO, O'Neill D'Cruz, Prielser G, Hambrook G, Worthington D. Plasmapheresis in a pregnant patient with multiple sclerosis. Arch Neurol 1990;47:11–12.
49. Watson WJ, Datz VL, Bowes WA. Plamapheresis during pregnancy. Obstet Gynecol 1990;75:566–576.
50. Orvieto R, Achiron R, Rotstein Z, Noy S, Bar-Hava I, Achiron A. Pregnancy and multiple sclerosis: a 2-year experience. Eur J Obstet Gynecol Reprod Biol 1999;82:191–194.
51. Haas J. High dose IVIG in the post partum period for prevention of exacerbations in MS. Mult Scler 2000;6:S18–S20.
52. Khan O, Zabad R, Caon C, Zvartau-Hind M, Tselis A, Lisak R. Comparative assessment of immunomodulating therapies for relapsing-remitting multiple sclerosis. CNS Drugs 2002;16:563–574.
53. Caon C, Khan OA. Use of immunomodulating therapy (IMT) during pregnancy in patients with multiple sclerosis (MS). J Neurol 2001;248(Supp 3):86.
54. Coyle PK, Johnson K, Pardo L, Stark Y. Pregnancy outcomes in patients with multiple sclerosis treated with glatiramer acetate. Neurology 2003;60:A60.
55. Walther EU, Hohfeld R. Multiple sclerosis: side effects of interferon beta therapy and their management. Neurology 1999;53:1622–1627.
56. Thompson AJ, Miller D, Youl B, et al. Serial gadolinium-enhanced MRI in relapsing/remitting multiple sclerosis of varying disease duration. Neurology 1992;42:60–63.

57. Birk K, Kalb RC. Multiple sclerosis and planning a family: fertility, pregnancy, childbirth, and parenting roles. In: Kalb RC, ed., Multiple sclerosis: a guide for families. Demos Vermande, New York, 1998, pp. 61–71.
58. Smeltzer SC. Reproductive decision making in women with multiple sclerosis. J Neurosci Nurs 2002;34:145–156.
59. Beck CT. Postpartum depression predictors inventory. Adv Neonatal Care 2003;3:47–48.
60. Chwastiak L, Ehde DM, Gibbons LE, Sullivan M, Bowen JD, Kraft GH. Depressive symptoms and severity of illness in multiple sclerosis: epidemiologic study of a large community sample. Am J Psychiatry 2002;159:1862–1868.
61. Poser S, Poser W. Multiple sclerosis and gestation. Neurology 1983;33:1422–1427.
62. Boeije HR, Duijnstee MS, Grypdonck MH. Continuation of caregiving among partners who give total care to spouses with multiple sclerosis. Health Soc Care Community 2003;11:242–252.
63. Zephir H, De Seze J, Stojkovic T, et al. Multiple sclerosis and depression: influence of interferon beta therapy. Mult Scler 2003;9:284–288.
64. Mohrbacher N, Stock J. The Breastfeeding Answer Book. La Leche League International, Schamberg, IL, 1997.
65. Nelson LM, Franklin GM, Jones MC, Multiple Sclerosis Study Group. Risk of multiple sclerosis exacerbation during pregnancy and breast-feeding. JAMA 1988;259:3441–3443.
66. Retzloff MG, Kobylarz EJ, Eaton C. Optic neuritis with transient total blindness during lactation. Obstet Gynecol 2001;98:902–904.
67. Caon C, Ching W, Tselis AC, Lisak R, Khan O. Oral prednisone taper has no effect on neurologic recovery following intravenous methlprednisolone for the treatment of an MS relapse. Neurology 2003;60(Suppl 1):A477–A478.
68. Keegan M, Pineda AA, McClelland RL, Darby CH, Rodriguez M, Weinshenker BG. Plasma exchange for severe attacks of CNS demyelination: predictors of response. Neurology 2002;58:143–146.
69. Johnson KP, Brooks BR, Cohen JA, et al. Copolymer 1 reduces relapse rate and improves disability in relapsing-remitting multiple sclerosis: results of a phase III multicenter, double-blind, placebo-controlled trial. Neurology 1995;45:1268–1276.
70. The PRISMS Group. Randomised, double-blind, placebo-controlled study of interferon beta-1a in relapsing remitting multiple sclerosis. Lancet 1998;352:1498–1504.
71. The IFNB Study Group. Interferon beta-1b in the treatment of MS: final outcome of the randomized controlled trial. Neurology 1995;37:611–619.
72. Jacobs JD, Cookfair DL, Rudick RA, et al. Intramuscular interferon beta-1a for disease progression in relapsing multiple sclerosis. Ann Neurol 1996;39:285–294.

9

Treatment of Progressive Multiple Sclerosis

Norman Wang, MD

INTRODUCTION

Treatment directed at the progressive phase of multiple sclerosis (MS) is the most difficult (Table 1). Immunosuppressive therapies, such as total lymphoid irradiation (TLI), cyclosporine, methotrexate, 2-chlorodeoxyadenosine (2-CdA), cyclophosphamide, mitoxantrone, azathioprine, interferon (IFN), steroids, intravenous immunoglobulin (IVIg), and plasma exchange have shown some positive clinical effects in progressive disease. However, all of these nonspecific immunosuppressants suffer from the same basic defect; they may temporarily halt a rapidly progressive downhill course, but it is difficult, or dangerous, to employ them for more than a few months to 1 or 2 years. Thus, because MS is an illness of decades, not months, immunosuppressive therapy is only at best a temporary solution.

TOTAL LYMPHOID IRRADIATION

TLI has potent immunosuppressive effects and is beneficial in patients with progressive MS (1). The absolute lymphocyte count is an indicator of therapeutic efficacy, with greater efficacy in patients with lower counts. Many patients begin reprogressing after initial therapy, and a major limitation is that use of TLI may preclude the use of other treatments that affect the immune system at a later time if the patient reenters the progressive phase.

CYCLOSPORINE

A large multicenter trial of cyclosporine in the United States (2) and a trial in London (3) found that cyclosporine has a beneficial, although modest, effect in ameliorating clinical disease progression. However, its clinical use is limited because of a narrow benefit-to-risk ratio.

From: *Current Clinical Neurology: Multiple Sclerosis*
Edited by: M. J. Olek © Humana Press Inc., Totowa, NJ

Table 1
Treatment Strategies for Multiple Sclerosis

Disease course/stage	Treatment
Monosymptomatic (e.g., optic neuritis)	Intravenous (IV) methylprednisolone, 100 mg/day for 5 days
Relapsing-remitting, no disease activity for several years and no magnetic resonance imaging (MRI) activity	IV corticosteroids if attacks occur
Relapsing-remitting, current disease	IV steroids plus Avonex (30 µg IM weekly) activity, and/or MRI activity or Betaseron (1 mL SC QD) or Copaxone (20 mg SC QD)
Relapsing-remitting, disease activity while on interferon (IFN) or Copaxone	Add monthly bolus of IV methyl-prednisolone, consider increasing IFN dose
Relapsing-remitting, accumulating disability (IFN/Copaxone/ steroid nonresponders)	IV monthly cyclophosphamide/steroid pulse therapy, consider IV mitoxantrone
Rapidly progressing disability	IV cyclophosphamide and corticosteroid eight day induction, followed by pulse maintenance
Very rapidly progressing disability	Plasma exchange
Secondary progressive	IV steroid monthly pulses or IV cyclophosphamide/steroid monthly pulses or methotrexate (PO or SC, 7.5 to 20 mg/week) with or without steroid pulses or consider addition of IFN-β if not already taking or consider IVIg monthly
Primary progressive	IV steroid pulses or methotrexate (PO or SC, 7.5 to 20 mg/week) with or without steroid pulses or Cladribine IV or SC or IVIg monthly or consider mitoxantrone or consider azathioprine

IM, intramuscularly; SC, subcutaneously; QD, every day; PO, administered orally.

METHOTREXATE

Methotrexate is a well-known immunomodulator used extensively in other conditions, such as rheumatoid arthritis. Weekly low-dose oral methotrexate (7.5 mg) was studied in a randomized, double-blind, placebo-controlled trial of 60 patients with chronic progressive MS *(4)*. Methotrexate positively affected measures of upper extremity function, such as the nine-hole peg test and a block-in box test; these tests are a sensitive measure of repeated use of digits. However, lower extremity function as measured by ambulation and disability scales were not affected. There was no clinically significant toxicity.

The safety of methotrexate also has been established in patients receiving 20 mg SC weekly *(5)*. Whether higher doses given intravenously or intrathecally would be more effective in MS is unclear.

CLADRIBINE

Cladribine (2-CdA, Leustatin), a potent immunosuppressive agent useful in the treatment of hairy cell leukemia, was reported to be of benefit in a study of patients with chronic progressive MS *(6)*. In this 1-year, double-blind trial, 48 matched pairs received 4 monthly courses of 2-CdA through a central venous catheter for a 7-day period. Seven out of 23 evaluable patients receiving placebo experienced a one point or more worsening in their Expanded Disability Status Scale (EDSS) score at 1 year, whereas only one out of 24 patients taking cladribine had worsened. Treated patients had improvement on disability scores, no increase in brain MRI lesions, and decreased cerebrospinal fluid (CSF) oligoclonal bands (OCBs), whereas the placebo group experienced the opposite in all of these categories. Side effects included two cases of herpes zoster, a fatal case of hepatitis (not clearly related to the treatment), and persistently lowered CD4 counts.

In a subsequent multicenter trial, 159 patients with progressive MS (30% of whom had primary-progressive MS [PPMS] and the remainder secondary-progressive MS [SPMS]) were randomly assigned to one of two doses of SC cladribine (0.07 mg/kg per day for 5 consecutive days every 4 weeks for either two or six cycles (total dose 0.7 mg/kg and 2.1 mg/kg, respectively) or to placebo *(7)*. There was no significant difference between the groups in terms of EDSS score during the course of the study. However, the results of magnetic resonance imaging (MRI) studies were significantly different between the treatment and placebo groups. At baseline, approximately 35% of patients in each group had enhanced T1 lesions on MRI; this remained unchanged in the placebo group, while decreasing to 10% and 6% in the low- and high-dose treatment groups, respectively. The cladribine groups also had a 90% reduction in the mean number of enhanced T1 lesions at month 6 that persisted for 24 months of follow-up, whereas the placebo group had a 33% and 50% reduction at the 6-month and final evaluation, respectively. Cladribine was generally well tolerated. The high-dose group reported more cases of upper respiratory infection, pharyngitis, back pain, arthralgia, and skin disorder, compared with the low-dose and placebo groups; no serious infections occurred. Dose-related decreases in the mean lymphocyte count occurred with cladribine therapy. A disadvantage of the SC method of administration is that the total lymphocyte and CD4 counts, as measures of effectiveness, do not fall for a number of months and may remain low for months after discontinuing therapy.

One explanation for the difference in outcome between these two studies in terms of the EDSS score is that the patients in the second study had relatively high EDSS scores at baseline (median score-6.0); the size and duration of the study were not powered to detect results in patients with this severity of disease *(7)*. In addition, a significant proportion had PPMS, and this subgroup did not respond as favorably on MRI as the SPMS.

A third study of 159 patients with progressive MS (70% SPMS, 30% PPMS) found that treatment with cladribine did not prevent brain atrophy compared with placebo *(8)*. Furthermore, the change in brain volume did not correlate with other MRI measures of disease (e.g., number and volume of enhancing lesions).

CYCLOPHOSPHAMIDE

Cyclophosphamide (Cytoxan) has been used for the treatment of MS since the early 1980s despite conflicting data. An early study compared an induction course of cyclophosphamide with steroid treatment and found impressive differences; however, in retrospect, the patients were all in a rapidly progressive phase of the illness *(9)*. By comparison, a Canadian study several years later found no effect from an induction course of cyclophosphamide; these patients and controls were more representative of the chronic progressive patients treated in other trials *(10)*.

Cyclophosphamide is most effective in patients younger than age 40 years, especially in those who have been in the progressive phase for <1 year. The drug is ineffective for PPMS.

Cyclophosphamide is administered in monthly bolus injections and maintained for a year or more, often concurrently with IV steroids. The duration of treatment is limited by the risk of bladder cancer, which appears to rise with time and may depend on the total accumulated drug dose.

MITOXANTRONE

Mitoxantrone is an anthracycline analog that is an effective chemotherapeutic agent for many cancers. The efficacy of mitoxantrone in MS was evaluated in a trial of 42 patients with active disease who were treated monthly with either IV methylprednisolone (1 g) plus IV mitoxantrone (20 mg) or IV methylprednisolone alone for 6 months *(11)*. Although the number of patients was small, there was a statistically significant reduction in the number of relapses and an increase in the number of patients free of attack associated with the combined therapy. In addition, 90% of the methylprednisolone/mitoxantrone group showed no new enhancing lesions on MRI vs only 31% in the methylprednisolone group.

These results prompted a multicenter, placebo-controlled, randomized, observer-blind trial of 194 patients with progressive MS that was completed in Europe *(12)*. Patients received IV treatment (5 mg/m^2 or 12 mg/m^2) every 3 months for 2 years. Treatment with mitoxantrone was associated with significant clinical benefits compared with placebo on multivariate analysis, reducing progression of disability and clinical exacerbations.

The risk of cardiotoxicity with mitoxantrone prevents prolonged usage, although 24 months of use in the randomized trial did not result in clinically significant cardiac dysfunction *(12)*. Mitoxantrone is now Food and Drug Administration

(FDA) approved for use in MS, but further studies are required to determine the optimal treatment protocols and frequency of long-term side effects.

AZATHIOPRINE

Azathioprine has been studied in both relapsing-remitting MS (RRMS) and chronic progressing MS (CPMS) since 1971. A meta-analysis of the results of five double-blind and two single-blind, randomized, control trials of azathioprine use in MS showed only a small difference after 2 years in favor of azathioprine *(13)*. The study concluded that the side-effect profile outweighs any small clinical gain.

INTERFERON

The efficacy of IFN has been well documented in patients with RRMS (*see* above). A small randomized trial of IFN-β-1a in PPMS found no benefit *(14)*.

On the other hand, IFN-β-1b is effective in patients with secondary progressive MS. In one study of such patients in 32 centers in Europe, for example, 358 patients received placebo and 360 received IFN-β-1a every other day subcutaneously for up to 3 years *(15)*. There was a 22% relative reduction in the proportion of patients with progression in the IFN-β-1b group compared with placebo. The time to becoming wheelchair-bound was also significantly delayed in the treatment group, equivalent to 12 months ($p < 0.01$). The placebo group had a mean 8% increase in MRI lesion volume, compared with a 5% decrease in the IFN-β-1b group.

The authors assert that the positive effect of treatment could not be ascribed merely to a reduction in disability as the result of relapses; there was also a direct effect on progression. Whether this results from suppression of some ongoing low-level inflammatory process could not be answered directly.

Side effects were manageable; 45 patients taking IFN-β-1b stopped because of adverse effects, compared with 15 taking placebo, but twice as many stopped because of inefficacy of treatment in the placebo group (*see* Side Effects of Interferons). Neutralizing antibodies were seen in 28% of patients (*see* Neutralizing Antibody Formation).

A North American study of IFN-β-1a b in secondary progressive MS found no effect on time to confirmed progression to disability, although significant benefit was shown on all other outcomes *(16)*. Two subsequent randomized, placebo-controlled studies of IFN-β-1a found similar results *(17,18)*. Subgroup analysis of one suggested that the maximal benefit occurred in women and in patients who were still experiencing relapses when treatment started *(17)*.

The reason for the disparity in the studies in terms of progression to disability is not clear. Factors that may be important include a shorter observation period (2 vs 3 years) and shorter duration of the prerandomization secondary progressive phase (2.2 vs 4 years) in the European study. In addition, there was a higher proportion of patients with prestudy relapses in the European study, a finding associated with improved outcomes in the most recent report *(17)*.

Additional hope for immunomodulatory therapy in patients with secondary progressive MS was provided by an MRI study that found that compared with placebo, treatment with IFN-β-1a for 3 years resulted in significant improvements in all MRI measures, particularly in patients with relapses in the 2 years prior to the study *(19)*.

These data have major implications for the treatment of MS. Secondary progressive disease is the single largest category of MS. The immunomodulatory drugs are now approved only for the treatment of relapsing MS; the FDA has approved IFN-β-1b (Betaseron) for use in patients with secondary progressive disease who continue to have relapses *(20)* and is considering approval of IFN-β-1b and IFN-β-1a for other patients with secondary progressive disease. These drugs may become standard therapy for secondary progressive MS, particularly for women and patients still experiencing relapses. Additional data may further clarify the appropriate use of these agents.

CORTICOSTEROIDS

Monthly bolus IV corticosteroids, typically 1000 mg of methylprednisolone, are used at many institutions for treatment of primary or secondary progressive MS alone or in combination with other immunomodulatory or immunosuppressive medications. A trial of methylprednisolone in secondary progressive MS was conducted, in which a total of 108 patients received either 500 mg or 10 mg of IV methylprednisolone every 8 weeks for 2 years *(21)*. Although there was no difference in the proportions of patients in each treatment group who experienced sustained progression of disability, the time to onset of sustained treatment failure was delayed in the high-dose group. Further studies are planned.

INTRAVENOUS IMMUNOGLOBULIN

Immunoglobulin may help patients with several autoimmune diseases, including chronic relapsing polyneuropathy and dermatomyositis, and also has been studied in MS. Its mechanism of action is unclear but may relate to antiidiotypic effects and suppression of tumor necrosis factor (TNF)- α. A randomized, placebo-controlled trial of monthly IVIg in RRMS involved 150 patients over 2 years *(22)*. IVIg was associated with fewer relapses (62 vs 116 with placebo) and a greater likelihood of being relapse-free (53 vs 36%. Only three patients receiving IVIg (4%) experienced side effects, including cutaneous reactions and depression; these manifestations were not unequivocally related to the IVIg.

Observations in animal models of MS revealed that IVIg could promote new myelin synthesis *(23)*. However, a double-blind, placebo-controlled study of 67 patients with an apparently irreversible motor deficit found that IVIg (0.4 g/kg for 5 days, then single infusions every 2 weeks for 3 months) did *not* reverse established weakness in MS *(24)*.

PLASMA EXCHANGE

Plasma exchange has been investigated in patients with acute central nervous system (CNS) inflammatory demyelinating disease who did not respond to steroid therapy *(25)*. Moderate or greater improvement in neurological disability occurred during eight of 19 (42%) courses of active treatment, compared with one of 17 (6%) courses of sham treatment. Improvement occurred early in the course of treatment and was sustained on follow-up. However, four of the patients who responded to the active treatment experienced new attacks of demyelinating disease during 6 months of follow-up.

BONE MARROW TRANSPLANT

Recent strategies have focused on more aggressive approaches to immunosuppression, such as autologous bone marrow transplantation (BMT). This approach has shown promise in experimental models of MS *(26,27)*. There has been one case report of a patient with MS who developed chronic myelogenous leukemia and was treated with allogeneic BMT *(28)*. Another patient with MS had a BMT after she failed to respond to corticosteroids, IFN-β, azathioprine, methotrexate, and/or cyclophosphamide *(29)*. The patient showed mild improvement in strength after autologous BMT but died 7 months after transplant from acute bronchopneumonia associated with cardiocirculatory insufficiency and elevated liver enzymes.

In one controlled trial, two patients with rapidly progressive disease were given cyclophosphamide followed by total body irradiation and methylprednisolone *(30)*. The patients then had an autologous stem cell transplantation. At the 2-month follow-up period, both patients improved clinically and were off of all immunosuppressive medications. Larger trials are awaited in order to evaluate the risk–benefit ratio of this approach.

ANTIINTEGRIN ANTIBODIES (NATALIZUMAB)

The formation of inflammatory lesions in patients with MS may involve lymphocytes and monocytes that gain access to the brain parenchyma from the circulation by first adhering to vascular endothelial cells *(31)*. The glycoprotein α-4 integrin is expressed on the surface of inflammatory lymphocytes and monocytes and may play a critical role in their adhesion to the vascular endothelium *(32,33)*.

These observations have led to investigations of α-4 integrin antagonists. Treatment with these agents in rodent models of MS resulted in reduced signs of disease activity and inflammation *(34–36)*. A small preliminary, placebo-controlled study in humans using the monoclonal antibody natalizumab, an α-4 integrin antagonist, also found that the drug reduced the frequency of new gadolinium (Gd)-enhancing lesions *(37)*.

These findings have now been extended in a larger and longer double-blind trial in which 213 patients with RRMS or relapsing secondary progressive MS were randomly assigned to receive 3 mg/kg or 6 mg/kg of IV natalizumab, or placebo, every 28 days for 6 months *(38)*. Both natalizumab groups had significant reductions in the mean number of new brain lesions on monthly Gd-enhanced MRI (9.6 for placebo vs 0.7 and 1.1 in the 3 mg/kg and 6 mg/kg natalizumab groups, respectively). This effect was evident 1 month after the first infusion and was sustained throughout the treatment period. In addition, there were significantly fewer relapses in the natalizumab groups (27, 13, and 14, respectively).

Although no direct comparative studies have been performed, these results suggest that natalizumab may be more effective than the IFNs or glatiramer acetate. Therapy with natalizumab was well tolerated, with a safety profile similar to that of placebo.

Longer term data and comparison studies, as well as the effect of natalizumab on the progression of disability, are necessary before firm recommendations can be made regarding the optimal use of this agent. Nevertheless, these data are promising.

REFERENCES

1. Cook SD, Devereux C, Troiano R, et al. Total lymphoid irradiation in multiple sclerosis. In: Rudick RA, Goodkin DE, eds, Treatment of Multiple Sclerosis: Trial Design, Results, and Future Perspectives. Springer Verlag, New York, 1992, p. 267.
2. The Multiple Sclerosis Study Group. Efficacy and toxicity of cyclosporine in chronic progressive multiple sclerosis: a randomized, double-blinded, placebo-controlled clinical trial.Ann Neurol 1990;27:591–605.
3. Rudge P, Koetsier JC, Mertin J, et al. Randomised double blind controlled trial of cyclosporin in multiple sclerosis (published erratum appears in J Neurol Neurosurg Psychiatry 1989;52[7]:932). J Neurol Neurosurg Psychiatry 1989;52:559–565.
4. Goodkin DE, Rudick RA, VanderBrug Medendorp S, et al. Low-dose (7.5 mg) oral methotrexate reduces the rate of progression in chronic progressive multiple sclerosis. Ann Neurol 1995; 37:30–40.
5. Olek MJ, Hohol MJ, Weiner HL. Methotrexate in the treatment of multiple sclerosis (letter; comment). Ann Neurol 1996;39:684.
6. Sipe JC, Romine JS, Koziol JA, et al. Cladribine in treatment of chronic progressive multiple sclerosis. Lancet 1994;344:9–13.
7. Rice GP, Filippi M, Comi G. Cladribine and progressive MS: clinical and MRI outcomes of a multicenter controlled trial. Cladribine MRI Study Group (in process citation). Neurology 2000;54:1145–1155.
8. Filippi M, Rovaris M, Iannucci G, et al. Whole brain volume changes in patients with progressive MS treated with cladribine (in process citation). Neurology 2000;55:1714–1718.
9. Hauser SL, Dawson DM, Lehrich JR, et al. Intensive immunosuppression in progressive multiple sclerosis. A randomized, three-arm study of high-dose intravenous cyclophosphamide, plasma exchange, and ACTH. N Engl J Med 1983;308:173–180.
10. The Canadian Cooperative Multiple Sclerosis Study Group. The Canadian cooperative trial of cyclophosphamide and plasma exchange in progressive multiple sclerosis. Lancet 1991; 337:441–446.
11. Edan G, Miller D, Clanet M, et al. Therapeutic effect of mitoxantrone combined with methyl-prednisolone in multiple sclerosis: a randomised multicentre study of active disease using MRI and clinical criteria. J Neurol Neurosurg Psychiatry 1997;62:112–118.
12. Hartung HP, Gonsette R, Konig N, et al. Mitoxantrone in progressive multiple sclerosis: a placebo-controlled, double-blind, randomised, multicentre trial. Lancet 2002;360:2018–2025.

13. Yudkin PL, Ellison GW, Ghezzi A, et al. Overview of azathioprine treatment in multiple sclerosis. Lancet 1991;338:1051–1055.
14. Leary SM, Miller DH, Stevenson VL, et al. Interferon beta-1a in primary progressive MS: an exploratory, randomized, controlled trial. Neurology 2003;60:44–51.
15. Placebo-controlled multicentre randomised trial of interferon beta-1b in treatment of secondary progressive multiple sclerosis. European Study Group on interferon beta-1b in secondary progressive MS. Lancet 1998;352:1491–1497.
16. Goodkin DE. North American Study Group. Interferon beta-1b in secondary progressive MS: clinical and MRI results of a 3-year randomized controlled trial. Neurology 2000;54:2352–.
17. Randomized controlled trial of interferon-beta-1a in secondary progressive MS: Clinical results. Neurology 2001;56:1496–1504.
18. Cohen JA, Cutter GR, Fischer JS, et al. Benefit of interferon beta-1a on MSFC progression in secondary progressive MS. Neurology 2002;59:679–687.
19. Li DK, Zhao GJ, Paty DW. Randomized controlled trial of interferon-beta-1a in secondary progressive MS: MRI results. Neurology 2001;56:1505–1513.
20. Berlex/Chiron Betaseron adds indication for secondary progressive multiple sclerosis. FDC Reports, Inc. Pharmaceutical Approvals Monthly 2003;8:3.
21. Goodkin DE, Kinkel RP, Weinstock-Guttman B, et al. A phase II study of i.v. methylprednisolone in secondary-progressive multiple sclerosis. Neurology 1998;51:239–245.
22. Fazekas F, Deisenhammer F, Strasser-Fuchs S, et al. Randomised placebo-controlled trial of monthly intravenous immunoglobulin therapy in relapsing-remitting multiple sclerosis. Austrian Immunoglobulin in Multiple Sclerosis Study Group. Lancet 1997;349:589–593.
23. Noseworthy JH, O'Brien PC, van Engelen BG, Rodriguez M. Intravenous immunoglobulin therapy in multiple sclerosis: progress from remyelination in the Theiler's virus model to a randomised, double-blind, placebo-controlled clinical trial. J Neurol Neurosurg Psychiatry 1994;57(Suppl):11–14.
24. Noseworthy JH, O'Brien PC, Weinshenker BG, et al. IV immunoglobulin does not reverse established weakness in MS (in process citation). Neurology 2000;55:1135–1143.
25. Weinshenker BG, O'Brien PC, Petterson TM, et al. A randomized trial of plasma exchange in acute central nervous system inflammatory demyelinating disease. Ann Neurol 1999;46:878.
26. van Gelder M, Kinwel-Bohre EP, van Bekkum DW. Treatment of experimental allergic encephalomyelitis in rats with total body irradiation and syngeneic BMT. Bone Marrow Transplant 1993;11:233–241.
27. Burt RK, Burns W, Ruvolo P, et al. Syngeneic bone marrow transplantation eliminates V beta 8.2 T lymphocytes from the spinal cord of Lewis rats with experimental allergic encephalomyelitis. J Neurosci Res 1995;41:526–531.
28. McAllister LD, Beatty PG, Rose J. Allogeneic bone marrow transplant for chronic myelogenous leukemia in a patient with multiple sclerosis. Bone Marrow Transplant 1997;19:395–397.
29. Kolar OJ, Emanuel DJ, Smith FO, et al. Bone marrow transplantation (BMT) in multiple sclerosis (MS). J Neurol Sciences 1997;150(Suppl):S50.
30. Burt RK, Traynor AE, Cohen B, et al. Autologous lymphocyte depleted hematopoietic stem cell transplantation for rapidly progressive multiple sclerosis; minimal toxicity from a cyclophosphamide/total body irradiation/methylprednisolone conditioning regimen. J Neurol Sciences 1997;150(Suppl):S116.
31. Hynes RO. Integrins: a family of cell surface receptors. Cell 1987;48:549–554.
32. Frenette PS, Wagner DD. Adhesion molecules. Part 1. N Engl J Med 1996;334:1526–1529.
33. Frenette PS, Wagner DD. Adhesion molecules. Part II: blood vessels and blood cells. N Engl J Med 1996;335:43–45.
34. Yednock TA, Cannon C, Fritz LC, et al. Prevention of experimental autoimmune encephalomyelitis by antibodies against alpha 4 beta 1 integrin. Nature 1992;356:63–66.
35. Kent SJ, Karlik SJ, Cannon C, et al. A monoclonal antibody to alpha 4 integrin suppresses and reverses active experimental allergic encephalomyelitis. J Neuroimmunol 1995;58:1–10.

36. Kent SJ, Karlik SJ, Rice GP, Horner HC. A monoclonal antibody to alpha 4-integrin reverses the MR-detectable signs of experimental allergic encephalomyelitis in the guinea pig. J Magn Reson Imaging 1995;5:535–540.

37. Tubridy N, Behan PO, Capildeo R, et al. The effect of anti-alpha4 integrin antibody on brain lesion activity in MS. The UK Integrin Study Group. Neurology 1999;53:466–472.

38. Miller DH, Khan OA, Sheremata WA, et al. A controlled trial of natalizumab for relapsing multiple sclerosis. N Engl J Med 2003;348:15–23.

10

Cyclophosphamide Therapy for Multiple Sclerosis

Derek R. Smith, MD

INTRODUCTION

Cyclophosphamide has long been a widely used alkylating agent in the treatment of malignancies, notably hematologic malignancies and, despite its long history, continues to find new uses in immune-mediated nonmalignant processes. Although cyclophosphamide has been studied as a treatment for multiple sclerosis (MS) for the past 30 years, it is only after successful trials of mitoxantrone with improved designs employing magnetic resonance imaging (MRI) as a surrogate marker that clinical researchers have become highly confident of the use of this class of drugs. Trial results suggest that it is efficacious in cases of worsening MS that have an inflammatory component as evidenced by relapses and/or gadolinium (Gd)-enhancing lesions on MRI or in patients in earlier stages of progression. There is no evidence of efficacy in primary-progressive (PPMS) or later secondary-progressive MS (SPMS). Although they are usually considered a general immunosuppressive agent, immunologic studies indicate that proliferating myelin-specific T-cells may be preferentially eliminated in MS. Side effects include nausea, alopecia, infertility, bladder toxicity, and risk of malignancy. Cyclophosphamide is usually given as every 4- to 8-week outpatient intravenous (IV) pulse therapy with or without corticosteroids and is usually well tolerated. Cyclophosphamide is recommended for patients with MS whose disease is not controlled by first-line agents and those with rapid worsening.

BACKGROUND

Cyclophosphamide is transformed in the liver to active alkylating metabolites, which then react with replicating DNA, destroying susceptible rapidly proliferating malignant and nonmalignant cells. It is widely used concurrently with other antineoplastic drugs for the treatment of leukemias and lymphomas, adenocarcinomas,

From: *Current Clinical Neurology: Multiple Sclerosis*
Edited by: M. J. Olek © Humana Press Inc., Totowa, NJ

and other malignancies. It is also used in marrow ablative regimes for both malignant and nonmalignant diseases. Cyclophosphamide has been used in numerous regimens for the treatment of immune-mediated diseases (1,2). Initially, out of concern for potential toxicities, cyclophosphamide use was restricted to the most aggressive immune-mediated diseases, such as Wegener's granulomatosis, polyarteritis nodosa, refractory polymyositis or inflammatory neuropathies, and primary central nervous system (CNS) vasculitis (3,4). A landmark study by Gorley et al. demonstrated that pulse cyclophosphamide therapy was much more effective than standard therapy in the treatment of lupus nephritis (5). This study demonstrated that cyclophosphamide could be well tolerated over time and highly effective in chronic immune-mediated diseases. It is the recommended form of therapy for the treatment of idiopathic nephrotic syndrome and for lupus nephritis, where it appears to have additive efficacy when give concomitantly with pulse methylprednisolone (6). Pulse cyclophosphamide is now regularly used in the treatment of severe systemic-onset juvenile rheumatoid arthritis (7), interstitial lung disease associated with collagen vascular diseases (8), and idiopathic thrombocytic purpura. Cyclophosphamide has been adopted in the treatment of numerous immune-mediated disorders of the peripheral nervous system (9).

CYCLOPHOSPHAMIDE TREATMENT
OF MULTIPLE SCLEROSIS

In the past, the rationale that led investigators to study cyclophosphamide as an MS treatment rested on the hypothesis that MS is an inflammatory, cell-mediated autoimmune disease affecting the CNS (10–12). The immunosuppressive effects of cyclophosphamide have proved to be effective for the treatment of other putative autoimmune diseases (1,2). More recently, it has become clear that a primary autoimmune hypothesis is not essential to the rationale for the use of immunosuppression, because inflammation is often the predominant cause of injury in viral infection. In this regard, Rodriguez et al. have investigated the effect of immunosuppression on CNS remyelination in a chronic virus-induced demyelinating disease (13). They have reported that treatment of animals with cyclophosphamide or anti-T-cell monoclonal antibodies enhanced new myelin synthesis, suggesting that factors associated with immune T-cells somehow impair remyelination and interference with the function of immune T-cells enhances CNS remyelination by oligodendrocytes.

Cyclophosphamide was first tested in MS in 1966 (14) and has since been used in selected patients with MS. Its use has gradually increased recently among clinicians who are confronted with persistent active inflammation in patients with MS treated with US Food and Drug Administration (FDA)-approved disease-modifying drugs, interferon (IFN)-β and glatiramer acetate. With FDA approval in 2000 of a related drug, mitoxantrone, for patients with worsening MS, the decision to treat patients with MS with drugs of this class has become standard practice (15,16). According to a recent survey regarding the use of immunosuppressive drugs, cyclophosphamide is being used by many neurologists for the treatment of MS *(17)*. There have been more than 40 published reports on the clinical and immunological effects of cyclophosphamide in MS (Tables 1 and 5), including many that indicate cyclophosphamide is efficacious in MS. Not all studies have shown positive effects. This has created differing opinions regarding its use, especially because two placebo-controlled trials conducted in the 1980s did not show positive effects *(18,19)*. Many questions remain unanswered regarding how cyclophosphamide should be used in the treatment of MS.

STAGES OF MULTIPLE SCLEROSIS

Later in the course of MS it has been proposed that a separate process of neurodegeneration may occur independent of active cell-mediated inflammation and thus may not be amenable to antiinflammatory therapies. With time, MS becomes less inflammatory, as measured by Gd-enhancing lesions on MRI *(20,21)*. It has been suggested that PPMS may represent an entirely different pathological process and thus respond differently to therapy *(22)*. Immunomodulatory drugs with proven efficacy in MS may not show efficacy in all clinical trials, depending on the patient populations being studied. This is best illustrated in studies of IFN-β-1b. Positive clinical effects were observed in the European trial of IFN-β-1b *(23)*, whereas there were no positive clinical effects in the North American trial IFN-β-1b trial *(24)*. Analyses of patient demographics demonstrate that those in the European trial were at an earlier stage of their disease. Cyclophosphamide results should be evaluated according to the stage of MS and the degree to which inflammation plays a role in the pathology of patients being treated. One reason for conflicting reports regarding the efficacy of cyclophosphamide in MS is that the patient populations treated were at different stages of their disease.

CLINICAL TRIALS OF CYCLOPHOSPHAMIDE IN MULTIPLE SCLEROSIS (TABLE 1)

In 1966, Aimard et al. described the successful arrest of a progressive case of MS using cyclophosphamide *(14)*. This led to an open uncontrolled clinical trial in which 30 patients with MS were treated with cyclophosphamide 200 mg/day IV for 4–6 weeks so that a total of 4–9 g of medication were administered. At the end of 2 years of follow-up, 50% of the patients were improved or stable *(25)*.

In 1969, Milac and Miller described their experience in treating 16 patients with oral cyclophosphamide *(26)*. Initially, patients were given sufficient cyclophosphamide to reduce their white blood cell count to 2000/mm³, but the rate of complications was considered too great at this level, so the dose was reduced to maintain the leukocyte count at 3000/mm³. The daily dose varied from 75 to 150 mg. Seven patients dropped out of the study because of adverse effects. In 1971, Wieczorek et al. reported that cyclophosphamide combined with azathioprine was efficacious in an open uncontrolled trial *(27)*. Gopel et al. reported a similar experience *(28)*. However, Cendrowski reported that the cyclophosphamide was no better than corti-

Table 1
Reports on the Clinical and Immunological Effects of Cyclophosphamide

Date	Author	No. of patients	Type of multiple sclerosis	Regimen	Comments
1966	Aimard	1	Progressive		Arrest of disease in patient with progressive multiple sclerosis (MS). First reported use.
1967	Girard	30	Progressive	200 mg/day IV for 4–6 weeks; 4–9 g total	50% improved or stable at 2 years. Open label.
1969	Millac	16	Progressive	Oral, 75–100 mg/day	Toxicity associated with low white blood cell (WBC) counts.
1973	Cendrowski	23	Relapsing and progressive	100–300 mg IV for 16–33 days plus 50 mg hydrocortisone	No difference in comparison to patients treated with adrenocorticotropic hormone (ACTH) or cortisol.
	Drachman	6	Acute attacks	4–5 mg/kg IV for 10 successive days	No effect observed on recovery from relapse.
1975	Hommes	32	Progressive	100 mg daily +50 mg prednisone bid; 8 g total over 20 days	Stabilization in 69% of patients. Open label, uncontrolled.
1977	Gonsette	110	Relapsing-remitting	IV over 2 weeks to achieve leukopenia of 2000 and lymphopenia of 1000. Dose = 1–12 g. No corticosteroids	Stabilization in 62% of patients over 2–4 years. Decrease in relapse rate. Open label, uncontrolled.
1980	Gonsette	134	Relapsing-remitting	Identical IV regimen as in 1977 report	Stabilization in relapse rate in 76% of patients. Open label, uncontrolled.
1980	Hommes		39 Chronic progressive	400 mg cyclophosphamide (CTX) plus 100 mg	8 g total. Stabilization in 69% of patients. Open label, uncontrolled. Factors associated with response: prednisone. patients with disease onset before 28 years of age, short duration of disease before

Year	Author	N	Type	Regimen	Comments
1981	Theys	21	Progressive	6–8 g given over 3–4 weeks	treatment, rapid progression of disease, low initial disability and HLA-DRw2 positivity. No effect in patients with moderately advanced MS over 2 years
1983	Hauser	20	Progressive	400–500 mg/day IV for 10–14 days plus ACTH	16/20 stabilized at 1 year vs 4/20 prescribed with ACTH and 9 of 18 prescribed with plasma exchange regimen. Randomized, control. No blinding or placebo control.
ACTH					
1987	Goodkin	27	Chronic progressive	Inpatient induction for 10–14 days with IV CTX/ACTH or outpatient induction with 700 mg/m² weekly for 6 weeks plus prednisone. Maintenance therapy of 700 mg/m² daily 2 months for 24 months	Stabilization in 59% of patients induced at 12 months vs. 17% in nonrandomized controls. Trend favoring maintenance therapy vs randomized controls. Nausea and vomiting a limiting side effect of maintenance therapy.
1987	Myers	14	Chronic progressive	Monthly therapy with 400–800 mg/m² oral or IV escalating to 1200–2000 mg/m² monthly; 5–13 doses given over 5–14 months to reduce B-cell and CD4⁺cells. With and without steroids.	Three improved, 9 unchanged, 2 worsened. Open label, uncontrolled. Regimen found too toxic for long-term use.
1987	Siracusa	14	Chronic progressive	Short course of intensive CTX until WBC count reached 3000	Five patients discontinued because of side effects. Patients stable, although not improved. Regimen believed to be too toxic without marked clinical benefit.

(continued)

Table 1 (*Continued*)
Reports on the Clinical and Immunological Effects of Cyclophosphamide

Date	Author	No. of patients	Type of multiple sclerosis	Regimen	Comments
1988	Carter	164	Progressive	2-week IV CTX/ACTH regimen	Eighty-one percent improved or stable at 1 year. Reprogression in 69% of patients at mean of 17.6 months. Improvement seen in younger patients with shorter disease duration. Open label, uncontrolled.
1988	Killian	14	Relapsing-remitting	Monthly 750 mg/m² IV pulses for 1 year	A trend showing decreased relapses in 6 treated patients vs 8 placebo patients ($p = 0.6$). Positive response in placebo patients treated in open label continuation study. Pilot-randomized, double-blind, placebo-controlled trial.
1989	Mauch	21	Chronic progressive	8 mg/kg IV at 4-day intervals until lymphocyte count was half the initial value. 1.9 g average total dose	20 out of 21 patients stable at 1 year vs 7 out of 21 patients receiving ACTH. Open label, nonrandomized controls.
1989	Canadian	55	Progressive	1 g IV on alternate days up to 9 g plus oral prednisone	No difference vs placebo ($n = 56$) or plasma exchange regime.($n = 57$). Randomized, double-blind, placebo controlled
1989	Trouillas	10	Progressive	IV (450 mg/day) for 20 days 3 weeks plus methyl-prednisolone (MP)	6 out of 10 stabilized at 3 years vs 9 out of 10 in plasma exchange regime vs. 0/10 in untreated or azathioprine controls. Open label, nonrandomized controls.

Year	Author	n	Disease type	Treatment	Outcome
1990	Millefiorini	15	Remitting-progressive	IV CTX followed by booster daily 2 months for 2 years	50% clinically stable at 2 years. No major side effects.
1990	D'Andrea	7	Relapsing-remitting	IV induction (11 doses 300 mg/m²) then daily 6 months for 3 years	Decrease relapse rate in all patients at 1 year; in subsequent 2 years 2 patients worse, others clinically stable.
1991	Likosky	22	Chronic progressive	IV (400–500 mg) 5 days/week until leukocyte count fell below 4000/mm³	No difference vs placebo (n = 21) at 12, 18, or 24 months. Randomized, single-blind, placebo-controlled
1993	Weiner	256	Progressive	Published IV CTX/ACTH induction vs. modified IV CTX/ACTH induction (600 mg/m² on days 1, 2, 4, 6, and 8) followed by 700 mg/m² IV pulses daily 2 months for 2 years or no prescription	No difference between published or modified induction (56% stable at 12 months); Benefit of booster vs no boosters at 24 and 30 months. Better response in patients Randomized, single-blinded, 40 years or younger. Non-treatment control for boosters.
1997	Weinstock-Guttman	17	Fulminant	IV 500 mg/m² plus IV MP for 5 days followed by maintenance therapy with CTX/methotrexate, MP or interferon (IFN)-β-1b	13 of 17 (75%) patients improved or stable at 12 months; 9 of 13 (69%) at 24 months Open label, uncontrolled, consecutive patients
1998	LaMantia	30	Chronic progressive	Every 2 month IV pulses (600 mg/m²) × 12 months with or without induction (300 mg/m² IV × 9 days)	At 12 months 75% stable if induction given; 35% stable if no induction. Increased response to treatment n remitting-progressive patients
1999	Gobbini	5	Refractory relapsing-remitting disease	Monthly pulses of CTX given for 12 months	MRI outcome: decrease in gadolinium (Gd)-enhancing lesions following pulse cyclophosphamide in all patients treated

(continued)

177

Table 1 (*Continued*)
Reports on the Clinical and Immunological Effects of Cyclophosphamide

Date	Author	No. of patients	Type of multiple sclerosis	Regimen	Comments
1999	Hohol	95	Progressive	Induction with 1 g IV MP for 5 days followed by IV pulse CTX/MP every 1 month for 1 year, every 6 weeks × 1 year and every 2 months for 1 year	Response to therapy linked to duration of progressive disease; a trend favoring responses in secondary vs primary progressive disease
2001	Zephir	111	Progressive	IV CTX/Mp 700 mg/m^2 monthly for 1 year	Response in patients with clinical attack in 2 years prior to therapy
2001	Perini	26	Secondary progressive	IV CTX/mp 800–1250 mg/m^2 monthly for 1 year then every 2 months × 1 year	Clinical improvement at 2 year/ reduction in Gd+lesions and T2 lesion volume
2001	Khan	14	Rapidly deteriorating refractory patients	Pulse CTX 1000 mg/m^2 given monthly plus 20 mg IV dexamethasone	Clinical improvement or stability in 14/14 patients at 6 months sustained at 18 months following treatment
2001	Patti	10	Rapidly progressive	Monthly pulses CTX 500 mg/m^2–1500 mg/m^2 for 18 months	Reduction in relapses, disability plus T2 MRI burden

Table 2
Factors Associated With a Response to Therapy

1 Rapidly progressive course
2 Gadolinium-positive lesions on magnetic resonance imaging
3 Relapses in the year before therapy
4 Less than 2 years in progressive phase
5 Younger age
6 Absence of primary progressive course

costeroids or adrenocorticotropic hormone (ACTH) alone *(29)*. In addition, Drachman found no effect of 4–5 mg/kg cyclophosphamide given for 10 successive days for the treatment of acute attacks *(30)*.

After these initial studies, Gonsette and Hommes reported positive effects in both patients with relapsing-remitting MS (RRMS) and PPMS treated with cyclophosphamide. Hommes et al. published three reports on his experience with cyclophosphamide in pilot studies of chronic progressive MS *(31–33)*. He treated 86 patients with a short course of cyclophosphamide (400 mg/day) plus prednisone (100 mg/day) given to induce a leukopenia below 2000/mm^3. Patients received a total dose of 8 g of cyclophosphamide and were treated in an uncontrolled open-label fashion. He reported on groups of 32 and 39 patients with varying times of follow-up and analyzed those factors associated with a response to therapy. He reported stabilization of disease for a period of 1 to 5 years in 69% of the patients. The factors that predicted a good response to therapy included disease onset before 28 years of age, short duration of disease before treatment, rapid progression of disease, low initial disability, and HLA-DRw2 positivity (Table 2). These factors were consistent with a report by Theys, who found no benefit of 6–8 g of cyclophosphamide given for 3 to 4 weeks in patients with moderately advanced MS *(34)*.

Gonsette et al. treated 201 patients with RRMS with cyclophosphamide and reported on groups of 110 patients with follow-up for 2 to 6 years *(35)* and 134 patients with follow-up for 2 to 10 years *(36)*. Patients were treated with IV cyclophosphamide without corticosteroids for a 1- to 2-week period and received between 1 and 2 g to maintain a leukopenia of 2000 and a lymphopenia of 1000 for 2–3 weeks. In summarizing their experience, Gonsette et al. reported a 75% decrease in the annual relapse rate in 70% of patients treated, compared to the relapse rate 1 to 2 years before treatment with the most pronounced effects in those with shortest disease and no effect in patients who were already severely handicapped. Of the patients, 30% failed to respond to cyclophosphamide. Stabilization as measured by time to next relapse was approximately 2.5 years. In addition, 60% of patients experienced improvement in neurologic signs and disability. The study was open label and uncontrolled. The authors discussed the known decrease in relapse rate that occurs in patients without treatment and stated that the decrease they observed was more than expected. They also reported that the effect of a short 2- to 3-week treatment was of limited duration (lasting 2 to 3 years) and discuss the need for a strategy to prolong the remission period.

A randomized, controlled study of the use of cyclophosphamide was reported in 1983 by Hauser et al. *(37)*. Patients with progressive MS were treated with a 2- to 3-week course of cyclophosphamide given intravenously 400–500 mg/day 1 to achieve leukopenia of $2000/mm^3$ plus ACTH and compared to a group that received ACTH alone or a group that received plasma exchange, ACTH, and oral cyclophosphamide. All patients were alopecic after the treatment. Although the study was a randomized and controlled trial, it was neither blinded nor placebo controlled. The results showed that 80% (16 out of 20) of the patients treated with cyclophosphamide were improved or stable at 1 year, compared to only 20% (4 out of 20) in the ACTH-treated group. The plasma exchange group showed an intermediate (50%) response. Positive clinical results were observed in terms of Expanded Disability Status Scale (EDSS), functional status scales, and numerous treatment failures. Analysis of the patient profiles demonstrates the patients were relatively young (35 years) and disease duration before treatment was between 2 and 3 years. It was reported that 11 of the 16 patients who were stable or improved at the 1-year period in the *New England Journal of Medicine* study experienced reprogression of their disease in the second or third year after treatment. Subsequent follow-up by Carter et al. of 164 patients treated with cyclophosphamide plus ACTH induction demonstrated that almost all patients began to reprogress, with the average time to reprogression being 18 months, and some patients reprogressed as soon as 6 months after cyclophosphamide therapy *(38)*.

The Northeast Cooperative Treatment Group *(39)* was formed to answer two questions regarding the use of cyclophosphamide in MS. First was a modified induction regimen with a fixed dose of cyclophosphamide equivalent to a published regimen in which dose was adjusted according to white count. Second, would an every-2-month booster (700 mg/m^2) therapy with pulses of cyclophosphamide prevent or delay reprogression? Patients were randomized into one of four groups and evaluated in a single blinded fashion. Patient groups received either the published or modified induction, followed by outpatient pulse therapy or no pulse therapy. There was no placebo group, and differences between the booster and nonbooster groups were blunted because both groups received an initial induction. The results demonstrated no difference between the published- vs the modified-induction regimen in either initial stabilization (56%) or subsequent progression in those not receiving boosters. A modest effect of boosters in delaying reprogression was observed at 24 and 30 months in patients receiving boosters ($p = 0.04$). Post hoc subgroup analyses showed an age effect with boosters delaying time to treatment failure in patients ages 18–40 years ($p = 0.003$) but not in patients ages 41–55 years ($p = 0.97$). In addition, patients with PPMS had a poorer prognosis than patients with SPMS ($p = 0.04$). Patients with recent-onset progression responded better to boosters ($p = 0.02$) than patients with progressive disease for more than 7 years ($p = 0.58$). In addition, Goodkin conducted a similar study in 27 patients with PPMS who were treated with every-2-month boosters of 700 mg/m^2 after induction and compared to nonrandomized controls in which a trend favoring boosters was observed *(40)*.

Two studies have been reported in which a placebo control group was used and no positive clinical effects observed with a 2-week induction regimen *(18,19)*. In the Canadian study, 55 patients with PPMS received 1 g of cyclophosphamide on alternate days until the white blood cell count fell below 4.5 or until 9 g were administered plus 40 mg prednisone orally for 10 days. The study was placebo controlled and single masked and included another treatment group that received plasma exchange. In the Kaiser study, 22 patients with PPMS received 400–500 mg cyclophosphamide IV 5 days per week until the leukocyte count fell below $4000/mm^3$ and were compared to a group receiving folic acid in a randomized, single-blind study. The results of these two studies and the 1983 *New England Journal of Medicine* study and the Northeast Cooperative Treatment Group have been extensively debated in the literature *(41–43)*. Placebo-controlled trials in MS have been subject to type 2 errors (false-negative). For example, a type 2 error occurred in a pilot study of mitoxantrone in progressive MS, which reported minimal efficacy and concluded that mitoxantrone was not worthy of further study in MS *(44)*. Analysis of the Canadian and Kaiser results suggests that patient groups that are not responsive to cyclophosphamide were different from patient groups reported to be responsive. The placebo-treated groups were stable. In the Kaisar study at 1 year, 70% of the placebo group was stable, and 53% were stable at 2 years. The Canadian study reported 67% of its placebo group stable at 2 years. In the Canadian study, 60% of the cyclophosphamide-treated patients were classified as chronic-progressive, whereas 40% were relapsing-progressive. The Canadian and Kaiser studies do not address the use of pulse cyclophosphamide therapy in MS, which is the most common regimen currently used in patients with MS.

Pulse Therapy and Magnetic Resonance Imaging Trials

Although there have been other reports of short 2- to 3-week courses of cyclophosphamide for the treatment of MS with both positive *(45,46)* and negative results *(47)*, most physicians currently use intermittent pulse therapy for the treatment of MS. Meyers treated 14 patients with escalating monthly doses to as high as 2000 mg/m^2, a regimen he found too toxic for long-term use *(48)*. Killian treated 14 patients with RMS with monthly pulses of 750 mg/m^2 for 1 year in a pilot-randomized, double-blind placebo-controlled trial that showed a positive trend ($p = 0.06$) in six treated vs eight placebo patients *(49)*. D'Andrea treated 7 patients with RRMS with every-6-month pulses after induction *(50)*, and Millefiorini treated 15 remitting-progressive patients with every-2-month boosters for 2 years after IV induction *(51)*, and both reported positive effects in open-label trials. Lamantia reported in 30 progressive patients a better response in relapsing-progressive patients and in those receiving induction plus boosters (600 mg/m^2) every 2 months for 12 months *(52)*.

With the widespread use of IFN-β and glatiramer acetate, physicians have been confronted with refractory patients and have reported positive results after treatment with cyclophosphamide in open-label studies *(52–56)*. These patients have been called "fulminant," "refractory relapsing-remitting," and "rapidly deteriorating refractory" patients. Weinstock-Guttman et al. reported that 75% of patients improved or were stable at 12 months after IV cyclophosphamide for 5 days followed by maintenance therapy. Khan et al. reported clinical improvement or stability in 14 consecutive patients given monthly cyclophosphamide pulses (1000 mg/m^2).

In the first MRI-based study of cyclophosphamide, McFarland's group at the National Institutes of Health (NIH) treated patients with RRMS who were not responsive to other immunomodulatory drugs with monthly pulses of cyclophosphamide (1000 mg/m^2). Patients were followed with monthly MRI and clinical evaluation for a mean of 28 months. All patients showed a rapid reduction in contrast-enhancing lesion frequency, and three patients showed a decrease in T2 lesion load within the first 5 months of starting cyclophosphamide treatment. The treatment was safe and well tolerated *(54)*. MRI studies in patients receiving cyclophosphamide before bone marrow transplantation demonstrate a marked decrease in Gd-enhancing lesions *(57)*. Perini et al. reported significant reduction of T2 lesions and Gd enhancement on MRI in 26 patients with SPMS given monthly IV cyclophosphamide pulses at 800–1250 mg/m^2 for 1 year and then every 8 weeks the second year *(58)*. Significant clinical improvement was also observed, and the treatment was safe and well tolerated. Zephir et al. reported on 111 consecutive patients with progressive disease (21 primary progressive and 90 secondary progressive) treated with pulse cyclophosphamide for 12 months *(59)*. They found that the response to cyclophosphamide was linked to whether patients with SPMS had superimposed relapses during the year before treatment. Patti et al. have recently reported on the effectiveness of a combination of cyclophosphamide and IFN-β in patients with rapidly progressive or "transitional" MS, characterized by frequent and severe attacks plus worsening on the disability status scale *(56)*. They treated 10 such patients with monthly pulses of IV cyclophosphamide (500 mg/m^2 to 1500 mg/m^2) to obtain a lymphopenia of between 600/mm^3 and 900/mm^3 for 12 consecutive months and then at 2-month intervals for a further 6 months and found a significant reduction the number of relapses, disability, and T2 MRI burden of disease. They found the treatment safe and well tolerated.

Combination Therapy Trial

A trial completed in 2003 evaluated the efficacy and safety of concomitant therapy with IFN-β-1a, cyclophosphamide, and methylprednisolone in patients with MS with active disease during IFN-β monotherapy *(60)*. This was a randomized, single-blind, parallel-group, multicenter trial in patients with MS with a history of active disease during IFN-β treatment. Patients were randomized to either cyclophosphamide 800 mg/m^2 plus methylprednisolone 1 g IV (CY/MP) or methylprednisolone once monthly for 6 months and then received IFN-β-1a monotherapy for an additional 18 months for a total of 24 months. The primary endpoint was change from baseline in the mean number of Gd-enhancing lesions. Secondary endpoints included the percentage of patients with Gd-enhancing lesions, change in T2 lesion

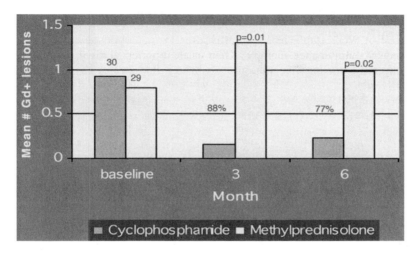

Fig. 1. Mean number of gadolinium (Gd)-enhancing lesions in patients with interferon (IFN)-β-resistant active multiple sclerosis (MS) randomized to either 6 months of monthly cyclophosphamide plus methylprednisolone infusions or 6 months of methylprednisolone only infusions. Cohort sizes are given over the baseline data, which is 1 month after an initial 3-day methylprednisolone course. Magnetic resonance imagings (MRIs) were obtained 1 month after infusion treatments. Patients treated with cyclophosphamide showed significantly fewer Gd-enhancing lesions vs. methylprednisolone alone at both 3 and 6 months. Percent reduction and *p* values are given.

burden, change in brain parenchymal fraction (BPF), time to treatment failure, and cumulative probability of relapse. Safety was assessed by the incidence of adverse events and the results of blood and urine testing.

A total of 59 patients were randomized to treatment: 30 to the CY/MP group and 29 to the MP group. Change from baseline scores in the number of Gd-enhancing lesions was significantly different between treatment groups at 3 ($p = 0.01$), 6 ($p = 0.04$), and 12 months ($p = 0.02$) (Fig. 1). The cumulative rate of treatment failure was significantly lower in the CY/MP group compared with the MP group (rate ratio, 0.30; 95% CI, 0.12 to 0.75; $p = 0.011$). CY/MP treatment was well tolerated. These results demonstrate that concomitant therapy with IFN-β-1a, cyclophosphamide and methylprednisolone decreased the number of Gd-enhancing lesions and slowed clinical activity in patients with active disease on IFN-β and is an option as rescue therapy for patients who are poorly responsive to IFN-β alone.

TREATMENT REGIMENS

As described, numerous treatment regimes have been employed, including oral administration, induction regimens given for a 2- to 3-week period, and pulse therapy given at various doses and intervals. These are summarized in Table 3 and

Table 3
Treatment Regimens

1. IV induction therapy: 600 mg/m^2 cyclophosphamide (CTX) given on days 1, 2, 4, 6, 8
   plus methylprednisolone (MP) given daily for 8 days
2. IV pulse therapy with CTX/MP after MP induction (1 g daily for 5 days): CTX pulses
   begun at 800 mg/m^2 with dose escalation designed to produce leukopenia of
   2000/mm^3; every 4 weeks for 12 weeks, every 6 weeks for 12, every 2 months for
   12 months.
   1 g MP given with CTX. Maximum dose 1600 mg/m^2
3. IV pulse therapy with CTX at a fixed dose: CTX pulses given at 800–1000 mg/m^2
   every 4–8 weeks for 12–24 months; given with or without MP
4. Combination therapy: IV pulse CTX therapy given concomitantly with INF-β
   or glatiramer acetate in nonresponders for various time periods

contained in Table 1. In the 1990s, an outpatient protocol was adopted by many centers beginning with 5 consecutive days of IV methylprednisolone (1 g/day) and a single dose (800 mg/m^2) of cyclophosphamide, followed by monthly pulses of cyclophosphamide/methylprednisolone given at increasing doses until a midmonth nadir of 1500–2000 total white blood cell/mm^3 was reached, from 800 mg/m^2 up to a maximum dose of 1600 mg/m^2. Pulses were given monthly for the first year, every 6 weeks during the second year, and every 3 months during the third year. This protocol was established so that treatment would not necessarily induce alopecia, and the doses of cyclophosphamide pulses were adjusted to uniformly affect white blood cells. A retrolective study of 95 consecutive patients treated by this protocol attempted to identify factors associated with clinical response and found length of time in the progressive stage linked to a positive response, with the suggestion that patients with PPMS were a nonresponsive subgroup *(61)*. In some instances of fulminant MS, induction therapy may be administered *(62)*. In some studies, including the NIH MRI study of Gobbini and McFarland, pulse cyclophosphamide was given without steroids with beneficial effect, whereas most groups have administered them together. Studies from the lupus literature suggest that the addition of steroids may be superior to cyclophosphamide alone *(5)* and may lessen the side effects. Long-term oral use is limited by greater risk of bladder toxicity.

TOXICITY

The adverse effects of cyclophosphamide are well known because the drug has been used for more than 30 years in the medical community (Table 4). Apart for alopecia, infertility, and nausea associated with the administration of the drug, the most frequent complication is hemorrhagic cystitis. This has been also seen in lupus nephritis protocols and has been the major reason why long-term oral cyclophosphamide has been avoided in MS. In addition, cases of bladder cancer have been observed in patients who have been treated long-term with cyclophosphamide. One should routinely obtain urine cytology at yearly intervals in patients treated with

Table 4
Side Effects

1	Nausea
2	Alopecia
3	Infertility
4	Infection
5	Bladder toxicity
6	Cancer risk

cyclophosphamide and recommend yearly cystoscopy after 2 years of therapy. In addition, patients are hydrated with 3 L of fluid on the day of treatment and the day after treatment. Gonadal failure occurs in both men and women receiving alkylating agents such as cyclophosphamide. Most of the available data concern the rate of ovarian failure in cancer survivors in whom alkylating agents were used as part of a multidrug regimen and at different doses than for immunologic disease. In a controlled trial in lupus nephritis *(5)*, a setting more relevant to MS, 23 of 46 women (50%) developed amenorrhea after receiving cyclophosphamide for 6 monthly courses then every 3 months for at least 2 more years beginning with a dose of 0.75 mg/m² then adjusting the dose based on the nadir. Risk factors for persistent amenorrhea and premature menopause include age >30 years and cumulative dose >300 mg/kg *(63,64)*. Numerous approaches have been considered to attempt to preserve ovarian function *(64)*. The rate of amenorrhea in women with MS treated with cyclophosphamide (approximately 40–80% in large series) appears similar to that reported for rheumatic diseases *(19,39)*. There are few data concerning the frequency of infertility in men with immune-mediated diseases treated with cyclophosphamide. An increased incidence of subsequent malignancies has been reported in patients both with cancer treated with cyclophosphamide and with rheumatic diseases *(65–67)*, and this may occur after therapy cessation. The magnitude of increased risk appears to increase as a function of total dose. Care must be taken when the cumulative lifetime dose exceeds 80–100 g *(65–67)*. Based on this, at a dose of 1000 mg/m², patients may receive approximately 50 doses during their lifetime. Some investigators have reported that cyclophosphamide is too toxic to administer because of side effects and patient discomfort *(24,68)*. This appears related to dosing schedules, concomitant use of steroids, and use of appropriate antiemetics, because most groups have reported cyclophosphamide generally well tolerated and easy to administer *(54–56,58,61)*.

IMMUNOLOGICAL EFFECTS

MS may be a Th1 type cell-mediated autoimmune disease *(10–12)*. Cyclophosphamide probably has selective effects on the immune system (Table 5).Cyclophosphamide enters the nervous system because it can be recovered from the cerebrospinal fluid (CSF) *(69,70)* and it reduces CSF myelin basic protein (MBP)

Table 5
Immunology

Date	Author	Comments
1980	Bahr	Cyclophosphamide appears in the spinal fluid after 3 weeks treatment with 400 mg/day.
1982	Ten Berge	Lymphopenia involving T- and B-cells; serum levels of immunoglobulin and primary and secondary antibody responses depressed.
1983	Brinkman	Alteration in lymphocyte populations in peripheral blood and CSF.
1983	Hommes	Cyclophosphamide present at same levels in serum and CSF.
1986	Wender	Decreased synthesis of CNSIg, though not as pronounced as with high doses of prednisone.
1987	Moody	47% reduction in CD4 cells, 22% reduction in CD8 cells; magntude of reduction of CD4 cells correlated with total dose received. B-cells reduced 50% and PHA responses reduced. No reduction in natural killer cells. Recovery of immune function occurred after 4 months.
1988	Lamers	Increased levels of CSF myelin basic protein (MBP) and intrathecally produced immunoglobulin (Ig) G reduced after treatment with cyclophosphamide and prednisone.
1989	Uitdehaag	Decreased CD4$^+$ cells after short-term therapy (8 g in 20 days) present as long as 13.5 years after treatment.
1997	Smith	Immune deviation after pulse cyclophosphamide/methylprednisolone treatment of multiple sclerosis: increased interleukin (IL)-4 production and associated esinophilia.
1998	Comabella	Elevated IL-12 in progressive multiple sclerosis correlates with disease activity and is normalized by pulse cyclophosphamide therapy.
1998	Takashima	Pulse cyclophosphamide plus methylprednisolone induces myelin-antigen-specific IL-4-secreting T-cells.

and intrathecally produced immunoglobulin (Ig) G *(71,72)*. Early studies demonstrated lymphopenia involving T- and B-cells *(73,74)*, with a more pronounced effect on CD4 cells *(75,76)*. These changes reversed after 4 months, although others reported changes as long as 13.5 years *(77)*. Patients treated with cyclophosphamide demonstrate increased IL-4 production and esinophilia *(78)*. Cyclophosphamide has a pronounced effect on interleukin (IL)-12, which may be linked to response to therapy *(79)*. Takashima et al. found that cyclophosphamide preferentially deviates myelin-reactive cells to those secreting IL-4 *(80)*. They reported an increased frequency of both MBP and proteolipid protein (PLP) cells secreting IL-4 in patients treated with cyclophosphamide. No such increase was observed in tetanus toxoid-secreting cells, and this change was not observed in patients treated with methylprednisolone. Cyclophosphamide therapy induced myelin antigen-specific Th2 responses.

CONCLUSIONS

Based on the body of literature, cyclophosphamide probably reduces inflammation in patients with MS with an active inflammatory component to their illness. This inflammatory component may not be prominent in later stages of progressive disease or in patients with PPMS. It is ineffective in later stages of the disease when there is less inflammation, as is true of other immune modulators. Because early inflammatory events correlate with later disability, strong antiinflammatory drugs, such as cyclophosphamide or mitoxantrone, may have an effect on later degenerative changes if given early in the disease to halt inflammation. However, drugs such as cyclophosphamide and mitoxantrone remain limited by their toxicity for widespread use in early stages of MS.

With the approval of mitoxantrone for worsening forms of MS, the question remains of the place of cyclophosphamide in this patient group. There have been no formal comparisons between mitoxantrone and cyclophosphamide. Because there are no reported studies of mitoxantrone in later stages of MS, one might expect that like cyclophosphamide, mitoxantrone may be less effective in later progressive MS. Mitoxantrone is easier to administer than cyclophosphamide but because of cardiac toxicity, can only be given for a 2-year period and cannot be given again if patients begin to reprogress. Sequential use of these agents has been done by some investigators, but toxicity profiles are unknown at this time. Cyclophosphamide has been tested as a rescue therapy in patients not responding to the IFNs *(60)*. Bone marrow transplantation, which is being tested in severe MS, involves treatment with cyclophosphamide. Cyclophosphamide can be administered for longer periods of time, although it too may be limited by cumulative dose considerations.

REFERENCES

1. Langford CA, Klippel JH, Balow JE, James SP, Sneller MC. Use of cytotoxic agents and cyclosporine in the treatment of autoimmune disease. Part 2: inflammatory bowel disease, systemic vasculitis, and therapeutic toxicity. Ann Intern Med 1998;129:49–58.
2. Langford CA, Klippel JH, Balow JE, James SP, Sneller MC. Use of cytotoxic agents and cyclosporine in the treatment of autoimmune disease. Part 1: rheumatologic and renal diseases. Ann Intern Med 1998;128:1021–1028.
3. Notermans NC, Lokhorst HM, Franssen H, et al. Intermittent cyclophosphamide and prednisone treatment of polyneuropathy associated with monoclonal gammopathy of undetermined significance. Neurology 1996;47:1227–1233.
4. Good JL, Chehrenama M, Mayer RF, Koski CL. Pulse cyclophosphamide therapy in chronic inflammatory demyelinating polyneuropathy. Neurology 1998;51:1735–1738.
5. Gorley M, Austin HR, Scott D, et al. Methylprednisolone and cyclophosphamide, alone or in combination, in patients with lupus nephritis. A randomized controlled trial. Ann Intern Med 1996;125:549–557.
6. Zimmerman R, Radhakrishnan J, Valeri A, Appel G. Advances in the treatment of lupus nephritis. Annu Rev Med 2001;52:63–78.
7. Wallace CA, Sherry DD. Trial of intravenous pulse cyclophosphamide and methylprednisolone in the treatment of severe systemic-onset juvenile rheumatoid arthritis. Arthritis Rheumatol 1997;40:1852–1855.

8. Schnabel A, Reuter M, Gross Wl. Intravenous pulse cyclophosphamide in the treatment of interstitial lung disease due to collagen vascular diseases. Arthritis Rheumatol 1998;41:1215–1220.

9. Gorson K, Ropper A, Weinberg D, Weinstein R. Treatment experience in patients with anti-MAG neuropathy. Muscle Nerve 2001;24:778–786.

10. Martin R, McFarland HF, McFarlin DE. Immunological aspects of demyelinating diseases. Annu Rev Immunol 1992;10:153–187.

11. Smith DR, Olek MJ, Balachov KE, Khoury SJ, Hafler DA, Weiner HL. Principles of immunotherapy. In: Clinical Neuroimmunology. Blackwell Science, Cambridge, MA, 1998, pp. 92–104.

12. Steinman L. Multiple sclerosis: a coordinated immunological attack against myelin in the central nervous system. Cell 1996;85:299–302.

13. Rodriguez M. Immunosuppression promotes CNS remyelination in chronic virus-induced demyelinating disease. Neurology 1992;42:276–277.

14. Aimard G, Girard PF, Raveau J. Multiple sclerosis and the autoimmunization process. Treatment by antimitotics. Lyon Med 1966;215:345–352.

15. Edan G, Miller D, Clanet M, et al. Therapeutic effect of mitoxantrone combined with methylprednisolone in multiple sclerosis: a randomized multicenter study of active disease using MRI and clinical criteria. J Neurol Neurosurg Psychiatry 1997;62:112–118.

16. Hartung HP, Gonsette RATM-SG, Mitoxantrone in progressive multiple sclerosis: a placebo-controlled, randomized, observer-blind phase III trial: clinical results and three-year follow-up. Neurology 1999;52(Supp 2):290.

17. Hommes OR, Weiner HL. Results of an international questionnaire on immunosuppressive treatment of multiple sclerosis. Mult Scler 2002;8:139–141.

18. Likosky WH, Fireman B, Elmore R. Intense immunosuppression in chronic progressive multiple sclerosis: the Kaiser study. J Neurol Neurosurg Psychiatry 1991;54:1055–1060.

19. The Canadian cooperative trial of cyclophosphamide and plasma exchange in progressive multiple sclerosis. The Canadian Cooperative Multiple Sclerosis Study Group. Lancet 1991;337:441–446.

20. Miller DH, Grossman RI, Reingold SC, McFarland HF. The role of magnetic resonance techniques in understanding and managing multiple sclerosis. Brain 1998;121:3–24.

21. Weiner HL, Guttmann CR, Khoury SJ, et al. Serial magnetic resonance imaging in multiple sclerosis: correlation with attacks, disability, and disease stage. J Neuroimmunol 2000;104:164–173.

22. Thompson AJ, Kermode AG, Wicks D, et al. Major differences in the dynamics of primary and secondary progressive multiple sclerosis. Ann Neurol 1991;29:53–62.

23. European Study Group on interferon beta-1b in secondary progressive MS. Placebo-controlled multicentre randomised trial of interferon beta-1b in treatment of secondary progressive multiple sclerosis. Lancet 1998;352:1491–1497.

24. Goodkin DE, and the North American Study Group on Laterferon Beta-1b in Secondary Progressive MS. The North American Study of Interferon Beta-1b in Secondary Progressive Multiple Sclerosis Presented at: The 52nd Annual Meeting of the American Academy of Neurology; May 1, 2000; San Diego, CA.

25. Girard PF, Aimard G, Pellet H. Immuno-depressive therapy in neurology. Press Med 1967;75:967–968.

26. Millac P, Miller H. Cyclophosphamide in multiple sclerosis. Lancet 1969;1:783.

27. Wieczorek V, Lehnert W, Brodkorb W. Experiences with immunosuppressive treatment of multiple sclerosis. Disch Ges Wesen 1971;26:1791–1794.

28. Gopel W, Benkenstein H, Banzhaf M. Immunosuppressive therapy of multiple sclerosis using cyclophosphamide and imuran. Report on 57 cases. Dtsch Gesundheitsw 1972;27:1955–1961.

29. Cendrowski W. Combined therapeutic trial in multiple sclerosis: hydrocortisone hemisuccinate with cyclophosphamide or cytosine arabinoside. Acta Neurol Belg 1973;73:209–219.

30. Drachman DA, Paterson PY, Schmidt RT, Spehlmann RF. Cyclophosphamide in exacerbations of multiple sclerosis. Therapeutic trial and a strategy for pilot drug studies. J Neurol Neurosurg Psychiatry 1975;38:592–597.

31. Hommes OR, Prick JJG, Lamers KJB. Treatment of the chronic progressive form of multiple sclerosis with a combination of cyclophosphamide and prednisone. Clin Neurol Neurosurg 1975;78:59–73.

32. Hommes OR, Lamers KJB, Reekers P. Prognostic factors in intensive immunosuppression on the course of chronic progressive multiple sclerosis. In: Bauer S, Poser S, Ritter G, eds. Progress in Multiple Sclerosis Research. Berlin, Springer Verlag, 1980, pp. 396–400.

33. Hommes OR, Lamers KJB, Reekers P. Effect of intensive immunosuppression on the course of chronic progressive multiple sclerosis. J Neurol 1980;223:177–190.

34. Theys P, Gosseye-Lissoir F, Ketelaer P, Carton H. Short-term intensive cyclophosphamide treatment in multiple sclerosis. A retrospective controlled study. J Neurol 1981;225 :119–133.

35. Gonsette R, Demonty L, Delmotte P. Intensive immunosuppression with cyclophosphamide in multiple sclerosis: follow-up of 110 patients for 2-6 years. J Neuroimmunol 1977;214:173 H. 181.

36. Gonsette RE, Demonty L, Delmotte P. Intensive immunosuppression with cyclophosphamide in remittent forms of multiple sclerosis. A follow up of 134 patients for 2–10 years. In: Bauer HJ, ed. Progress in Multiple Sclerosis Research, Springer-Verlag, New York1980.

37. Hauser SL, Dawson DM, Lehrich JR, et al. Intensive immunosuppression in progressive multiple sclerosis: a randomized, three-arm study of high dose intravenous cyclophosphamide, plasma exchange and ACTH. N Engl J Med 1983;308:173–180.

38. Carter JL, Hafler DA, Dawson DM, Orav J, Weiner HL. Immunosuppression with high-dose IV cyclophosphamide and ACTH in progressive multiple sclerosis: cumulative 6-year experience in 164 patients. Neurology 1988;38(2):9–14.

39. Weiner HL, Mackin GA, Orav EJ, et al. Intermittent cyclophosphamide pulse therapy in progressive multiple sclerosis: final report of the Northeast Cooperative Multiple Sclerosis Treatment Group. Neurology 1993;43:910–918.

40. Goodkin DE, Plencer S, Palmer SJ, Teetzen M, Hertsgaard D. Cyclophosphamide in chronic progressive multiple sclerosis: maintenance vs. nonmaintenance therapy. Arch Neurol 1987;44:823–827.

41. Noseworthy JH, Ebers GC, Roberts R. Cyclophosphamide and MS [letter to the editor]. Neurology 1994;44:579–581.

42. Noseworthy JH, Vandervoort MK, Penman M, et al. Cyclophosphamide and plasma exchange in multiple sclerosis [letter to the editor]. Lancet 1991;337:1540–1541.

43. Weiner HH, Dawson DM, Hafler DA, Macklin GA, Orav EJ. Cyclophosphamide and plasma exchange in multiple sclerosis [letter to the editor]. Lancet 1991;337:1033–1034.

44. Noseworthy JH, Vandervoort MK, Karlik SJ, et al. An open-trial evaluation of mitoxantrone in the treatment of progressive MS. Neurology 1993;43:1401–1406.

45. Mauch E, Kornhuber HH, Pfrommer U, Hahnel A, Laufen H, Krapf H. Effective treatment of chronic progressive multiple sclerosis with low-dose cyclophosphamide with minor side effects. Euro Arch Psychiatry Neurological Sci 1989;238:115–117.

46. Trouillas P, Neushwander P, Nighoghossian N, Adeleine P, Tremisi P. Immunosuppression intensive dans la sclerose en plaques progressive etude ouverte comparant trois groupes: cyclophosphamide, cyclophosphamide-plasmaphereses et temoins resultats a trois ans. Rev Neurol 1989;145:369–377.

47. Siracusa GF, Amato MP, Fratiglioni L, Sita D, Amaducci L. Short-term intensive cyclophosphamide treatment in progressive multiple sclerosis. Ital J Neurol Sci 1987;8:589–592.

48. Myers LK, Seyer JM, Stuart JM, Kang AH. Suppression of murine collagen-induced arthritis by nasal administration of collagen. Immunology 1997;90:161–164.

49. Killian JM, Bressler RB, Armstrong RM, Huston DP. Controlled pilot trial of monthly intravenous cyclophosphamide in multiple sclerosis. Arch Neurol 1988;45:27–30.

50. D'Andrea F, D'Aurizio C, Marini C, Prencipe M. Cyclophosphamide in relapsing remitting multiple sclerosis. Ital J Neurol Sci, 1990;11:271–274.

51. Millefiorini E, Di Giovanni M, Bernardi S, Grasso MG, DiGiampietro A, Gambi D. 24-month follow-up of multiple sclerosis patients treated with cyclophosphamide. Ital J Neurol Sci 1990;11:605–607.

52. La Mantia L, Eoli M, Salmaggi A, Torri V, Milanese C. Cyclophosphamide in chronic progressive multiple sclerosis: a comparative study. Ital J Neurol Sci 1998;19:32–36.

53. Weinstock-Guttmann B, Kinkel RP, Cohen JA, Ransohoff RR, Rudick RA. Treatment of "transitional MS" with cyclophosphamide and methylprednisolone (CTX/MP) followed by interferon β. Neurology 1997;48:S45.006.

54. Gobbini MI, Smith ME, Richert ND, Frank JA, McFarland HF. Effect of open label pulse cyclophosphamide therapy on MRI measures of disease activity in five patients with refractory relapsing-remitting multiple sclerosis. J Neuroimmunol 1999;99:142–149.

55. Khan OA, Zvartau-Hind M, Caon C, et al. Effect of monthly intravenous cyclophosphamide in rapidly deteriorating multiple sclerosis patients resistant to conventional therapy. Mult Scler, 2001;7:185–188.

56. Patti F, Cataldi ML, Nicoletti F, Reggio E, Nicoletti A, Reggio A. Combination of cyclophosphamide and interferon-beta halts progression in patients with rapidly transitional multiple sclerosis. J Neurol Neurosurg Psychiatry 2001;71:404–407.

57. Mancardi GL, Saccardi R, Filippi M, et al. Autologous hematopoietic stem cell transplantation suppresses Gd-enhanced MRI activity in MS. Neurology 2001;57:62–68.

58. Perini P, Marangoni A, Tzinteva E, Ranzato F, Tavolato B, Gallo P. Two years therapy of secondary progressive multiple sclerosis (SPMS) with pulse intravenous cyclophosphamide/methylprednisolone. Clinical and MRI data. Mult Scler 2001;7:S62.

59. Zephir H, Senechal O, Stojkovic T, et al. Treatment of progressive multiple sclerosis with cyclophosphamide. Rev Neurol 2002;158:65–69.

60. Smith DR, Weinstock-Guttmann B, Cohen J, et al. Design of randomized, blinded, MRI trial of pulse cyclophosphamide rescue therapy in B-IFN resistant active MS. Presented at American Academy of Neurology 53rd Annual Meeting. Philadelphia, 2001.

61. Hohol MJ, Olek MJ, Orav EJ, L. et al. Treatment of progressive multiple sclerosis with pulse cyclophosphamide/methylprednisolone: response to therapy is linked to the duration of progressive disease. Mult Scler 1999;5:403–409.

62. Case records of the Massachusetts General Hospital. Weekly clinicopathological exercises. Case 26-1998. A 15-year-old girl with hemiparesis, slurred speech, and an intracranial lesion. N Engl J Med 1998;339:542–549.

63. Boumpas DT, Austin HA, Vaughan EM, Yarboro CH, Klippel JH, Balow JE. Risk for sustained amenorrhea in patients with systematic lupus erythematosus receiving intermittent pulse cyclophosphamide therapy. Ann Intern Med 1993;119:366–369.

64. Slater CA, Liang MH, McCune JW, Christman GM, Laufer MR. Preserving ovarian function in patients receiving cyclophosphamide. Lupus 1999;8:3–10.

65. Moore MJ. Clinical pharmacokinetics of cyclophosphamide. Clin Pharmacokinet 1991;20:194–208.

66. Radis CD, Kahl LE, Baker GL, et al. Effects of cyclophosphamide on the development of malignancy and on long-term survival of patients with rheumatoid arthritis. A 20-year followup study. Arthritis Rheum 1995;38:1120–1127.

67. Talar-Williams C, Hijazi YM, Walther MM, et al., Cyclophosphamide-induced cystitis and bladder cancer in patients with Wegener granulomatosis. Ann Intern Med 1996;124:477–484.

68. Myers LW, Fahey JL, Moody DJ, Mickey MR, Frane MV, Ellison GW. Cyclophosphamide "pulses" in chronic progressive multiple sclerosis. Arch Neurol 1987;44:828–832.

69. Hommes OR, Aerts F, Bahr U, Schulten HR. Cyclophosphamide levels in serum and spinal fluid of multiple sclerosis patients treated with immunosuppression. J Neurol Sci 1983;58:297–303.

70. Bahr U, Hommes OR, Aerts F. Determination of cyclophosphamide in urine, serum and cerebrospinal fluid of multiple sclerosis patients by field desorption mass spectrometry. Clinica Chimica Acta 1980;103:183–192.

71. Wender M, Tokarz E, Michalowska G, Wajgt A. Therapeutic trials of multiple sclerosis and intrathecal IgG production. Ital J Neurol Sci 1986;7:205–208.

72. Lamers KJ, Uitdehaag BM, Hommes OR, Doesburg W, Wevers RA, von Geel WJ, The short-term effect of an immunosuppressive treatment on CSF myelin basic protein in chronic progressive multiple sclerosis. J Neurol Neurosurg Psychiatry 1988;51:1334–1337.

73. Ten Berge RJ, van Walbeek HK, Schellekens PT. Evaluation of the immunosuppressive effects of cyclophosphamide in patients with multiple sclerosis. Clin Exp Immunol 1982;50:495–502.

74. Brinkman CJ, Nillesen WM, Hommes OR. T-cell subpopulations in blood and cerebrospinal fluid of multiple sclerosis patients: effect of cyclophosphamide. Clin Immunol Immunopathol 1983;29:341–348.

75. Moody DJ, Kagan J, Liao D, Ellison GW, Myers LW. Administration of monthly-pulse cyclophosphamide in multiple sclerosis patients. Effects of long-term treatment on immunologic parameters. J Neuroimmunol 1987;14:161–173.

76. Mickey MR, Ellison GW, Fahey JL, Moody DJ, Myers LW. Correlation of clinical and immunological states in multiple sclerosis. Arch Neurol 1987;44:371–375.

77. Uitdehaag BM, Nillesen WM, Hommes OR., Long-lasting effects of cyclophosphamide on lymphocytes in peripheral blood and spinal fluid. Acta Neurol Scand 1989;79:12–17.

78. Smith DR, Balashov KW, Hafler DA, Khoury SJ, Weiner HL. Immune deviation following pulse cyclophosphamide/methylprednisolone treatment of multiple sclerosis: increased interleukin-4 production and associated eosinophilia. Ann Neurol 1997;42:313–318.

79. Comabella M, Balashov K, Issazadeh S, Smith DR, Weiner HL, Khoury SJ. Elevated interleukin-12 in progressive multiple sclerosis correlates with disease activity and is normalized by pulse cyclophosphamide therapy. J Clin Invest 1998;102:671–678.

80. Takashima H, Smith DR, Fukaura H, Khoury SJ, Hafler DA, Weiner HL. Pulse cyclophosphamide plus methylprednisolone induces myelin-antigen-specific IL-4-secreting T cells in multiple sclerosis patients. Clin Immunol Immunopathol 1998;88:28–34.

11

Repair and Neuroprotective Strategies in Multiple Sclerosis

Fernando Dangond, MD

INTRODUCTION

Multiple sclerosis (MS) is a demyelinating and inflammatory disease of the central nervous system (CNS). The destruction of the oligodendrocyte-derived myelin lamellae leads to loss of nerve insulation and results in impairment of fast saltatory conduction. Axons and neurons are also damaged and lost in the disease process *(1)*, and cell repopulation is hampered by the inability of mature neurons to undergo cell division. An attractive approach for reestablishing electrochemical circuits in MS would be to restore the function or number of myelin-generating oligodendrocytes in early lesions, to act as bridges that guide and promote axonal regeneration.

MS lesions contain inflammatory cells, astrocytic scarring, myelin debris, myelin-engulfing macrophages, degraded extracellular matrix, naked axons, oligodendrocyte progenitor or stem cells, and a tumefactive nature resulting from blood–brain barrier (BBB) breakdown. Cytotoxic factors released by immune cells and the attack by antibodies and complement all act in concert, leading to the devastating white-matter lesions *(2)*. The dynamic nature and heterogeneity of this complex milieu must be understood in more detail to better guide neuroprotective and repair attempts *(3)*, and new technologies are being applied to elucidate the responsible pathways *(4,5)*. In this chapter, the current knowledge of potential repair approaches, pitfalls, and challenges for research that lie ahead for achieving protection or regeneration in MS are discussed.

MYELIN REPAIR

Because of environmental influences and the presence of established regulatory mechanisms within cells in charge of generating myelin sheaths, remyelination at MS lesion sites is not expected to be governed by exactly the same processes that operate in developmental myelination. The endogenous remyelination that occurs

From: *Current Clinical Neurology: Multiple Sclerosis*
Edited by: M. J. Olek © Humana Press Inc., Totowa, NJ

in MS is incomplete. The poorly remyelinated axon has myelin sheaths of reduced length and thickness *(6)*. This incomplete remyelination in MS could be the result of decreased progenitor cell numbers, impaired migration, or poor axonal receptiveness *(7)*. Proproliferative signals from the axon or glia to the oligodendrocytes may also fail and lead to poor remyelination. For instance, the molecule Jagged1 inhibits process outgrowth and differentiation by oligodendrocytes that express the Notch1 receptor *(8)*. Inability of neural or glial cells to maintain downregulation of Jagged1 would, in theory, be deleterious in MS lesions.

Remyelination occurs spontaneously in animal models of demyelination and is associated with improved neurological function *(9–11)*. The Theiler's murine encephalomyelitis virus (TMEV) SJL/J model exhibits a chronic progressive demyelinating disease and minimal spontaneous remyelination. The TMEV virus is harbored by oligodendrocytes, which are eventually destroyed during the ensuing inflammatory process. If immunosuppressed with cyclophosphamide or via genetic manipulation, however, TMEV-infected animals have enhanced myelin repair and partial functional recovery. Axonal preservation is key in ensuring that myelin repair has a positive functional outcome in this model. Other experimental models of demyelination used to study remyelination in MS include toxin (cuprizone or lysolecithine)-induced and myelin antigen-induced demyelination. Interestingly, although antibodies against myelin proteins, such as myelin oligodendrocyte glycoprotein (MOG), play an important role in demyelination in experimental autoimmune encephalomyelitis (EAE) *(12)* and are found within MS lesions *(13,14)*, other antibodies have been found to have promyelinating properties in EAE and in TMEV-induced demyelination *(15–17)*.

Mature oligodendrocytes provide trophic support to axons and protect neurons from apoptosis *(18,19)*. It is believed that during an autoimmune attack which targets myelin, progenitor cells can mature and migrate to areas of tissue damage to replace damaged oligodendrocytes. Identification of markers of oligodendrocytes as they mature in vivo is an essential piece of the puzzle that must be understood before a rational strategy for myelin repair is implemented. Oligodendrocyte progenitor cells (OPCs) express the O-2A marker, are found along the subventricular and ventricular zones, and are capable of differentiating into mature oligodendrocytes *(7)*. Although O-2A cells are also able to differentiate into type 2 astrocytes in vitro, their ability to differentiate into astrocytes in vivo is in question. The QKI RNA-binding proteins have been recently described as markers of actively myelinating oligodendrocytes in rat brain *(20)*. The platelet-derived growth factor-α (PDGF-α) receptor has also been used to identify OPCs in adult human brain and in MS lesions *(21)*. During this differentiation and migration process, these cells acquire an elaborate morphology and express various cell surface markers. Although the study of these markers is beginning and has been fraught with difficulties in correlating in vitro with *in situ* data, it is expected that understanding the details of this differentiation and its maintenance at the genetic regulation level will yield important therapeutic options for MS. Mature oligodendrocytes express myelin basic protein (MBP), proteolipid protein (PLP), myelin associated glyco-protein (MAG), and MOG, whereas less mature cells express CNP and Gal-C. The presence of adult progenitor cells within the MS lesions has been demonstrated *(21)*, but inflammation itself may promote the migration of OPCs *(22)*. However, questions arise regarding whether the primary cells leading to partial remyelination of the MS plaque are recruited OPCs or actually represent spared oligodendrocytes or OPCs already residing within or near the lesion zone. Studies of human spinal cords with MS reveal that the numbers of mature oligodendrocytes is diminished in chronic lesions and that OPCs are present in a quiescent state *(23)*, indicating a loss of dynamic recruitment of these cells to areas of damage *(24,25)*.

The CNS exhibits a natural capacity for remyelination as part of a general defense and repair mechanism after injury. Oligodendrocyte precursors repopulate areas of lysolecithin-induced demyelination in experimental rats *(26)*. Clearly, stud-ies in EAE have shown that spontaneous remyelination correlates with recovery *(9)*. After MS-related optic neuritis (ON), which results in prolongation of the visual evoked potentials (VEPs), a gradual shortening of the VEPs is seen over several months, presumably resulting from remyelination events *(27)*. This remyelination is seen shortly after acute demyelination occurs, and OPCs are actively involved in this process. This remyelination is incomplete, despite the evidence that repair at the molecular level is being promoted. For instance, genomic studies have shown that growth factor and repair genes are recruited after CNS injury *(28)*.

The use of antibodies that promote remyelination *(29)* has also been proposed as a treatment for MS *(30)*. Antibodies against glatiramer acetate (Copaxone) enhance remyelination of axons in a rat model *(31)*. Copaxone also reduces the degree of axonal loss in the mouse model of EAE *(32)*. Antibody-dependent complement damage to myelin could be inhibited in vivo by currently used therapies such as intravenous (IV) immunoglobulin (IVIg), by a protective effect already dem-onstrated in vitro *(33)*.

NEURONAL AND GLIAL PROTECTION

Growth factors such as fibroblast growth factor 2 (FGF2) and platelet-derived growth factor (PDGF) have been implicated in priming of cells in charge of remyelinating areas of damage *(34)*. Others have shown that glial growth factor 2 (GGF2) *(35)*, ciliary neurotrophic factor (CNTF), leukemia inhibitory factor (LIF), cardiotrophin 1, and oncostatin M have promyelinating function *(36)*. Insulin-like growth factor 1 (IGF-1) has been shown to promote remyelination by some investi-gators *(37)* but not others *(38)*. IGF-1 may, in addition, have antiapoptotic proper-ties for oligodendrocytes *(39)*.

Antioxidant therapies, because of their ability to interfere with pathways that culminate in apoptosis, will likely be included in the neuroprotection armamen-tarium for EAE *(40)*. For instance, metallothionein-II has antioxidant, antiinflam-matory, neuroprotective, and oligodendrocyte-generating action in the Lewis rat model of EAE *(41)*. The author has demonstrated that the histone deacetylase

(HDAC) inhibitor small molecule drug Trichostatin A (TSA) has antiinflammatory properties and ameliorates MOG-induced EAE *(42)*. In addition, TSA has neuroprotective action, which, in part, results from inhibition of caspase activation (i.e., an antiapoptotic role). In vitro studies with TSA have demonstrated that indeed this drug is neuroprotective, inhibits caspase activation, and prevents neuronal death induced by prooxidants *(43)*. Interestingly, the histone deacetylase inhibition properties of the anticonvulsant drug valproic acid may underlie its in vitro neuroprotective function *(44)*. Furthermore, HDAC inhibitors enhance production of the immunosuppresive and regulatory factor TGF-β1 *(45)*, and regulatory T-cells have been proposed to exert neuroprotection in EAE *(46)*.

Neurotransmitters have also been implicated in oligodendrogliogenesis. The role of the muscarinic, dopamine, and α-amino-3-hydroxy-5-methylisoxazole-4-propionic acid (AMPA)/kainate receptors is being studied *(47)*, and antiglutamatergic drugs ameliorate EAE *(48)*. Others have shown that the antibiotic minocycline blocks caspase activation and also has neuroprotective function in EAE *(49–51)*. A combination of drugs with purported neuroprotective effects will likely lead to rational approaches to preventing disability in MS.

Axonal loss correlates with disability in the EAE model *(52)*. It has become clear that even in acute MS lesions there is axonal and neuronal loss *(1,53)* and that, at least in part, this loss results from programmed cell death. Therefore, attempts at protecting neurons and the existing pools of progenitor cells should be aimed at counteracting the predominant proapoptotic pathways involved in the disease. The fas and TNF-α proapoptotic pathways are primary effectors for neuronal death in EAE. Downstream cascades culminate in activation of caspases 8, 9, and 3, effectors in the signaling of cell death. Recent studies in EAE have shown that overexpression of the prosurvival gene Bcl2 protects mice primed to develop EAE *(54)*. Methods of enhancing prosurvival pathways (i.e., neurotrophin-triggered transduction signals) are also being investigated *(55)*.

Neuronal growth factor (NGF) enhances neural growth and also has the ability to switch the T-cell phenotype from Th1 (proinflammatory) to Th2 (prohumoral, modulatory) *(56)*. This strategy may be beneficial in neuroprotection, because the Th2 cytokine interleukin (IL)-10 reduces CNS tissue loss after contusion in experimental models *(57)*. However, even factors that play proinflammatory roles, such as IL-1β, may trigger remyelination *(37)*. Most likely, the combined and rational use of neurotrophins and cytokines will be beneficial to any attempts to preserve integrity of neurons and oligodendrocytes.

Besides resulting in damage to oligodendrocytes and neurons, tissue destruction by infiltrating immune cells eventually leads to extracellular matrix (ECM) disintegration and gliosis. Matrix metalloproteinases (MMPs) from perivascular macrophages have been implicated in the proteolytic damage to MS BBB and brain tissue, leading to a milieu that counteracts myelin or axonal repair *(58)*, and, therefore, inhibitors of these molecules have been proposed for the treatment of MS *(59)*. Similarly, ECM proteoglycans participate differentially in plaque tissue, delimiting the border zones and presumably affecting repair ability at the center of the lesion *(60)*. The role of axon-glial interactions is crucial to homeostasis in the white matter, and understanding these interactions may lead to better approaches at preventing chronic demyelination (i.e., creating the ideal environment for tissue repair to occur). Furthermore, understanding the key molecules that participate in axonal guidance after injury will be important for any repair strategies.

CELL TRANSPLANTATION

The use of cell transplants is increasingly being proposed to repopulate areas of brain damage in MS, stroke, and neurodegenerative disorders *(61)*. Unfortunately, the use of progenitor cells is limited by serious ethical and technical considerations related to their potential use in humans. Their general use in animal models to highlight their potential is discussed.

Embryonic or Adult Neural Stem Cells and Hematopoietic Stem Cells

These cells are pluripotent and can be expanded and differentiated in vitro. Unfortunately, multiple limitations exist for their use, including the inability to direct their migration, the multifocality of lesions, and the presence of ongoing inflammation in MS. Furthermore, it is unknown if transplanted stem cells may, in some individuals, trigger a more aggressive autoimmune reaction, resulting in disease worsening, or if concomitant treatment with immune modulators or immunosuppressors may alter the ability of transplanted cells to repopulate lesion areas. Another caveat is the current inability to monitor the progress of repopulation by stem cells or their ability to repair myelin in vivo. Studies in rats have shown that neural stem cells injected intrathecally become engrafted into the lesioned spinal cord and differentiate into oligodendrocytes and astrocytes, with some behaving as Schwann cells near the adjacent nerve roots *(62)*. Neural stem cells isolated from adult brain biopsies could potentially be used for repopulating neurons in areas of tissue damage. Importantly, recent data suggest that stem cell transplantation is protective in EAE *(63)* and suppresses inflammation in MS *(64)*, but more studies regarding its long-term effects are needed.

Oligodendrocyte Progenitor Cells

OPCs from both newborn and adult mouse brains have been used for transplantation experiments and are ideal for myelin repair because of their preserved migratory and mitotic capabilities. Oligodendrocyte precursors can have beneficial effects in a canine myelin mutant model, whether transplanted in neonate or adult animals *(65)*. Recent reports have shown that in rats, it is also possible to deliver genetically transduced oligodendrocyte precursors into the ventricles and document their spreading throughout different brain regions *(66)*. This technique shows the versatility of the cells and their ability to penetrate transependymally to potential areas of damage.

Schwann Cells

Because these cells can be isolated from the sural nerve of a patient with MS and can be grown in vitro *(67,68)*, it is feasible to transplant them into the brain to accomplish remyelination *(69)*. A potential advantage, which remains speculative, would be that an autoimmune response may not be triggered by the autologous graft. Schwann cells have the ability to remyelinate areas of lysolecithin-induced demyelination in mouse spinal cord *(70)*. Recently, a Yale study led by Dr. Timothy Vollmer transplanted Schwann cells into the brain of three patients with MS (summary available at http:://www.myelin.org). This study showed that Schwann cell transplantation into the CNS is safe, but no evidence of long-term engraftment could be proved with the available techniques.

Olfactory Ensheathing Cells

Recently, the use of transplants of olfactory ensheathing cells (OECs), glial cells that wrap around the axons of the first cranial nerve, has been proposed as an alternative for delivering myelinating cells into MS lesions *(71,72)*. However, these techniques are fraught with multiple barriers, including the realization that the use of too many cells could be paradoxically deleterious *(73)*, bringing into question how it would be possible to learn to titrate the numbers of cells for the treatment of individual lesions. OECs exhibit characteristics of Schwann cells and astrocytes and could be obtained from the nasal mucosa of a patient with MS for autologous transplantation. OECs remyelinate the spinal cord of adult rats *(74)* and restore functions, such as breathing and climbing, in these animals *(75)*.

LESSONS LEARNED FROM NEUROPROTECTION STUDIES IN ISCHEMIA, INFECTION, TOXICITY, AND INJURY: POTENTIAL APPLICATION TO THE EAE MODEL

Both MS and EAE are influenced by inflammatory molecules, hormonal changes, excitotoxicity, and oxidant stress mechanisms. Manipulation of these pathways, some of which culminate in neuronal apoptosis, will likely lead to neuroprotection across CNS diseases that course with degeneration or inflammation. The following sections describe neuroprotective mechanisms in animal models of ischemia, infection, excitotoxicity, and injury, because some may have potential relevance to the EAE model.

Immune System Modulation

The promotion of regulatory immune cells that can penetrate the CNS and induce neuroprotection is achievable in animal models. For instance, activated myelin-specific regulatory T-cells can have neuroprotective properties in an animal model of CNS axotomy *(76)* via their ability to secrete neurotrophins *(77)*. Therapies that reduce TNF-α also have neuroprotective effects. For instance, cytokines, such as IL-10, reduce the production of TNF-α and exert neuroprotection via this pathway, as demonstrated in models of spinal cord injury *(78)*. SB239063, a p38 mitogen-activated protein kinase (p38MAPK) inhibitor, reduces the production of IL-1 and TNF-α and has neuroprotective effects in a focal ischemic stroke rat model *(79)*. Immunosuppressants, such as FK506, which binds the intracellular proteins FKBPs, also have neuroprotective properties in rat models of ischemia *(80)*. Furthermore, cyclosporin A inhibits calcium-induced mitochondrial damage and prevents axonal loss in traumatic injury models *(81)*. Finally, NR58-3.14.3, a broad-spectrum chemokine inhibitor, exerts neuroprotection in a rat model of brain ischemia-reperfusion injury *(82)*.

Blockade of Excitotoxicity or Calcium Entry

Intracortical injections of *N*-methyl-D-aspartate (NMDA) results in tissue damage that can be ameliorated by oral triflusal, and the underlying mechanism may involve attenuation of expression of inducible nitric oxide synthase (iNOS) expression and proinflammatory molecules, such as TNF-α, IL-1β, and COX-2 *(83)*. Ifenprodil and eliprodil are noncompetitive NMDA receptor antagonists that inhibit calcium channel currents and protect brain tissue from experimentally induced hippocampal ischemia in gerbils *(84)*. It has also been demonstrated that the combined use of antagonists for the excitotoxicity receptors AMPA (GYKI-52466) and NMDA (MK-801) achieves better neuroprotection than the use of each agent alone *(85)*. MK-801 ameliorates hippocampal degeneration induced in hamsters by the measles virus *(86)*. Drugs that inhibit glutamate release presynaptically, such as 2-chloroadenosine, also exert neuroprotection in kainic acid-injured rat striatum *(87)*. Unfortunately, drugs that block excitotoxic pathway receptors, such as AMPA, have not been successful in human trials, resulting, in part, from poor water solubility and renal toxicity *(88)*.

Strategies to counteract downstream pathways that mediate the effects of glutamate are also neuroprotective. These include blockade of the glutamate-induced calpain activity with the calpain inhibitor MDL-28170 and blockade of the NOS enzyme with its antagonist NG-nitro-L-arginine *(89)*. Apolipoprotein E (apo E) also protects neurons against NMDA excitotoxicity in vitro *(90)*. In a rat model of kainic acid-induced neurodegeneration, estradiol or estradiol plus progesterone prevents hilar neuronal loss when injected simultaneously with kainic acid in ovariectomized animals *(91)*. Estrogen-induced neuroprotection is related to its antioxidant properties *(92,93)* by acting as a free radical scavenger and preventing the intracellular accumulation of peroxides. Estrogen treatment is also effective in ameliorating EAE *(94,95)*.

Blockade of Calcium or Sodium Channels

Calcium channel blockers reduce the extent of brain or spinal cord ischemia in animal models *(96,97)*. Flunarizine is a calcium channel blocker that at low doses can prevent ischemia-induced brain injury in fetal sheep *(98)*. Similarly, the selective N-type calcium channel blocker ziconotide reduces ischemia-induced spinal cord injury *(99)*.

The rise in intracellular sodium is intimately linked to calcium entry and increased cellular energy demands. Thus, sodium channel blockers may also be used as neuroprotective agents. Indeed, drugs that redistribute regional cerebral blood flow and block sodium channels such as vinpocetine (ethyl apovincaminate) have been shown in experimental models to exert neuroprotection *(100)*. Antiepileptic drugs that modulate sodium channels, such as lamotrigine, riluzole, verapamil, and diphenylhydantoin, are neuroprotective in slices of hippocampus injured by the sodium channel activator veratridine *(101)*. In addition, the sodium-potassium adenosine triphosphate (ATP)ase pump, which extrudes intracellular sodium, and drugs that reduce extracellular sodium can be manipulated to exert neuroprotection *(102)*. Blockade of the sodium-hydrogen exchanger may result in reduction in intracellular acidosis and thus lead to neuroprotection *(102)*.

Drugs With Mitochondrial Effects

Creatine monohydrate has neuroprotective effects, when injected subcutaneously, in a transient cerebral hypoxia-ischemia model. Creatine may work by maintaining energy metabolism (prevent energy failure), preventing calcium overload, counteracting mitochondrial permeability transition pore opening, enhancing cytoplasmic high-energy phosphates *(103)*, and exerting antioxidant effects *(104)*.

Antioxidants and Metal-Ion Chelators

Studies in immature brains *(105)* have shown that administration of α-phenyl-*N-tert*-butylnitrone (PBN), a known superoxide scavenger, attenuates both H_2O_2- and NMDA-mediated toxicity. However, desferrioxamine (DFX), an iron chelator, is only effective when given before the administration of H_2O_2. TPEN, a metal chelator with higher affinities for a broad spectrum of transition metal ions, protects against H_2O_2 toxicity but not against NMDA-induced damage.

Neurotransmitter-Mediated Protection

Neurotransmitters from specific regions of the brain can also exert neuroprotective effects on neurons. For instance, dopamine serves as a trophic factor to striatal neurons, protecting them against glutamate receptor-mediated excitotoxicity *(106)*. Potentiators of γ-aminobutyric acid (GABA) receptor-mediated ion fluxes, such as isoflurane, also have neuroprotective properties *(107)*.

Vitamins and Neuroprotection

Vitamin D hormone (1,25-dihydroxyvitamin D[3]) modulates L-type voltage-sensitive Ca^{2+} channels (L-VSCCs) and confers neuroprotection in stroke animal models and in hippocampal slice cultures *(108)*. Antioxidants such as vitamin E exert neuroprotection via their ability to modulate activity of the transcription factor NF-κB (NF-κB), which is implicated in survival pathways *(109)*. Ascorbic acid may reduce NMDA toxicity via blocking of calcium influx, resulting in reduced nitrous oxide induction *(110)*.

The Role of Trophic Factors in Neuroprotection

Cell populations may have different responses to excitotoxic or oxidant insult by upregulating the expression of neurotrophic factors that may be disease- or brain region-specific. Glial-derived neurotrophic factor (GDNF) and neurotrophins 3 and 4 become upregulated following intrastriatal injection of glutamate receptor agonists *(111)*. FGF2 mRNA is upregulated in astrocytes after brain injury and, when tested in animal models of stroke or excitotoxic damage, has neuroprotective action. This action results, in part, from its ability to modulate ROS detoxifying enzymes and calcium homeostasis and promote neurogenesis *(112)*. Finally, GM1 gangliosides and their semisynthetic component LIGA20 activate the Trk neurotrophin receptors in cerebellar granule cells and thus prevent glutamate induced injury *(113)*.

CONCLUSIONS

MS has puzzled investigators for its complexity and heterogeneity. Genomic techniques such as DNA microarrays, proteomics, and the study of single nucleotide polymorphisms (SNPs), are now increasingly being used to decipher potential molecular clues of this multifactorial disease *(4,5)*. The unveiling of these disease-associated biomarkers and pathways will likely translate into identifying potential targets of treatment. Recognizing patients with MS who are at risk for oligodendrocyte apoptosis, for instance, will help tailor individual myelin repair techniques exclusively for this group of patients. Identification of molecular pathways involved in neural protection could be harnessed for the early rescue of neurons to prevent disability in MS. Therefore, the identification of genetic polymorphisms associated with clinical disability and neuronal damage is key to identifying targets of treatment. An example is the apoE ε4 allele, which has been correlated with enhanced MS severity *(114,115)* and enhanced susceptibility to developing MRI T1 holes *(116)*.

Animal research brings important insight into mechanisms playing a role in disease processes, but, unfortunately, extrapolating beneficial effects of animal treatments into human disease, especially in the field of MS, has been disappointing. A more thorough understanding of how truly versatile stem cells are for their use in human neurodegenerative diseases is needed. This includes a better understanding of how stem cells are influenced by the tissue milieu into which they are transplanted, the optimal routes of delivery, and the potential occurrence of untoward effects. Knowledge of these pitfalls will facilitate strategies for making the environment permissive for remyelination attempts. Methods for monitoring degree of remyelination in humans are also needed; magnetization transfer ratios (MTRs) in experimental models of demyelination have shown that indeed magnetic resonance techniques may be used for this purpose *(117)*, but more accurate techniques that detect remyelination at the cellular level are required. The application of known neuroprotective drugs to the EAE model will yield new information regarding novel strategies to prevent neuronal and axonal loss. Finally, the exploration of the use of embryonic stem cells as repair and protective agents in humans is complicated by serious ethical and technical considerations.

REFERENCES

1. Trapp BD, Ransohoff R, Rudick R. Axonal pathology in multiple sclerosis: relationship to neurologic disability. Curr Opin Neurol 1999;12:295–302.
2. Noseworthy JH, Lucchinetti C, Rodriguez M, Weinshenker BG. Multiple sclerosis. N Engl J Med 2000;343:938–952.
3. Paz Soldan MM, Rodriguez M. Heterogeneity of pathogenesis in multiple sclerosis: implications for promotion of remyelination. J Infect Dis 2002;186(Suppl 2):S248–S253.
4. Dangond F. From Genetics to Genomics and Proteomics. New technologies in myelin research. In: Dangond F, ed., Disorders of Myelin in the Central and Peripheral Nervous Systems. Butterworth-Heinemann, Boston, 2002, p. 355–363.
5. Iglesias AH, Camelo S, Hwang D, Villanueva R, Stephanopoulos G, Dangond F. Microarray detection of E2F pathway activation and other targets in multiple sclerosis peripheral blood mononuclear cells. J Neuroimmunol 2004;150:163–177.
6. Blakemore WF. Pattern of remyelination in the CNS. Nature 1974;249:577.
7. Stangel M, Hartung HP. Remyelinating strategies for the treatment of multiple sclerosis. Prog Neurobiol 2002;68:361–376.
8. John GR, Shankar SL, Shafit-Zagardo B, et al. Multiple sclerosis: re-expression of a developmental pathway that restricts oligodendrocyte maturation. Nat Med 2002;8:1115–1121.
9. Murray PD, McGavern DB, Sathornsumetee S, Rodriguez M. Spontaneous remyelination following extensive demyelination is associated with improved neurological function in a viral model of multiple sclerosis. Brain 2001;124:1403–1416.
10. Smith EJ, Blakemore WF, McDonald WI. Central remyelination restores secure conduction. Nature 1979;280:395–396.
11. Smith KJ, Blakemore WF, McDonald WI. The restoration of conduction by central remyelination. Brain 1981;104:383–404.
12. Linington C, Bradl M, Lassmann H, Brunner C, Vass K. Augmentation of demyelination in rat acute allergic encephalomyelitis by circulating mouse monoclonal antibodies directed against a myelin/oligodendrocyte glycoprotein. Am J Pathol 1988;130:443–454.
13. Raine CS, Cannella B, Hauser SL, Genain CP. Demyelination in primate autoimmune encephalomyelitis and acute multiple sclerosis lesions: a case for antigen-specific antibody mediation. Ann Neurol 1999;46:144–160.
14. Genain CP, Cannella B, Hauser SL, Raine CS. Identification of autoantibodies associated with myelin damage in multiple sclerosis. Nat Med 1999;5:170–175.
15. Miller DJ, Bright JJ, Sriram S, Rodriguez M. Successful treatment of established relapsing experimental autoimmune encephalomyelitis in mice with a monoclonal natural autoantibody. J Neuroimmunol 1997;75:204–209.
16. Rodriguez M, Lennon VA. Immunoglobulins promote remyelination in the central nervous system. Ann Neurol 1990;27:12–17.
17. Rodriguez M, Miller DJ, Lennon VA. Immunoglobulins reactive with myelin basic protein promote CNS remyelination. Neurology 1996;46:538–545.
18. Wilkins A, Chandran S, Compston A. A role for oligodendrocyte-derived IGF-1 in trophic support of cortical neurons. Glia 2001;36:48–57.
19. Taniike M, Mohri I, Eguchi N, Beuckmann CT, Suzuki K, Urade Y. Perineuronal oligodendrocytes protect against neuronal apoptosis through the production of lipocalin-type prostaglandin D synthase in a genetic demyelinating model. J Neurosci 2002;22:4885–4896.
20. Wu HY, Dawson MR, Reynolds R, Hardy RJ. Expression of QKI proteins and MAP1B identifies actively myelinating oligodendrocytes in adult rat brain. Mol Cell Neurosci 2001;17:292–302.

21. Scolding N, Franklin R, Stevens S, Heldin CH, Compston A, Newcombe J. Oligodendrocyte progenitors are present in the normal adult human CNS and in the lesions of multiple sclerosis. Brain 1998;121:2221–2228.
22. Tourbah A, Linnington C, Bachelin C, Avellana-Adalid V, Wekerle H, Baron-Van Evercooren A. Inflammation promotes survival and migration of the CG4 oligodendrocyte progenitors transplanted in the spinal cord of both inflammatory and demyelinated EAE rats. J Neurosci Res 1997;50:853–861.
23. Wolswijk G. Chronic stage multiple sclerosis lesions contain a relatively quiescent population of oligodendrocyte precursor cells. J Neurosci 1998;18:601–609.
24. Wolswijk G. Oligodendrocyte survival, loss and birth in lesions of chronic-stage multiple sclerosis. Brain 2000;123:105–115.
25. Wolswijk G. Oligodendrocyte precursor cells in the demyelinated multiple sclerosis spinal cord. Brain 2002;125:338–349.
26. Gensert JM, Goldman JE. Endogenous progenitors remyelinate demyelinated axons in the adult CNS. Neuron 1997;19:197–203.
27. Jones SJ, Brusa A. Neurophysiological evidence for long-term repair of MS lesions: implications for axon protection. J Neurol Sci 2003;206:193–198.
28. Carmody RJ, Hilliard B, Maguschak K, Chodosh LA, Chen YH. Genomic scale profiling of autoimmune inflammation in the central nervous system: the nervous response to inflammation. J Neuroimmunol 2002;133:95–107.
29. Rodriguez M, Miller DJ. Immune promotion of central nervous system remyelination. Prog Brain Res 1994;103:343–355.
30. Warrington AE, Bieber AJ, Ciric B, et al. Immunoglobulin-mediated CNS repair. J Allergy Clin Immunol 2001;108:S121–S125.
31. Ure DR, Rodriguez M. Polyreactive antibodies to glatiramer acetate promote myelin repair in murine model of demyelinating disease. FASEB J 2002;16:1260–1262.
32. Gilgun-Sherki Y, Panet H, Holdengreber V, Mosberg-Galili R, Offen D. Axonal damage is reduced following glatiramer acetate treatment in C57/bl mice with chronic-induced experimental autoimmune encephalomyelitis. Neurosci Res 2003;47:201–207.
33. Stangel M, Compston A, Scolding NJ. Oligodendroglia are protected from antibody-mediated complement injury by normal immunoglobulins ("IVIg"). J Neuroimmunol 2000;103:195–201.
34. Frost EE, Nielsen JA, Le TQ, Armstrong RC. PDGF and FGF2 regulate oligodendrocyte progenitor responses to demyelination. J Neurobiol 2003;54:457–472.
35. Marchionni MA, Cannella B, Hoban C, et al. Neuregulin in neuron/glial interactions in the central nervous system. GGF2 diminishes autoimmune demyelination, promotes oligodendrocyte progenitor expansion, and enhances remyelination. Adv Exp Med Biol 1999;468:283–295.
36. Stankoff B, Aigrot MS, Noel F, Wattilliaux A, Zalc B, Lubetzki C. Ciliary neurotrophic factor (CNTF) enhances myelin formation: a novel role for CNTF and CNTF-related molecules. J Neurosci 2002;22:9221–9227.
37. Mason JL, Suzuki K, Chaplin DD, Matsushima GK. Interleukin-1beta promotes repair of the CNS. J Neurosci 2001;21:7046–7052.
38. Cannella B, Pitt D, Capello E, Raine CS. Insulin-like growth factor-1 fails to enhance central nervous system myelin repair during autoimmune demyelination. Am J Pathol 2000;157:933–943.
39. Mason JL, Ye P, Suzuki K, D'Ercole AJ, Matsushima GK. Insulin-like growth factor-1 inhibits mature oligodendrocyte apoptosis during primary demyelination. J Neurosci 2000;20:5703–5708.
40. Hooper DC, Bagasra O, Marini JC, et al. Prevention of experimental allergic encephalomyelitis by targeting nitric oxide and peroxynitrite: implications for the treatment of multiple sclerosis. Proc Natl Acad Sci U S A 1997;94:2528–2533.
41. Penkowa M, Hidalgo J. Treatment with metallothionein prevents demyelination and axonal damage and increases oligodendrocyte precursors and tissue repair during experimental autoimmune encephalomyelitis. J Neurosci Res 2003;72:574–586.

42. Camelo S, Iglesias AH, Hwang D, et al. The Histone deacetylase inhibitor trichostatin A ameliorates murine experimental encephalomyelitis, a model of multiple sclerosis. Am Assoc Neuropathol Mtg, Platform Presentation, Cleveland, OH, 2004.

43. Ryu H, Lee J, Olofsson BA, et al. Histone deacetylase inhibitors prevent oxidative neuronal death independent of expanded polyglutamine repeats via an Sp1-dependent pathway. Proc Natl Acad Sci U S A 2003;100:4281–4286.

44. Jeong MR, Hashimoto R, Senatorov VV, et al. Valproic acid, a mood stabilizer and anticonvulsant, protects rat cerebral cortical neurons from spontaneous cell death: a role of histone deacetylase inhibition. FEBS Lett 2003;542:74–78.

45. Moreira JM, Scheipers P, Sorensen P. The histone deacetylase inhibitor Trichostatin A modulates CD4+ T cell responses. BMC Cancer 2003;3:30.

46. Kohm AP, Carpentier PA, Miller SD. Regulation of experimental autoimmune encephalomyelitis (EAE) by CD4+CD25+ regulatory T cells. Novartis Found Symp 2003;252:45–52.

47. Belachew S, Rogister B, Rigo JM, Malgrange B, Moonen G. Neurotransmitter-mediated regulation of CNS myelination: a review. Acta Neurol Belg 1999;99:21–31.

48. Gilgun-Sherki Y, Panet H, Melamed E, Offen D. Riluzole suppresses experimental autoimmune encephalomyelitis: implications for the treatment of multiple sclerosis. Brain Res 2003;989:196–204.

49. Nessler S, Dodel R, Bittner A, et al. Effect of minocycline in experimental autoimmune encephalomyelitis. Ann Neurol 2002;52:689–690.

50. Brundula V, Rewcastle NB, Metz LM, Bernard CC, Yong VW. Targeting leukocyte MMPs and transmigration: minocycline as a potential therapy for multiple sclerosis. Brain 2002;125:1297–1308.

51. Popovic N, Schubart A, Goetz BD, Zhang SC, Linington C, Duncan ID. Inhibition of autoimmune encephalomyelitis by a tetracycline. Ann Neurol 2002;51:215–223.

52. Wujek JR, Bjartmar C, Richer E, et al. Axon loss in the spinal cord determines permanent neurological disability in an animal model of multiple sclerosis. J Neuropathol Exp Neurol 2002;61:23–32.

53. Peterson JW, Bo L, Mork S, Chang A, Trapp BD. Transected neurites, apoptotic neurons, and reduced inflammation in cortical multiple sclerosis lesions. Ann Neurol 2001;50:389–400.

54. Offen D, Kaye JF, Bernard O, et al. Mice overexpressing Bcl-2 in their neurons are resistant to myelin oligodendrocyte glycoprotein (MOG)-induced experimental autoimmune encephalomyelitis (EAE). J Mol Neurosci 2000;15:167–176.

55. Ebadi M, Bashir RM, Heidrick ML, et al. Neurotrophins and their receptors in nerve injury and repair. Neurochem Int 1997;30:347–374.

56. Villoslada P, Hauser SL, Bartke I, et al.Human nerve growth factor protects common marmosets against autoimmune encephalomyelitis by switching the balance of T helper cell type 1 and 2 cytokines within the central nervous system. J Exp Med 2000;191:1799–1806.

57. Takami T, Oudega M, Bethea JR, Wood PM, Kleitman N, Bunge MB. Methylprednisolone and interleukin-10 reduce gray matter damage in the contused Fischer rat thoracic spinal cord but do not improve functional outcome. J Neurotrauma 2002;19:653–666.

58. Maeda A, Sobel RA.. Matrix metalloproteinases in the normal human central nervous system, microglial nodules, and multiple sclerosis lesions. J Neuropathol Exp Neurol 1996;55:300–309.

59. Rosenberg GA. Matrix metalloproteinases and neuroinflammation in multiple sclerosis. Neuroscientist 2002;8:586–595.

60. Sobel RA, Ahmed AS. White matter extracellular matrix chondroitin sulfate/dermatan sulfate proteoglycans in multiple sclerosis. J Neuropathol Exp Neurol 2001;60:1198–1207.

61. Savitz SL, Malhotra A, Gupta G, Rosenbaum DM. Cell transplants offer promise for stroke recovery. J Cardiovasc Nurs 2003;18:57–61.

62. Wu S, Suzuki Y, Noda T, et al. Immunohistochemical and electron microscopic study of invasion and differentiation in spinal cord lesion of neural stem cells grafted through cerebrospinal fluid in rat. J Neurosci Res 2002;69:940–945.

63. Pluchino S, Quattrini A, Brambilla E, et al. Injection of adult neurospheres induces recovery in a chronic model of multiple sclerosis. Nature 2003;422:688–694.
64. Muraro PA, Ingoni RC, Martin R. Hematopoietic stem cell transplantation for multiple sclerosis: current status and future challenges. Curr Opin Neurol 2003;16:299–308.
65. Archer DR, Cuddon PA, Lipsitz D, Duncan ID. Myelination of the canine central nervous system by glial cell transplantation: a model for repair of human myelin disease. Nat Med 1997;3:54–59.
66. Learish RD, Brustle O, Zhang SC, Duncan ID. Intraventricular transplantation of oligodendrocyte progenitors into a fetal myelin mutant results in widespread formation of myelin. Ann Neurol 1999;46:716–722.
67. Van den Berg LH, Bar PR, Sodaar P, Mollee I, Wokke JJ, Logtenberg T. Selective expansion and long-term culture of human Schwann cells from sural nerve biopsies. Ann Neurol 1995;38:674–678.
68. Rutkowski JL, Kirk CJ, Lerner MA, Tennekoon GI.. Purification and expansion of human Schwann cells in vitro. Nat Med 1995;1:80–83.
69. Harrison BM. Remyelination by cells introduced into a stable demyelinating lesion in the central nervous system. J Neurol Sci 1980;46:63–81.
70. Baron-Van Evercooren A, Gansmuller A, Duhamel E, Pascal F, Gumpel M. Repair of a myelin lesion by Schwann cells transplanted in the adult mouse spinal cord. J Neuroimmunol 1992;40:235–342.
71. Boyd JG, Skihar V, Kawaja M, Doucette R. Olfactory ensheathing cells: Historical perspective and therapeutic potential. Anat Rec 2003;271B:49–60.
72. Franklin RJ. Remyelination by transplanted olfactory ensheathing cells. Anat Rec 2003; 271B:71–76.
73. Lakatos A, Smith PM, Barnett SC, Franklin RJ. Meningeal cells enhance limited CNS remyelination by transplanted olfactory ensheathing cells. Brain 2003;126:598–609.
74. Barnett SC, Alexander CL, Iwashita Y, et al. Identification of a human olfactory ensheathing cell that can effect transplant-mediated remyelination of demyelinated CNS axons. Brain 2000;123 (Pt 8):1581–1588.
75. Li Y, Decherchi P, Raisman G. Transplantation of olfactory ensheathing cells into spinal cord lesions restores breathing and climbing. J Neurosci 2003;23:727–731.
76. Moalem G, Leibowitz-Amit R, Yoles E, Mor R, Cohen IR, Schwartz M. Autoimmune T cells protect neurons from secondary degeneration after central nervous system axotomy. Nature Medicine 1999;5:49–55.
77. Moalem G, Gdalyahu A, Shani Y, et al. Production of neurotrophins by activated T cells: implications for neuroprotective autoimmunity. J Autoimmun 2000;15:331–345.
78. Bethea JR, Nagashima H, Acosta MC, et al. Systemically administered interleukin-10 reduces tumor necrosis factor-alpha production and significantly improves functional recovery following traumatic spinal cord injury in rats. J Neurotrauma 1999;16:851–863.
79. Barone FC, Irving EA, Ray AM, et al. Inhibition of p38 mitogen-activated protein kinase provides neuroprotection in cerebral focal ischemia. Med Res Rev 2001;21:129–145.
80. Brecht S, Schwarze K, Waetzig V, et al. Changes in peptidyl-prolyl cis/trans isomerase activity and fk506 binding protein expression following neuroprotection by fk506 in the ischemic rat brain. Neuroscience 2003;120:1037–1048.
81. Buki A, Okonkwo DO, Povlishock JT. Postinjury cyclosporin A administration limits axonal damage and disconnection in traumatic brain injury. J Neurotrauma 1999;16:511–521.
82. Beech JS, Reckless J, Mosedale DE, Grainger DJ, Williams SC, Menon DK. Neuroprotection in ischemia-reperfusion injury: an antiinflammatory approach using a novel broad-spectrum chemokine inhibitor. J Cereb Blood Flow Metab 2001;21:683–689.
83. Acarin L, Gonzalez B, Castellano B. Decrease of proinflammatory molecules correlates with neuroprotective effect of the fluorinated salicylate triflusal after postnatal excitotoxic damage. Stroke 2002;33:2499–2505.
84. Bath CP, Farrell LN, Gilmore J, et al. The effects of ifenprodil and eliprodil on voltage-dependent Ca2+ channels and in gerbil global cerebral ischaemia. Eur J Pharmacol 1996;299:103–1120.

85. Arias RL, Tasse JR, Bowlby MR. Neuroprotective interaction effects of NMDA and AMPA receptor antagonists in an in vitro model of cerebral ischemia. Brain Res 1999;816:299–308.

86. Andersson T, Schwarcz R, Love A, Kristensson K. Measles virus-induced hippocampal neurodegeneration in the mouse: a novel, subacute model for testing neuroprotective agents. Neurosci Lett 1993;154:109–112.

87. Arvin B, Neville LF, Pan J, Roberts PJ. 2-chloroadenosine attenuates kainic acid-induced toxicity within the rat striatum: relationship to release of glutamate and Ca2+ influx. Br J Pharmacol 1989;98:225–235.

88. Akins PT, Atkinson RP. Glutamate AMPA receptor antagonist treatment for ischaemic stroke. Curr Med Res Opin 2002;18(Suppl 2):S9–S13.

89. Brorson JR,. Marcuccilli CJ, Miller RJ. Delayed antagonism of calpain reduces excitotoxicity in cultured neurons. Stroke 1995;26:1259–1266.

90. Aono M, Lee Y, Grant ER, et al. Apolipoprotein E protects against NMDA excitotoxicity. Neurobiol Dis 2002;11:214–220.

91. Azcoitia I, Fernandez-Galaz C, Sierra A, Garcia-Segura LM. Gonadal hormones affect neuronal vulnerability to excitotoxin-induced degeneration. J Neurocytol 1999;28:699–710.

92. Behl C, Skutella T, Lezoualc'h F, et al. Neuroprotection against oxidative stress by estrogens: structure-activity relationship. Mol Pharmacol 1997;51:535–541.

93. Bae YH, Hwang JY, Kim YH, Koh JY. Anti-oxidative neuroprotection by estrogens in mouse cortical cultures. J Korean Med Sci 2000;15:327–336.

94. Bebo BFJ, Fyfe-Johnson A, Adlard K, Beam AG, Vandenbark AA, Offner H. Low-dose estrogen therapy ameliorates experimental autoimmune encephalomyelitis in two different inbred mouse strains. J Immunol 2001;166:2080–2089.

95. Trooster WJ, Teelken AW, Kampinga J, Loof JG, Nieuwenhuis P, Minderhoud JM. Suppression of acute experimental allergic encephalomyelitis by the synthetic sex hormone 17-alpha-ethinylestradiol: an immunological study in the Lewis rat. Int Arch Allergy Immunol 1993;102:133–140.

96. Barone FC, Price WJ, Jakobsen P, Sheardown MJ, Feuerstein G. Pharmacological profile of a novel neuronal calcium channel blocker includes reduced cerebral damage and neurological deficits in rat focal ischemia. Pharmacol Biochem Behav 1994;48:77–85.

97. Barone FC, Lysko PG, Price WJ, et al. SB 201823-A antagonizes calcium currents in central neurons and reduces the effects of focal ischemia in rats and mice. Stroke 1995;26:1683–1690.

98. Berger R, Lehmann T, Karcher J, Garnier Y, Jensen A. Low dose flunarizine protects the fetal brain from ischemic injury in sheep. Pediatr Res 1998;44:277–282.

99. Burns LH, Jin Z, Bowersox SS. The neuroprotective effects of intrathecal administration of the selective N-type calcium channel blocker ziconotide in a rat model of spinal ischemia. J Vasc Surg 1999;30:334–343.

100. Adam-Vizi V. [Neuroprotective effect of sodium channel blockers in ischemia: the pathomechanism of early ischemic dysfunction]. Orv Hetil 2000;141:1279–1286.

101. Ashton D, Willems R, Wynants J, Van Reempts J, Marrannes R, Clincke G. Altered Na(+)-channel function as an in vitro model of the ischemic penumbra: action of lubeluzole and other neuroprotective drugs. Brain Res 1997;745:210–221.

102. Agrawal SK, Fehlings MG. Mechanisms of secondary injury to spinal cord axons in vitro: role of Na+, Na(+)-K(+)-ATPase, the Na(+)-H+ exchanger, and the Na(+)-Ca2+ exchanger. J Neurosci 1996;16:545–552.

103. Brustovetsky N, Brustovetsky T, Dubinsky JM. On the mechanisms of neuroprotection by creatine and phosphocreatine. J Neurochem 2001;76:425–434.

104. Adcock KH, Nedelcu J, Loenneker T, Martin E, Wallimann T, Wagner BP. Neuroprotection of creatine supplementation in neonatal rats with transient cerebral hypoxia-ischemia. Dev Neurosci 2002;24:382–338.

105. Almli LM, Hamrick SE, Koshy AA, Tauber MG, Ferriero DM. Multiple pathways of neuroprotection against oxidative stress and excitotoxic injury in immature primary hippocampal neurons. Brain Res Dev Brain Res 2001;132:121–129.

106. Amano T, Ujihara H, Matsubayashi H, et al. Dopamine-induced protection of striatal neurons against kainate receptor-mediated glutamate cytotoxicity in vitro. Brain Res 1994;655:61–69.
107. Bickler PE, Warner DS, Stratmann G, Schuyler JA. gamma-Aminobutyric acid-A receptors contribute to isoflurane neuroprotection in organotypic hippocampal cultures. Anesth Analg 2003;97:564–571.
108. Brewer LD, Thibault V, Chen KC, et al. Vitamin D hormone confers neuroprotection in parallel with downregulation of L-type calcium channel expression in hippocampal neurons. J Neurosci 2001;21:98–108.
109. Behl C. Vitamin E protects neurons against oxidative cell death in vitro more effectively than 17-beta estradiol and induces the activity of the transcription factor NF-kappaB. J Neural Transm 2000;107:393–407.
110. Bell JA, Beglan CL, London ED. Interaction of ascorbic acid with the neurotoxic effects of NMDA and sodium nitroprusside. Life Sci 1996;58:367–371.
111. Alberch J, Perez-Navarro E, Canals JM. Neuroprotection by neurotrophins and GDNF family members in the excitotoxic model of Huntington's disease. Brain Res Bull 2002;57:817–822.
112. Alzheimer C, Werner S. Fibroblast growth factors and neuroprotection. Adv Exp Med Biol 2002;513:335–351.
113. Bachis A, Rabin SJ, Del Fiacco M, Mocchetti I. Gangliosides prevent excitotoxicity through activation of TrkB receptor. Neurotox Res 2002;4:225–234.
114. Fazekas F, Strasser-Fuchs S, Kollegger H, et al. Apolipoprotein E epsilon 4 is associated with rapid progression of multiple sclerosis. Neurology 2001;57:853–857.
115. Chapman J, Sylantiev C, Nisipeanu P, Korczyn AD. Preliminary observations on APOE epsilon4 allele and progression of disability in multiple sclerosis. Arch Neurol 1999;56:1484–1487.
116. Fazekas F, Strasser-Fuchs S, Schmidt H, et al. Apolipoprotein E genotype related differences in brain lesions of multiple sclerosis. J Neurol Neurosurg Psychiatry 2000;69:25–28.
117. Deloire-Grassin MS, Brochet B, Quesson B, et al. In vivo evaluation of remyelination in rat brain by magnetization transfer imaging. J Neurol Sci 2000;178:10–16.

12

Future Therapies for Multiple Sclerosis

Michael J. Olek, DO

INTRODUCTION

Future immunotherapy for immune-mediated neurologic diseases is in a state of rapid development. The current therapeutic arsenal consists of a mixture of older and new agents whose uses are actively being redefined. Our current understanding of mechanisms of action of established medications and developing approaches will be discussed in relation to disease pathogenesis models. Also, we will present a framework for incorporating current and future therapies into rational treatment strategies and will be addressed together with a review of relevant clinical studies. Mechanisms of immunotherapy and clinical strategies will be discussed in the context of multiple sclerosis (MS).

MECHANISTIC STRATEGIES FOR IMMUNE INTERVENTION

Most researchers would now agree that a T-cell mediated cellular immune response is central to the pathogenesis of MS. Although MS has not formally been proven to be a cell-mediated autoimmune disease directed against central nervous system (CNS) myelin, it is this hypothesis on which most investigators base their therapeutic strategies. Animal models for these more common neurologic immune mediated diseases have been developed. The approaches of immunotherapy or immunomodulation that are being applied to MS derive from treatment of experimental autoimmune encephalomyelitis (EAE), which has become the primary animal model for MS and from the application to MS of immunosuppressant and/or immunomodulatory drugs used for cancer, transplantation and other organ-specific inflammatory conditions. Whether EAE is a true model for MS remains an open question, but the application of immunotherapeutic strategies to MS has often stemmed from their success in EAE *(1)*. Furthermore, independent of its relationship to MS, EAE has become one of the prime immunologic paradigms for studying cellular mechanisms of experimental autoimmune disease used by immunologists. Animal models for the other neurologic immune mediated diseases will likely also serve a useful purpose in understanding the role of new therapeutic approaches in these diseases. There are a number of ways in which immune intervention can affect

From: *Current Clinical Neurology: Multiple Sclerosis*
Edited by: M. J. Olek © Humana Press Inc., Totowa, NJ

T-cell biology. Our current understanding of T-cell activation is that T-cells recognize antigens in the context of the major histocompatibility complex (MHC). Activation requires appropriate costimulatory signals by an antigen presenting cell. In MS, activated T-cells then migrate to the nervous system where they recognize the myelin antigen to which they were sensitized, release inflammatory cytokines, and initiate the destruction of the myelin sheath. Figure 1 depicts mechanisms by which immunotherapy may affect the autoimmune process in multiple sclerosis.

Anergy and Apoptosis

If disease is initiated by an antigen reactive T-cell then one strategy is to block the activation of such a cell by inducing anergy. As shown in Fig. 1, the triggering of a myelin reactive cell in MS may involve antigen presentation of a cross reactive antigen such as a virus or stimulation of the autoreactive T-cell by other mechanisms such as a superantigen *(2)*. The induction of anergy implies that the myelin reactive cell is paralyzed in a way that it is not functional and cannot therefore be activated to cause damage in the nervous system. Anergy can be induced if the myelin reactive cells encounter free antigen or an antigen is presented by a cell that does not have costimulatory properties such as B7. Of note is that orally administered antigens can induce anergy if free antigen enters the blood stream *(3)*. The B7/CD28 interaction is required for a disease-inducing T-cell (TH$_1$ type) to be activated. Alternately, some conditions (e.g., repeated exposure of activated cells to high doses of antigen) to agonists of some tumor necrosis factor (TNF) superfamily receptors *(4)*, or to superantigen can result in programmed cell death or apoptosis *(5)*. This strategy could be used to eliminate autoreactive cells and may also play a role in oral tolerance *(6)*.

Receptor Blockade

Three classes of receptor can be targeted for blockade: (1) adhesion molecules, (2) the T-cell recptor/major histocompatibility complex (TCR/MHC) complex, and (3) costimulatory molecules. In MS, myelin reactive T-cells include those with reactivity against proteolipid protein (PLP), myelin basic protein (MBP) or other

---

Fig. 1. (*opposite page*) Immune mechanisms and strategies of immunotherapy in MS.The major steps of the pathogenetic cascade are shown: (1) activation of autoreactive T-cells in the periphery/anergy induction, (2) transmigration of proinflammatory T-cells and monocytes through the blood–brain barrier/receptor blockade leading to autoreactive T-cells, (3) generation of regulatory cells to inactivate myelin-reactive cells or secrete cytokines that suppress inflammation at the target organ, and (4) effector stage of the disease, with damage of oligodendrocytes, myelin sheath and axons. A possible further stage, the resolution of lesions by regulatory mechanisms and remyelination, is not highlighted separately. *Abbr:* APC, antigen presenting cell; TNF, tumor necrosis factor; TCR, T-cell receptor; ICAM, intracellular adhesion molecule; MHC, major histocompatibilty complex; MMP-matrix metaloProtease; IL, interleukin ;VCAM, vascular cell adhesion molecule; IFN, interferon; LFA, leukocyte function antigen; TGF, transforming growth factor.

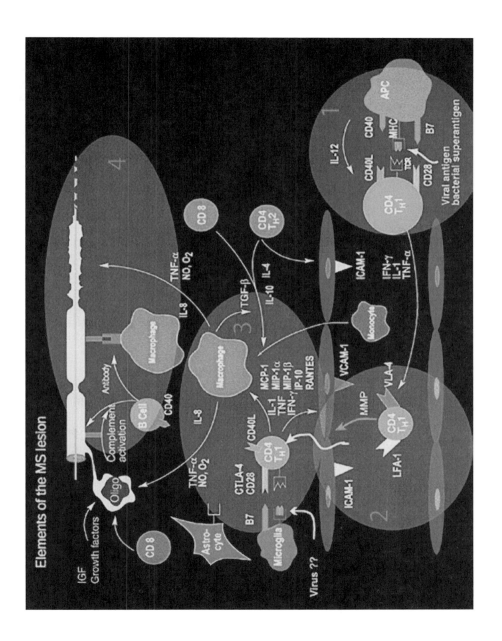

Elements of the MS lesion

211

myelin antigens such as myelinoligodendrocyte glycoprotein (MOG), myelin-associated glycoprotein (MAG), or other undefined antigens *(7)*. These cells can be blocked with compounds that affect their ability to migrate into the nervous systems by interfering with their adhesion to endothelial cell surfaces. In addition, receptor blockade by antagonists for components of the MHC/TCR complex or costimulatory molecules could prevent myelin specific cells from being activated.

Regulatory T-Cells and Immune Deviation

Although the biology of regulatory or suppressor T-cells is not completely understood, there are two types of regulatory T-cells that have been characterized and found effective in the EAE model and can be applied for the treatment of neurologic immune mediated diseases. One is an anti-clonotypic or an anti-idiotypic T-cell that reacts with antigen specific autoreactive T-cells *(8)*. These cells may be generated during T-cell vaccination. The second is an antigen specific regulatory T-cell. These regulatory T-cells can migrate to the CNS or cervical lymphatics where they encounter antigen and secrete antiinflammatory cytokines such as IL-4, IL-10 and transforming growth factor (TGF)-α that suppress inflammation *(9,10)*. These cells can be generated by oral toleration. As more is learned about immune mechanisms of inflammation and regulation, it appears there is a balance between TH_1 and TH_2 type responses. Disease inducing cells, or TH_1 type cells, can secrete inflammatory cytokines such as IL-2, TNF, and interferon (IFN)-γ which recruit other T-cells and macrophages that induce inflammation. Regulatory TH_2 type cells secrete cytokines that suppress inflammation. Strategies to block TH_1 type cytokines or administer or enhance TH_2 type cytokines are being developed. Similarly, anti-clonotypic T-cells may also function by secreting antiinflammatory cytokines.

Although it is possible to interrupt an immune response in the EAE model with the aforementioned strategies of immune manipulation, not all of these strategies are easily translated into humans. For example, not all compounds cross the blood–brain barrier and some compounds need to be administered by intravenous or subcutaneous injection over prolonged periods of time. In animal models, the time of immunization and disease induction is known so that therapeutic agents can be given at critical points in the immune response. In MS, the intermittent chronic activation of the immune system makes such time dependent targeted therapy difficult. Furthermore, one of the difficulties with immune-specific therapies is that, although the specific therapy may suppress animal models of disease in which inbred strains are used, patients represent an outbred population. Thus, individual patients may recognize different portions of an autoantigen and use a relatively nonrestricted set of T-cell receptors.

ANTIGEN-SPECIFIC IMMUNOTHERAPY

Antigen-specific modulation of the immune response is an attractive approach for treating an autoimmune disease (Table 1). The difficulty with any antigen-specific therapy, however, is the presumption that one knows the autoantigen that patho-

Table 1
Antigen Specific Immunotherapy

1. Glatiramer acetate (Copaxone)
2. T-cell receptor
3. Antigen-MHC complexes
4. Oral tolerance

genic T-cells attack and that there is only one autoantigen being attacked. Furthermore, once a tissue is inflamed, multiple reactivities may develop and inflammatory cells that are not specific for myelin antigens could play an important role in the ongoing disease process. The spreading of autoimmune responses has been shown in EAE and diabetes models. In rheumatoid arthritis, even though it is initiated by T-cells, joint inflammation and destruction may become T-cell independent processes. In addition, γ-δ T-cells reactive to heat shock proteins may be secondarily generated and participate in CNS inflammation and damage.

Glatiramer Acetate (Copaxone)

Glatiramer acetate (GA) (Copaxone) is a random polymer designed initially based on the amino acid composition of MBP. The mechanism by which Copaxone may work in humans is unknown. It could function by generating regulatory cells as this has been shown in animals treated with altered myelin peptides *(11,12)*. Altered myelin peptides will likely also reach clinical trials. In addition, proliferation of MBP specific T-cell clones has also been reported to be suppressed by Copaxone and it theoretically could interfere with binding of MBP or other peptides to the MHC cleft *(13,14)*.

Experimental studies in EAE have shown that orally administered GA can suppress disease and that the mechanism of suppression is identical to that when administered subcutaneously *(15)*. A multinational trial of oral GA (the CORAL study) has recently been completed. Patients ($n = 1650$) with clinically definite relapsing-remitting (RR) MS and one or more attacks in the year prior to entry were randomized to 5 or 50 mg of either GA or placebo tablets, given daily for 56 weeks, and were evaluated every 2 months. Magnetic resonance imaging (MRI) scans were done at baseline and at completion of the study. A subset of those patients had MRIs every 2 months. The primary outcome measure was the total number of relapses per group. This study has been completed recently, and although the results have not been published, a statistically significant effect was not observed, although the group receiving the higher dose demonstrated a tendency toward a therapeutic benefit. New formulations of oral GA are currently being developed for future testing. A study of GA in primary-progressive MS (PPMS), carrying the acronym PROMISE, was launched approximately 2.5 years ago. The results of this study are eagerly awaited. The oral GA trial in RRMS was found to be negative (no benefit) although the results have not been published to date.

T-Cell Vaccination and T-Cell Receptor Therapy

In animal models, restricted T-cell receptor usage by MBP reactive cells has been demonstrated and it is possible to suppress EAE by vaccinating or immunizing with MBP reactive clones or T-cell receptor peptides *(8,16,17)*. This approach induces regulatory cells that interact with the injected clones or peptides. It has been shown that the mechanism for this protection involves both an "anti-activated T-cell" response which is short lived, and anti-clonotypic T-cell responses, which are longer lived. Moreover, animal experimentation has suggested the safety of T-cell vaccination using either fixed or irradiated T-cell clones. Two phase 1 studies of T-cell vaccination have been performed in MS patients. In the first, four subjects with progressive MS were given a total of seven inoculations of attenuated, autologous T-cell clones isolated from the cerebrospinal fluid (CSF) *(18)*. These cells were not antigen-specific. There were no untoward side effects and immunologic studies suggested that the inoculation of autologous T-cell activated clones was associated with partial, short-term immunosuppression as evidences by down-regulation of subsequent stimulation via the CD2 pathway of activation. In addition, the autologous mixed lymphocyte response, which is reduced in about half of the patients with MS, was enhanced for a short period of time after the T-cell vaccination. In a second study, six patients were inoculated with MBP specific T-cells *(19)*. It was found that T-cell responses to the inoculants developed and there was a depletion of MBP reactive cells in the recipients. Furthermore, CD8[+] anti-clonotypic T-cell lines were isolated from treated patients that recognized the CD4[+] MBP-specific T-cells. In addition to using T-cell clones to vaccinate, in a phase 1 trial investigators have inoculated MS patients with immunogenic regions of the T-cell receptor that recognizes immunodominant regions of MBP; changes in MBP reactive cells have been reported. The conceptual problem with T-cell vaccination and T-cell receptor therapy is that, in MS, T-cell receptor usage of MBP reactive cells is not likely to be as restricted as in animals. Furthermore, there are reactivities to other myelin antigens such as PLP in MS *(20)*. Thus, T-cell vaccination or T-cell receptor therapy may be too specific, downregulating only a small proportion of autoreactive cells. Although a subcategory of patients could theoretically benefit from such a therapy treatment, it would have to be administered very early in the disease course. There is a possibility that treatment may not be effective over time in a chronic disease such as MS.

Anergy Induction

An alternative approach to inactivating autoreactive T-cells is to use free antigen, antigen coupled to autologous cells, or antigen-MHC complexes. This approach induces anergy and has been used successfully in the EAE model. It is well known that intravenous administration of soluble antigen can lead to tolerogenic signals to the immune system. Investigators attempted phase I trials to induce tolerance to MBP by injecting MBP into MS patients but were unsuccessful and, in some instances, sensitized patients. Although less specific than T-cell receptor therapy, because all cells reacting to a particular antigen are suppressed, anergy induction does not address the issue that there is reactivity to more than one myelin antigen in MS. However, it is theoretically possible to anergize against a number of different myelin antigens. An important issue for clinical use is how often the treatment would need to be given, by what route, and whether sensitization could occur with repeated treatment. Similar issues are raised by approaches which attempt to induce apoptosis of autoreactive cells and which are as yet less developed.

Oral Tolerance

Oral tolerance refers to the long recognized observation that proteins that pass through the gastrointestinal tract generate systemic hyporesponsiveness. Thus, if animals are fed a protein such as ovalbumin or MBP and are subsequently immunized, the immune response against the fed antigen is reduced. Oral tolerance evolved to allow the mucosal immune system (gut-associated lymphoid tissue [GALT]) to absorb proteins without becoming sensitized to them. In recent years, a great deal has been learned about the mechanism of oral tolerance and the use of oral tolerance has been successfully applied to several animal models of autoimmune diseases including animal models of MS, arthritis, uveitis, diabetes, thyroiditis, myasthenia, and in transplantation *(21)*. Oral tolerance is also being tested clinically in the human disease states of MS, rheumatoid arthritis, uveitis, and juvenile diabetes. Depending on the amount of antigen fed, orally administered antigens result in the generation of active suppression or anergy. Low doses favor active suppression whereas higher doses favor anergy or apoptosis *(3,6)*. The doses and strategy being used in clinical trials are aiming to generate regulatory T-cells that suppress inflammation at the target organ. Antigens that pass through the gut preferentially generate TH_2 type cells that secrete IL-4, IL-10, and TGF-β. Such cells leave the gut and migrate to the organ that contains the fed antigen. The regulatory cells are then stimulated to release antiinflammatory cytokines. Oral tolerance can be conceptualized as a natural drug delivery system in which physiologic antiinflammatory cytokines are delivered to the target organ by one's own cells, depending on the fed protein. Thus, it is not necessary to know what the autoantigen is in an autoimmune disease in order for oral toleration to be effective. In this regard, it has been shown that MBP or PLP induced EAE in the mouse can be suppressed by MBP feeding *(22)*. Recombinant human proteins and the use of compounds that enhance the generation of TH_2 type regulatory cells may enhance the biologic effects of oral tolerance. Of note is that in animals, IFN-β enhances the protection by orally administered myelin antigens *(24)*.

ANTIGEN-NONSPECIFIC IMMUNOMODULATION

A number of approaches of antigen-nonspecific immunotherapy are have been shown to be successful in animal models and are being considered for clinical trials (Table 2). They illustrate approaches that are designed to affect the immune system in a number of different ways. They are listed as having minimal to moderate systemic toxicity.

Table 2
Antigen-Nonspecific Immunomodulation

1. Interferons
   a. α (IFN- βa-n3 [Alferon] and Interferon- βa-2a [Roferon])
   b. β (Avonex, Betaseron, Rebif)
   c. τ
2. Drugs to alter lymphocyte traffic
   a. Selective Anti-adhesion Molecule MAbs (anti-VLA-4 MAb [Antegren])
   b. Matrix metalloproteinase inhibitors
   c. Antivirals
   d. Nitric oxide synthase inhibitors
3. Monoclonal antibodies
   a. Campath
   b. Anti-CD-40/Anti-CD2/Anti-CD4/Anti-T12/and others
   c. CNTO 1275
   d. Zenapax
   e. Antegren
   f. Rituxan
   g. WA-J695
4. IL-2 toxin
5. TGF-β/IL-4/IL-10
6. TNF antagonists (Pentoxifylline/anti-TNF MAbs)
7. Immunoglobulin
8. Plasmaphoresis
9. Unclassified
   a. Hormone therapy (estrogen, testosterone)
   b. Anticholesterol medications (Statin drugs)—(Lipitor, Zocor)

Abbr: IFN, interferon; MAbs, monoclonal antibodies; IL, interleukin; TGF, transforming growth factor; TNF, tumor necrosis factor.

Interferons

IFN-α, -β, and -τ are type I interferons that appear to act through the same receptor. It is not yet clear whether there are immunologically significant differences in the way they activate this receptor. The intracellular events following receptor binding are being rapidly elucidated. Whereas IFN-β has been shown to affect the course of relapsing-remitting MS, the important question of its mechanism of action at the level of cellular interactions is currently unknown *(24)*. The possibilities are as follows: (1) IFN-γ augments immune responses and has been shown to increase MS attacks *(25)*. IFN-β decrease IFN-γ production by activated lymphocytes *(26)*. (2) IFN-β may help reverse a suppressor cell defect that has been described in MS *(27)*, although the defect is more common in progressive MS patients *(28)*. (3) Viral infections have been associated with increased MS attacks *(29)* and IFN-β could be working through its antiviral effects, although there is no evidence from the trial that IFN-β worked by this mechanism *(24)*. (4) As described in Fig. 1, a balance between TH$_1$ and Th$_2$ type immune responses may be important in MS and IFN-β may favor the generation of TH₂ type responses *(30)*. (5) IFN-β has been shown to down regulate IL-2 receptor on lymphocytes of treated MS patients, and thus may act to block the expansion phase of an immune response *(31)*. (6) IFN-β can stimulate IL-10 production by macrophages which can suppress immune responses *(32)*. Oral IFN-τ was shown to be effective in EAE *(33)*. An open-label phase I clinical trial in humans revealed safety up to a dose of 1.8 mg administered daily for 29 days *(34)*. There was also a dose dependent rise in IL-10. No neutralizing antibodies were detected. A large multi-center phase II trial will begin enrollment in July 2004.

Drugs to Alter Lymphocyte Traffic

It is known that there is rapid trafficking of cells from the peripheral immune system into the CNS in MS *(35)*. In this regard, total lymphoid irradiation had an ameliorating effect on progressive MS and only involved manipulation of the peripheral immune system. EAE can be suppressed by monoclonal antibodies (MAbs) and other drugs that alter traffic of the cells into the nervous system *(36,37)* and such compounds are being considered for treatment of MS. Such treatment has the advantage of not being dependent on antigen specificity of the migrating cells. However, one potential difficulty with this approach is that it is given at a specific point in time when the disease is active in animals and such time-dependent therapy is difficult in MS. The degree to which it could be applied to the chronic progressive type of MS remains to be seen.

Anti-Integrin Antibodies (Natalizumab/Antegren)

The formation of inflammatory lesions in patients with MS may involve lymphocytes and monocytes that gain access to the brain parenchyma from the circulation by first adhering to vascular endothelial cells *(38)*. The glycoprotein α4 integrin is expressed on the surface of inflammatory lymphocytes and monocytes and may play a critical role in their adhesion to the vascular endothelium *(39,40)*. These observations have led to investigations of α4 integrin antagonists. Treatment with these agents in rodent models of multiple sclerosis resulted in reduced signs of disease activity and inflammation *(41–43)*. A small preliminary, placebo-controlled study in humans using the monoclonal antibody natalizumab, an α4 integrin antagonist, also found that the drug reduced the frequency of new gadolinium-enhancing lesions *(44)*. These findings have now been extended in a larger and longer double-blind trial in which 213 patients with relapsing-remitting or relapsing-secondary-progressive MS were randomly assigned to receive 3 mg/kg or 6 mg/kg of intravenous (IV) natalizumab, or placebo, every 28 days for 6 months *(45)*. Both natalizumab groups had significant reductions in the mean number of new brain lesions on monthly gadolinium-enhanced MRI (9.6 for placebo vs 0.7 and 1.1 in the 3 mg/kg and 6 mg/kg natalizumab groups, respectively). This effect was evident 1 month after the first infusion and was sustained throughout the treatment period. In addition, there were significantly fewer relapses in the natalizumab groups *(44,45)*. Whereas no direct comparative studies have been performed, these results suggest that natalizumab may be more effective than the interferons or glatiramer acetate. Therapy with natalizumab was well tolerated, with a safety profile similar to that of placebo. On the basis of the above study results, Biogen-Idec is sponsoring two large multi-center double-blind placebo-controlled trials with Antegren. One trial uses IV Antegren as monotherapy monthly for 2 years. The other study combines Antegren with Avonex. One-year data has been submitted to the Food and Drug Administration (FDA) and early approval will be determined in late 2004.

Monoclonal Antibodies

Phase I studies of anti-T-cell MAb infusions have been undertaken in MS studying the immunologic affects of three anti-T-cell MAbs: anti-CD2, anti-CD4, and anti-T12 *(46,47)*. Investigators reported that anti-T-cell monoclonal antibody infusions suppressed in vitro measures of the human immune response. Specifically, an anti-CD2 monoclonal decreased T-cell activation by phytohemagglutinin, and anti-CD4 MAb infusions abolished pokeweed mitogen-induced immunoglobulin synthesis without lysis of the $CD4^+$ T-cell populations. With repeated infusions, human anti-mouse antibodies were found in the circulation. Although most of the human anti-mouse antibodies were not immunoglobulin isotype-specific, significant anti-idiotypic activity was observed after repeated infusions. Other investigators reported that anti-CD3 infusions were associated with significant toxic effects in MS patients *(48)*. Although the clinical usefulness of currently available anti-T-cell murine MAbs in chronic disease such as MS is hampered by human anti-mouse antibodies, there are a number of potential approaches to solve the problem. First is the use of humanized MAbs with a human Fc and mouse Fab region. A second approach is to attach a toxin to the murine MAb, resulting in both a greater elimination of targeted T-cell population and potentially preventing human anti-mouse antibodies. More extensive studies with anti-CD4 have been carried out by Steinman and colleagues (unpublished data) at Stanford using a humanized anti-CD4 MAb, with a larger trial undertaken at the Institutes of Neurology at Queen's Square, London. At Stanford, patients with chronic progressive MS were treated with a chimeric anti-CD4 antibody with a humanized Fc region *(1)*. Results of the large trial were essentially negative despite very marked reduction in $CD4^+$ cells *(49,50)*. Possible explanations are that MS becomes a T-cell independent disease late in the course or that regulatory T-cells were also removed by this therapy. The effects of anti-CD52 (Campath 1H), a lymphocyte depleting humanized MAb, on brain and spinal cord atrophy were investigated in a crossover trial of 25 patients with SPMS and an EDSS score between 4.0 and 6.0. Patients received intravenous Campath 1H 20 mg for 3 to 4 hours for 5 consecutive days and were followed for 18 months. Campath 1H markedly reduced the mean number and volume of Gd^+ lesions from baseline over the course of the study. Despite these findings, 13 of 25 patients had substantial decreases in brain volume. Of the 14 patients with data available, the mean spinal cord area was reduced from 94 mm^2 at baseline to 87.6 mm^2 at 18 months ($p < 0.001$) *(51)*.

In a multi-arm, multiple dose, 6-month phase 2 trial (47 treated, 12 placebo) *(52)*, the recombinant humanized immunoglobulin G$_1$ monoclonal antibody ATM-027 was shown to deplete Vβ 5.2/5.3+ T-cells, reduce the expression of T-cell receptors, and reduce T-cell reactivity to some myelin antigens. This treatment was without apparent toxicity. Serial studies showed a minor degree of reduced MRI activity (perhaps 10-30%), but not to a level of statistical significance. Prolonged (18 months) Vβ 5.2/5.3+ T-cell depletion was observed in a second, small study of 14 patients *(53)*.

IL-2 Toxin

IL-2 toxin targets activated cells and has been shown to be effective in some animal models. It is being tried in diseases such as rheumatoid arthritis and in multiple sclerosis.

TGF-β

This naturally suppressive cytokine that has been shown to suppress animal models of autoimmune diseases including EAE and arthritis *(54)*. As discussed previously, it mediates the effect of regulatory cells generated by oral tolerance. Trials of injectable TGF-β have been initiated in MS. There has been some interest in trying IL-4 or IL-10 similarly.

TNF Antagonists

Because TNF may be a mediator of tissue damage in MS, investigators are considering treatment with TNF antagonists in MS. This includes the use of pentoxifylline, a drug which favors Th2 type responses and downregulates TNF production *(55)* and the use of anti-TNF monoclonal antibodies. Such antibodies have shown some usefulness in rheumatoid arthritis *(56)*.

Immunoglobulin

Intravenous immunoglobulins (IVIg) mechanism of action is unclear but may relate to anti-idiotypic effects *(57)*. One hypothesis based on animal work, which serves as basis for an IVIg trial in MS, is that it can promote remyelination *(58)*. A detailed discussion is presented in the next section.

Plasmaphoresis

This process removes plasma proteins and replaces them with colloid and will be discussed in the next section.

Unclassified

The results of an open pilot study of estradiol in MS *(59)* and a report describing the immunomodulating effects of cholesterol-lowering statins *(60)* have fueled support for definitive large-scale MS trials *(61)*.

Table 3
Antigen-Nonspecific Immunosuppression

1. Azathioprine (Imuran)
2. Cyclophosphamide (Cytoxan)
3. Mycophenolate Mofetil (Cellcept)
4. Cyclosporine
5. Methotrexate
6. Mitoxanthrone (Novantrone)
7. Total lymphoid irradiation (TLI)
8. Cladribine
9. Bone marrow transplant

ANTIGEN-NONSPECIFIC IMMUNOSUPPRESSION

Table 3 lists immunosuppressive agents which have been used in neurologic immune mediated diseases. The mechanisms of immunosuppression of these agents are likely multiple. One shared component is probably a direct cytotoxic effect on pathogenic leukocytes. However, this cannot explain the entire effect as severely leukopenic treated patients with very active autoimmune disease have been seen. Therefore, other mechanisms should be involved. Data suggests that some pulse cyclophosphamide treated chronic progressive MS patients have a shift to from Th1 to Th2 type cytokine production *(30)*. On the other hand, in diseases characterized by hypergammaglobulinemia and exaggerated B-cell responses these functions seem to be selectively reduced by cyclophosphamide therapy *(62)*. An explanation for these findings is that proliferating cells are selectively vulnerable to the cytotoxic effects of cyclophosphamide as is the case in in vitro studies. In addition, monocyte functions and cytokine production are inhibited and this may impact both antigen presentation and effector mechanisms. Azathioprine has similar effects to cyclophosphamide except that cytokine production seems to be spared. The main effects of cyclosporine seem to be the result of a down regulation of IL-2 and IL-2 receptor and thus lymphocyte activation. Mycophenolic acid (Cellcept) is also being studied in MS patients and results are pending. Mitoxantrone (Novantrone) is a potent immunosuppressant agent given intravenously every 3 months that was recently approved for use in worsening relapsing-remitting and secondary-progressive MS. A detailed discussion can be found in Chapter 9. Although mitoxantrone is now FDA approved for use in MS, a 2003 report of the Therapeutics and Technology Subcommittee of the American Academy of Neurology recommended that, because of its toxicity and the somewhat limited evidence of benefit, mitoxantrone should be reserved for patients with rapidly advancing disease who have failed other therapies *(63)*.

CORTICOSTEROIDS

Corticosteroids have been used in autoimmune disease since the 1940s but their mechanism of action remains poorly understood. Similarly to type I interferons, the intracellular events following glucocorticoid receptor binding are being elucidated. The principle immunomodulatory effects seem to involve binding of the activated glucocorticoid receptor to immunoregulatory transcription factors, thus preventing them from activating genes, as well as\ increasing expression of inhibitors of these transcription factors *(64)*. At the level of cellular interaction there are effects on leukocyte circulatory kinetics, functional capabilities, and cytokine production, all of which probably play a role in their therapeutic benefit. The benefits of intravenous corticosteroids in acute inflammation in MS likely result from decreasing the entry of cells into the brain and by preventing proliferation and perhaps inducing apoptosis of activated cells. These agents deplete CD4+ cells, decrease cytokine release including TNF and IFN-γ, and decrease class II expression *(65)*. In animal models, glucocorticoids have been shown to cause a shift from Th1 to Th2 cytokine production *(66)*. In humans, DTH-type responses are suppressed after only 2 weeks of therapy. In MS, steroids have also been shown to decrease IgG synthesis in the CNS and reduce CSF antibodies to MBP and oligoclonal bands. The factors underlying the difference in response to oral vs intravenous glucocorticoids brought out in the optic neuritis trial are unknown *(67,68)*. Intravenous methylprednisolone (IVMP) is often used for the treatment of MS relapses. The effects of IVMP on BPV were studied in a randomized, single-blinded trial of 88 patients with RRMS and EDSS scores of less than or equal to 5.5. Patients received regular pulses of IVMP (1 g per day for 5 days, with an oral prednisone taper) and the same treatment for relapses as required ($n = 43$) or IVMP (same regimen) only for relapses ($n = 45$). Over the 5-year study, pulsed doses of IVMP were administered every 4 months for the initial 3 years and then every 6 months thereafter. At baseline, mean BPV was 1254.8 (±71.8) mL and 1263.4 (±66.4) mL in the two treatment groups, respectively ($p = NS$). At 5 years, the absolute change from baseline in BPV was +2.6 mL in the pulsed IVMP group compared with –74.5 mL in the relapse-only group ($p = 0.003$). Thus, pulsed IVMP prevented progressive brain atrophy in this study, although randomized, double-blind, placebo-controlled trials are needed before definitive conclusions can be made *(69)*.

PRINCIPLES FOR CLINICAL APPLICATION OF THERAPIES

The following principles are important for immunotherapy and can serve as a framework from within which to view the various treatment modalities that are currently being used and tested (Table 4). In essence, a treatment hierarchy is given with the least toxic therapy given first. Some of the new therapies now available to MS patients are beginning to make an impact on immunotherapy of other neurological immune-mediated diseases. Advances in MRI and a clearer understanding of how the immune system functions have made an impact on developing therapy for MS.

First-Line Therapy

IFN-βs (Avonex, Betaseron, Rebif) and Glatiramer Acetate (Copaxone) represent a class of first-line drugs for the treatment of MS. Some forms of antigen-specific therapy such as T-cell or T-cell receptor vaccination could also represent

Table 4
Approach to Immunotherapy for Neurological
Immune Mediated Diseases

1. First-line therapy
2. Corticosteroid usage
   a. Acute exacerbations
   b. Chronic therapy
3. Second-line immunosuppression to halt refractory or progressive disease
   a. Immunosuppressants
   b. Plasma exchange/IVIg
   c. Bone marrow transplant
4. Reinstitution of first-line therapy
5. Combination and pulse therapy
6. Neuroprotection
7. Disease monitoring

first-line therapy. Ultimately, drugs such as Copaxone must be compared to IFN-β in terms of efficacy, ease of administration, and side-effect profile. Based on the results of the recent CHAMPS trial, Avonex has been approved for patients with a clinically isolated syndrome (CIS) and an abnormal MRI. In addition, the cost of treatment will be an important factor in therapy if there are no major differences in efficacy or toxicity profile between first-line drugs. These immune modifying medications are discussed in detail in Chapter 7.

Appropriate Use of Steroids

Steroid Use in Exacerbations

Based on what is currently known about IFN-β and other relatively nontoxic drugs that could be given early in the course of MS, it is expected that patients will continue to have relapses. Thus, short courses of IV methylprednisolone are given when a significant relapse occurs to speed recovery. Given what was reported in the optic neuritis study, IV methylprednisolone may have a prolonged salutory effect on the course of MS. Acute attacks are either not treated or are treated with a short course of corticosteroids. Indications for treatment of a MS relapse include functionally disabling symptoms with objective evidence of neurological impairment. Thus, mild sensory attacks are typically not treated. In the past adrenocorticotropic hormone and oral prednisone were primarily used. More recently, physicians are treating with short courses of IV methylprednisolone (500–1000 mg daily for 3–7 days) with or without a short prednisone taper *(65)*. Optic neuritis may occur during the course of MS or be one of the initial symptoms. A recent trial of optic neuritis demonstrated that patients treated with oral prednisone alone were more likely to suffer recurrent episodes of optic neuritis as compared to those treated with methylprednisolone followed by oral prednisone *(67,68)*. These results now make intravenous methylprednisolone the primary treatment used for optic neuritis and has further supported its use for major attacks. Furthermore, as part of the optic neuritis study, it was found that treatment with a 3-day course of high-dose methylprednisolone reduced the rate of development of MS over a 2-year period *(70)*. The protective effect was most apparent in patients at highest risk for MS, those with multiple focal brain MRI abnormalities. Although these results need to be confirmed in a larger series of patients, they support the use of high-dose IV methylprednisolone for acute MS attacks. High-dose IV methylprednisolone appears to be accompanied by relatively few side effects in most patients although a number of side effects have been reported including mental changes, unmasking of infections, gastric disturbances, and an increased incidence of fractures. Anaphylactoid reactions and arrhythmia may also occur.

Chronic Steroid Usage

The goal is to achieve the lowest possible dose that will maintain quiescence of disease to avoid the long term side effects of steroids. Monthly pulses of intravenous methylprednisolone for the treatment of relapsing-remitting progressive and progressive MS has been investigated and shown to have some benefit. Long-term side effects of corticosteroids include cataracts, osteoporosis, aseptic bone necrosis, Cushing's syndrome, hypertension, and exacerbation of diabetes. Corticosteroids are discussed in detail in Chapter 9.

Second-Line Immunotherapy to Halt Refractory or Progressive Disease

Although some patients may respond to first-line treatments, it is expected that others will be refractory to therapy or enter a progressive stage. In these instances, immunotherapy or immunosuppression with stronger medication may be warranted depending on the individual case. Drugs in this category would be classified as second- or third-line treatment depending on the risk–benefit ratio of the therapy. Second- or third-line therapy could find utility even if such treatment could only be given effectively on a short-term basis if such treatment allowed reinstitution of first-line therapy. The neurologic immune mediated diseases being discussed all have progressive forms and experienced clinicians vary in their preferences for which agents to use for these. Treatment directed at the progressive phase is the most difficult because the immune mediated diseases may be harder to affect once a progressive stage has been initiated. For this reason, there is a trend toward using these agents either prior to or earlier during the progressive stage in some autoimmune diseases such as rheumatoid arthritis.

Immunosuppressive Agents

Cyclophosphamide (CTX) total lymphoid radiation (TLI), Cellcept, Novantrone, cyclosporin, azathioprine, methotrexate, and cladribine have shown some positive clinical effects in neurologic immune mediated diseases. Cytoxan is discussed in detail in Chapter 10. TLI has potent immunosuppressive effects and a double-blind study of lymphoid irradiation reported benefit in patients with progressive MS (reviewed in ref. *71*). The absolute lymphocyte count appeared to be a crude indication of therapeutic efficacy, with greater efficacy in patients with lower counts. Many patients started progressing again after initial therapy and a major limitation of the use of TLI is whether it, or other treatments that similarly affect the immune system, can be given to those who reenter the progressive phase despite therapy. Mycophenolate-mofetil (MMF/Cellcept) is an inhibitor of inosine monophosphate dehydrogenase, which is necessary for *de novo* purine biosynthesis in lymphocytes.The drug is being successfully and increasingly used for prevention of organ transplant rejection. Beneficial effects in the treatment of autoimmune diseases have been shown in Crohn's disease. The inhibition of lymphocytes by the drug may therefore result in improvement in patients with refractory MS. In this open surveillance trial, we treated seven patients with chronic progressive or relapsing MS. The patients were informed about the drug and its attendant risks, and all gave informed consent before initiation of treatment. Entry criteria in this trial included the diagnosis of MS, disease-progression in terms of EDSS despite established treatment, and no other diseases such as infections or liver or kidney disorders. All patients received the usual dose employed in the treatment of transplanted patients (2 g/day). The administration of MMF led to improvement or stopped progression in five cases. Three of the five patients emphasized improved movement, although EDSS did not change. One of the five patients had to reduce the dose from 2 to 1.5 g per day because of frequent infections, one discontinued the treatment owing to uncontrolled nausea. Two patients without beneficial effects stopped the drug through nausea and/or nonresponse. MRI findings before and at least 6 months after treatment start were available in two patients and showed fewer lesions and no change, respectively. The four patients, who still receive MMF, are feeling well without progression and would like to continue this therapy. In all seven patients treated there was no deterioration concerning EDSS. Although the beneficial effects in five patients demonstrate that MMF may be of value in the treatment of MS, this open-label study does not allow a final conclusion. The question of whether more responsive patients would be found in an unselected group requires further study *(72)*. A large multicenter trial of cyclosporin in the United States *(73)* and a trial in London *(74)* suggest that cyclosporin has a beneficial, albeit modest effect in ameliorating progressive MS, but it has not found clinical use because of the narrow benefit-to-risk ratio. Azathioprine has been the subject of a large number of studies in MS (reviewed in ref. *75*) and meta-analysis of the results of all published blind, randomized controlled trials showed a statistically significant benefit in reducing frequency of relapses over a 3-year period, but minimal effect on disability *(76)*. Methotrexate has found widespread use in the treatment of autoimmune diseases, such as rheumatoid arthritis, which has led to its use in neurologic immune-mediated disease. A double-blind trial of 7.5 mg/week of oral methotrexate in 60 chronic-progressive MS patients showed a significant beneficial effect on measures of upper extremity disability *(77)*. Further experience may help clinicians to avoid a drawback to the use of methotrexate, which is its ability to induce an irreversible hepatotoxicity. Cladribine, an immunosuppressive agent approved for the treatment of hairy cell leukemia, showed positive effects in a recent trial in which 7 of 23 placebo treated patients vs 1 of 24 cladribine treated patients had a worsening of one point or more on the EDSS scale at 1-year follow-up *(78)*. The effects of cladribine, a lymphocytotoxic agent, on whole-brain volume were studied in a randomized, double-blind, placebo-controlled trial of 159 patients with progressive MS and an EDSS score from 3.0 to 6.5. Patients received one of three regimens: (1) eight courses of placebo; (2) two courses of cladribine (0.07 mg/kg daily subcutaneously for 5 consecutive days, total dose = 0.7 mg/kg) followed by six courses of placebo; or (3) six courses of cladribine (0.07 mg/kg daily subcutaneously for 5 consecutive days, total dose = 2.1 mg/kg) followed by two courses of placebo. At baseline, brain volume was 1042 (±18.8) mL, 1053 (±18.1) mL, and 1082 (±19.9) mL, respectively, in the three treatment groups. Cladribine did not significantly affect brain volume over time. At 12 months, the mean reduction from baseline in brain volume was 0.4% with placebo, 0.4% with the lower dose of cladribine, and 1.5% with the higher dose of cladribine *(79,80)*.

Plasmaphoresis and Intravenous Immune Globulin

These approaches have been used in fulminant neurological-immune mediated diseases with variable success which has led to some extension of their use into more chronic diseases. IVIg is easier and generally safer to use than plasmaphoresis, but both remain expensive. IVIg showed promise in early MS trials *(81)*. Immune globulin may help patients with a number of autoimmune diseases, including chronic relapsing polyneuropathy and dermatomyositis, and has also been studied in relation to MS. Its mechanism of action is unclear but may relate to anti-idiotypic effects and suppression of TNF-α. A randomized, placebo-controlled trial of monthly IVIg in RRMS involved 150 patients over 2 years *(81)*. IVIg was associated with fewer relapses (62 vs 116 with placebo) and a greater likelihood of being relapse-free (53 vs 36%). Only 3 patients receiving IVIg (4%) experienced side effects including cutaneous reactions and depression; these manifestations were not unequivocally related to the IVIg. Observations in animal models of MS revealed that IVIg could promote new myelin synthesis *(58)*. However, a double-blind, placebo-controlled study of 67 patients with an apparently irreversible motor deficit found that IVIg (0.4 g/kg for 5 days, then single infusions every 2 weeks for 3 months) did not reverse established weakness in MS *(83)*. Plasma exchange has been investigated in patients with acute central nervous system inflammatory demyelinating disease who did not respond to steroid therapy *(84)*. Moderate or greater improvement in neurological disability occurred during 8 of 19 (42%) courses of active treatment compared with 1 of 17 (6%) courses of sham treatment. Improvement occurred early in the course of treatment and was sustained on follow-up. However, 4 of the patients who responded to the active treatment experienced new attacks of demyelinating disease during 6 months of follow-up.

Bone Marrow Transplantation

Recent strategies have focused on more aggressive approaches to immunosuppression such as autologous bone marrow transplantation (BMT) or stem cell transplantation (SCT). This approach has shown promise in experimental models of MS *(85,86)*. In a study assessing safety, 26 patients with severe MS were treated with autologous SCT; one patient had a flare of MS during treatment with granuloyte-colony stimulating factor for stem cell mobilization, one patient had a syndrome of fevers and progressive neurologic deterioration and died 2 years after high-dose immunosuppressive therapy, and there was a relatively high rate of bladder complications and engraftment syndrome (a noninfectious syndrome of fever, rash, and fatigue) *(87)*. A second uncontrolled study of SCT in 21 patients with rapidly progressive MS also found a high rate of engraftment syndrome *(88)*. Patients with high pretransplantation disability scores did not appear to benefit from SCT and the study was unable to assess whether there was benefit in the subgroup of patients with lower baseline disability scores. A recent article on stem cell research in MS involved 14 patients with severe MS (EDSS 4–6.5) receiving autologous hematopoietic SCT. The median follow-up was 3 years. The probability of progression-free survival was 85.7% and the probability of activity-free disease was 46.4%. The number of relapses 1-year prior was 48 and the number of relapses at the end of the 3 years was 2. On MRI there was a 20.2% reduction in T2 lesion burden and a 13.75% reduction in corpus callosal volume. No T1 enhanced lesions were seen after transplantation. After 36 months the EDSS was stable in eight, improved in four, and worsened in two patients. No deaths or grade III/IV complications occurred *(89)*. Larger controlled trials are awaited in order for the risk–benefit ratio of this approach to be calculated.

Reinstitution of First-Line Therapy

The principle of second- or third-line therapy may be used to induce remission of disease activity with an immunosuppressive agent, followed by reinstitution of first-line therapy, nontoxic therapy to maintain quiesence. The degree to which subsequent first-line therapy will be effective is unknown. Furthermore, a major problem that confronts clinicians is being able to determine when a remission has indeed occurred.

Combination and Pulse Therapy

Until the pathogeneses of neurological immune-mediated diseases are precisely understood, it is unlikely that a single treatment will be effective in all patients. The principle of combination therapy has found utility in cancer treatment and is becoming an important principle for the therapy of MS and other neurological-immune mediated diseases. Rationales for combining different mechanistic approaches exist. Combining systemic immune deviation with immune deviation of antigen-specific cells or molecular blockades are interesting possibilities. Pulse steroids or relatively nontoxic immunomodulation may find utility in conjuction with other antigen-specific forms of therapy. As it becomes clear which mechanistic strategies work best, more rational combinations can be designed. Because some forms of therapy cannot safely be given chronically, intermittent pulse therapy with

Table 5
Combination Trials in Multiple Sclerosis

1. Avonex and Mitoxantrone	16. Betaseron and Methotrexate
2. Avonex and Fludarabine	17. Betaseron and Copaxone
3. Avonex and Methotrexate	18. Betaseron and Mitoxantrone
4. Avonex and Cytoxan	19. Betaseron and Azathioprine
5. Avonex and Provigil	20. Rebif and Cytoxan
6. Avonex and CellCept	21. Rebif and Corticosteroids
7. Avonex and Prednisone and Azathioprine	22. Rebif and Azathioprine
8. Avonex and Azathioprine	23. Rebif and Copaxone
9. Avonex and Antegren (SENTINEL)	24. High-dose cyclophosphamide and total
10. Avonex and corticosteroids or meth-	body irradiation with stem cell or bone
otrexate	marrow rescue
11. Avonex and IVIg	25. Copaxone and Albuterol
12. Avonex and Copaxone (CombiRx)	26. Copaxone and Antegren
13. Avonex and Selegiline	27. Copaxone and Mitoxantrone
14. Avonex and Minocycline	28. Mitoxantrone plus either interferon or
15. Betaseron and Cytoxan	Copaxone

drugs that affect the immune system may become an important principle for therapy. Current combination trials in MS are listed in Table 5.

An open-label study was performed to evaluate the safety and efficacy of combination therapy with weekly oral methotrexate (20 mg) and IFN-β-1a in 15 patients with MS who had experienced exacerbations while receiving IFN-β monotherapy. Nausea was the only major side effect. A 44% reduction in the number of gadolinium-enhanced lesions seen on MRI scan was observed during combination therapy ($p = 0.02$). There was a trend toward fewer exacerbations. This combination therapy appears to be safe and well tolerated, and should be studied in a controlled trial *(90)*. A recent pilot trial of combining Avonex and Copaxone enrolled 33 subjects with relapsing-remitting MS, an MRI consistent with MS, and an EDSS between 0 and 5.5 who had been taking Avonex for 6 months or more. Previous results proved safety of the combination. This report showed additional safety as well as no evidence for increased risk in terms of new lesion load. The number and volume of gadolinium enhanced lesions showed a decline from baseline to 6 months, as well as from 6–12 months, suggestive of increased efficacy. Larger trials are in progress *(91)*.

Neuroprotection

A potential benefit of the neuroprotective agent riluzole on cervical cord atrophy was suggested in a pilot study of 16 patients with PPMS and EDSS scores from 3.0 to 7.5. After receiving no treatment for the first year, patients were treated with riluzole 100 mg daily during the second year. MRI scans were analyzed in a blinded fashion. At baseline, mean spinal cord area was 66.7 mm^2, which was reduced to

65.4 mm^2 (–2.0% median change) at 1 year. After treatment with riluzole during the second year, little further change was seen in mean spinal cord area (65.2 mm^2, –0.2% median change vs first year) (92).

Disease Monitoring

The major problems confronting therapy of neurological immune-mediated diseases are unpredictable courses and the length of time over which disability accumulates. Even for treatments that have proven efficacy, it may be difficult to determine in an individual patient whether the treatment is having a therapeutic effect unless the disease becomes truly quiescent clinically or the patient improves on therapy. In some instances it is clear that a patient is either a responder or nonresponder to a particular treatment. We have occasionally seen such positive clinical effects in younger patients with rapidly progressive, steroid unresponsive MS treated with pulse cyclophosphamide. The hope is that surrogate markers, which are linked to the underlying disease process, will allow a more rational approach to assessing therapy apart from clinical assessment. MRI has provided such a surrogate marker in MS and was one of the major factors in the approval of IFN-β for the treatment of relapsing remitting MS (93). Even though MRI is not a perfect correlate of disease activity, it may ultimately serve as the best objective measure of ongoing disease in the nervous system given that it is now known that MS is chronically active even when clinical activity is not present (94,95). However, apart from formal clinical trials, MRIs are costly and impractical to perform on a frequent basis in a general neurology practice. There is a large body of evidence showing abnormalities of immune function in MS including activated T-cells, loss of suppressor influences, the presence of activated myelin-reactive T-cells in the peripheral blood and abnormal cytokine patterns. One intriguing recent observation is that the cytokine TNF-α may correlate with disease activity and disease disability (96,97). TNF-α can be measured in whole peripheral blood following stimulation with PHA and TNF-α message can be measured in frozen blood samples. TNF-α may play a role in the disease process as it is an important inflammatory cytokine that can result in damage of CNS myelin. Ultimately, however, immune measures such as TNF must be correlated with response to therapy as measured by clinical and MRI criteria. As with other recombinant protein drugs used for the treatment of a number of diseases, antibodies commonly develop to IFN-β products during the treatment of patients with MS. Neutralizing antibodies (NAbs) are a subset of antibodies that reduce or diminish the biologic activity of IFN-β. Individual Phase III clinical trials and direct comparison studies with IFN-β-1b (Betaseron), intramuscular (IM) IFN-β-1a (Avonex), and subcutaneous IFN-β-1a (Rebif) have shown that NAbs develop more frequently during treatment with IFNβ-1b than IFN-β-1a and that between the two IFN-β-1a products, NAbs develop more frequently during treatment with subcutaneous IFN-β-1a than IM IFN-β-1a. Data from clinical trials of IFNβ products indicate that clinical efficacy of IFN-β is reduced in NAb-positive patients. In light of these data, the immunogenicity of IFN-β products should be considered prior to initiating treatment with IFN-β. Also, ongoing laboratory

Table 6
Current Clinical Trials in Multiple Sclerosis

1.	3,4 DiAminoPyridine/4-AminoPyridine (Fampridine)	34.	Low-fat diet with fatty acids
2.	Acupuncture	35.	Lymphocytapheresis
3.	Albuterol (Proventil)	36.	Marijuana derivatives
4.	α-Lipoic acid	37.	Methotrexate
5.	Altered Peptide Ligand (NBI-5788)	38.	Methylprednisolone
6.	Antibiotic therapy	39.	Micellar paclitaxel (PAXCEED)
7.	Anesthetic cream (EMLA)	40.	Mitoxantrone (Novantrone)
8.	Aspirin	41.	Modafinil (Provigil)
9.	Azathioprine (Imuran)	42.	Monoclonal antibodies (Campath, anti-CD-40, CNTO 1275, Zenapax, Antegren, Rituxan, WA-J695)
10.	Baclofen		
11.	Bone marrow/peripheral stem cell transplant	43.	Mycophenolate mofetil (CellCept)
12.	CTLA 4-Ig	44.	Myelin basic protein peptide
13.	Cyclophosphamide (Cytoxan)	45.	Pain medication (Advil, Aleve, Tylenol)
14.	Dexrazoxane (Zinecard)	46.	Phosphodiesterase inhibitor (Ibudilast)
15.	Dextromethorphan/quinidine	47.	Phosphodiesterase-4 inhibitor (Rolipram)
16.	Donezepil HCL (Aricept)	48.	Pirfenidone (Deskar)
17.	Estriol	49.	Pixantrone
18.	Fluoxetine (Prozac)	50.	Plasma exchange
19.	Gabapentin (Neurontin)	51.	Prednisone
20.	Ginkgo biloba	52.	Rehabilitation
21.	Glatiramer acetate (Copaxone)	53.	Riluzole (Rilutek)
22.	Immunoglobulin (IVIg)	54.	Rosiglitazone maleate (Avandia)
23.	Inosine	55.	Schwann cell transplantation
24.	Insulin-like growth factor-1 (IGF-1)	56.	Sildenafil citrate (Viagra)
25.	IFN-α-n3 (Alferon)	57.	Cholesterol-lowering medications (Statin drugs-Zocor/Lipitor)
26.	IFN-α-2a (Roferon)		
27.	IFN-β-1a (Avonex, Rebif)	58.	T-cell receptor peptide
28.	IFN-β-1b (Betaseron)	59.	T-cell vaccination
29.	IFN-τ (oral)	60.	Teriflunomide
30.	IL-1 receptor blocker (anakinra; Kineret)	61.	Testosterone
31.	IL12 monoclonal antibodies	62.	Thalamic stimulation
32.	Laquinimod	63.	Valacyclovir (Valtrex)
33.	Levitracetam (Keppra)	64.	Yoga

monitoring of patients treated with higher-dose IFN-β is recommended for early detection of NAbs *(98)*. Apart from formal studies, the treating neurologist must decide on therapy based on clinical assessment and accumulation of disability. Furthermore, a decision must be made as to whether a person has responded to therapy or whether additional treatment should be given. These decisions are generally made based on the frequency with which the patient is having attacks and level of progression. MS therapy remains a dynamic everchanging field. The explosion of new trials have stimulated and accelerated immunologic research in this field and has lead to the development of new trials compounds. Current clinical trials are listed in Table 6.

REFERENCES

1. Steinman L, Lindsey JW, Alters S, Hodgkinson S. From treatment of experimental allergic encephalomyelitis to clinical trials in multiple sclerosis. In: Bach JF, ed., Monoclonal Antibodies and Peptide Therapy in Autoimmune Diseases. Marcel Dekker Inc., New York, 1993, pp. 253–260.
2. Brocke S, Gaur A, Piercy C, et al. Induction of relapsing paralysis in experimental autoimmune encephalomyelitis by bacterial superantigen. Nature 1993;365:642–644.
3. Friedman A, Weiner HL. Induction of anergy or active suppression following oral tolerance is determined by frequency of feeding and antigen dosage. PNAS 1994;in press.
4. Abbas A. Die and let live: eliminating dangerous lymphocytes. Cell 1996;84: 655–657.
5. Webb S, Morris C, Sprent J. Extrathymic tolerance of mature T-cells : Clonal elimination as a consequence of immunity. Cell 1990;63:1249–1256.
6. Chen Y, Inobe J, Marks R, Gonella P, Kuchroo VK, Weiner HL. Peripheral deletion of antigen reactive T-cells in oral tolerance. Nature 1995;376:177–180.
7. Kerlero de Rosbo N, Milo R, Lees MB, Burger D, Bernard CC, Be-Nun A. Reactivity to myelin antigens in multiple sclerosis. JCI 1993;92:2602–2608.
8. Ben-Nun A, Wekerle H, Cohen IR. Vaccination against autoimmune encephalomyelitis using attenuated cells of a T lymphocyte line reactive against myelin basic protein. Nature 1981; 292:60–61.
9. Khoury SJ, Hancock WW, Weiner HL. Oral tolerance to myelin basic protein and natural recovery from experimental autoimmune encephalomyelitis are associated wtih down-regulation of inflammatory cytokines and differential upregulation of TGF-β, IL-4 and PGE expression in the brain. J Exp Medicine 1992;46:1355–1364.
10. ChenY, Kuchroo VK, Inobe J, Hafler DA, Weiner HL. Regulatory T cell clones induced by oral tolerance: suppression of autoimmune encephalomyelitis. Science 1994;265: 1237–1240.
11. Nicholson L, Greer J, Sobel RA, Lees MB, Kuchroo VK. An altered peptide ligand mediates immune deviation and prevents EAE. Immunity 1995;3:397–405.
12. Brocke S, Gijbels K, Allegretta M, et al. Treatment of EAE with a peptide analogue of MBP. Nature 1996;379:343–346.
13. Racke MK, Martin R, McFarland H, Fritz RB. Copolymer-1-induced inhibition of antigen-specific T-cell activation: Interference with antigen presentation. J Neuroimmunol 1992;37:75–84.
14. Teitelbaum D, Milo R, Arnon R, Sela M. Synthetic copolymer-1 inhibits human T-cell lines specific for myelin basic protein. PNAS 1992;89:137–141.
15. Teitelbaum D, Arnon R, Sela M. Immunodetection of experimental autoimune encehalomyelitis by oral administration of copolymer 1. Proc Natl Acad Sci USA 1999;96;3842–3847.
16. Howell MD, Winters ST, Olee T, Powell HC, Carlo DJ, Brostoff SW. Vaccination against experimental allergic encephalomyelitis with T cell receptor peptides. Science 1989;246:668–670.
17. Vandenbark AA, Hashim G, Offner H. Immunization with a synthetic T-cell receptor V-region peptide protects against experimental autoimmune encephalomyelitis. Nature 1989;341:541–544.
18. Hafler DA. T Cell Vaccination in Multiple Sclerosis: A Preliminary Report. Clin Immunol Immunopathol 1992;62:307–313.
19. Zhang J, Medaer R, Stinissen P, Hafler D, Raus J. MHC-restricted depletion of human myelin basic protein-reactive T cells by T cell vaccination. Science 1993;261:1451–1454.
20. Zhang J, Markovic-Plese S, Lacet B, Raus J, Weiner HL, Hafler DA. Increased frequency of IL-2 responsive T cells specific for myelin basic protein and proteolipid protein in peripheral blood and cerebrospinal fluid of patients with multiple sclerosis. J Exp Med 1994;179:973–984.
21. Weiner HL, Friedman A, Miller A, et al. Oral Tolerance: Immunologic mechanisms and treatment of murine and human organ specific autoimmune diseases by oral administration of autoantigens. Ann Rev Immunol 1994;12:809–837.

22. Al-Sabbagh A, Miller A, Santos LM, Weiner HL. Suppression of PLP induced EAE in the SJL mouse by oral administration of MBP. Neurology 1994;24:2104–2109.

23. Al-Sabbagh A, Nelson PA, Weiner HL. Beta interferon enhances oral tolerance to MBP and PLP in experimental autoimmune encephalomyelitis. Neurology 1994;44:A242(abstract)..

24. Arnason BGW. Interferon beta in multiple sclerosis. Neurology 1993;43:641–643.

25. Hirsch RL, Panitch HS, Johnson KP. Lymphocytes from multiple sclerosis patients produce elevated levels of gamma interferon in vitro. J Clin Immunol 1985;5:386–389.

26. Noronha A, Toscas A, Jansen MA. IFN-β downregulates T cell activation and IFN-γ production: implications for MS. J Neuroimmunol 1993;46:145–153.

27. Antel JP, Brown-Bania M, Reder A, Cashman N. Activated suppressor cell dysfunction in multiple sclerosis. J Neuroimmunol 1986;137:137–141.

28. Noronha A, Toscas A, Jensen MA. Interferon beta augments suppressor cell function in multiple sclerosis. Ann Neurol 1990;27:207–210.

29. Sibley WA, Bamford CR, Clark K. Clinical viral infections and multiple sclerosis. Lancet 1985;1:1313–1315.

30. Smith D, Balshov K, et al. Increased IL-4 secretion and decreased gamma-IFN secretion in multiple sclerosis patients treated with cyclophosphamide or beta-interferon. The 9th International Congress of Immunology, San Francisco, California, July, 1995.

31. Rudick R, et al. In vitro and in vivo inhibition of mitogen driven T cell activation by recombinant interferon beta. Neurology 1993;43:2080–2087.

32. Porrini A, Gambi D, Reder AT. Interferon effects on IL-10 secretion; mononuclear cell response to IL-10 is normal in multiple sclerosis patients. J Neuroimmunol 1995;61:27–34.

33. Soos JM, Mujtaba MG, Subramaniam PS, Streit WJ, Johnson HM. Oral feeding of interferon tau can prevent the acute and chronic relapsing forms of experimental allergic encephalomyelitis. J Neuroimmunol 1997;75:43–50.

34. Olek MJ, Smith DR, Cook SL, Khoury SJ, Weiner HL. Phase I study of oral recombinant ovine interferon-tau in relapsing-remitting multiple sclerosis. AAN, Philadelphia, May 2001, S11.005.

35. Hafler DA, Weiner HL. In vivo labeling of peripheral blood T-cells using monoclonal antibodies: rapid traffic into cerebrospinal fluid in multiple sclerosis. Ann Neurol 1987;22:90–93.

36. Yednock TA, Cannon C, Fritz L, et al. Prevention of experimental autoimmune encephalomyelitis by antibodies against α4β1 integrin. Nature 1992;356:63–66.

37. Archelos JJ, Jung S, Maurer M, et al. Inhibition of experimental autoimmune encephalomyelitis by an antibody to the intercellular adhesion molecule ICAM-1. Ann Neurol 1993;34:145–154.

38. Hynes RO. Integrins: a family of cell surface receptors. Cell 1987; 48:549.

39. Frenette PS, Wagner DD. Adhesion molecules—Part 1. N Engl J Med 1996;334:1526–1529.

40. Frenette PS, Wagner DD. Adhesion molecules—Part II: Blood vessels and blood cells. N Engl J Med 1996;335:43–45.

41. Yednock TA, Cannon C, Fritz LC, Sanchez-Madrid F, Steinman L, Karin N. Prevention of experimental autoimmune encephalomyelitis by antibodies against alpha 4 beta 1 integrin. Nature 1992;356:63–66

42. Kent SJ, Karlik SJ, Cannon C, et al. A monoclonal antibody to alpha 4 integrin suppresses and reverses active experimental allergic encephalomyelitis. J Neuroimmunol 1995;58:1–10.

43. Kent SJ, Karlik SJ, Rice GP, Horner HC. A monoclonal antibody to alpha 4-integrin reverses the MR-detectable signs of experimental allergic encephalomyelitis in the guinea pig. J Magn Reson Imaging 1995;5:535–540.

44. Tubridy N, Behan PO, Capildeo R, et al. The effect of anti-alpha4 integrin antibody on brain lesion activity in MS. The UK Antegren Study Group. Neurology 1999;53:466–472.

45. Miller DH, Khan OA, Sheremata WA, et al. A controlled trial of natalizumab for relapsing multiple sclerosis. N Engl J Med 2003;348:15–23.

46. Hafler DA, Fallis RJ, Dawson DM, Schlossman DF, Reinherz EL, Weiner HL. Immunologic responses of progressive multiple sclerosis patients treated with anti-T-cell monoclonal antibody. Neurology 1986;36:777–784.

47. Hafler DA, Ritz J, Schlossman SF, Weiner HL. Anti-CD4 and anti-CD2 monoclonal antibodies infusions in humans: immunosuppressive effects and human anti-mouse responses. J Immunol 1988;141:131–138.
48. Weinshenker BG, Bass B, Karlik S, Ebers GC, Rice GPA. An open trial of OKT3 in patients with multiple sclerosis. Neurology 1991;41:1047–1052.
49. Lindsey J, Hodgkinson S, Mehta R, Mitchell D, Enzmann D, Steinman L. Repeated treatment with chimeric anti-CD4 antibody in multiple sclerosis. Ann Neurol 1994;36:183–189.
50. Barkhof, F, Thompson A, Hodgkinson S, et al. Double-blind, placebo-controlled, MR monitored exploratory trial of chimeric anti-CD4 antibodies in MS. The 11th European Congress on Multiple Sclerosis, Jerusalum, Israel, Sept. 1995.
51. Paolillo A, Coles AJ, Molyneux PD, et al. QuantitativeMRI in patients with secondary progressive MS treated with monoclonal antibody Campath 1H. Neurology 1999;53:751–757.
52. Killestein J, Olsson T, Wallstrom E, et al. Antibody-mediated suppression of Vbeta5.2/5.3$^+$ T cells in multiple sclerosis: results from an MRI-monitored phase II clinical trial. Ann Neurol 2002;51:467–474.
53. Olsson T, Edenius C, Ferm M, et al. Depletion of Vbeta5.2/5.3 T cells with a humanized antibody in patients with multiple sclerosis. Eur J Neurol 2002;9:153–164.
54. Santambrogio L, Hochwald GM, Saxena B, et al. Studies on the mechanisms by which transforming growth factor-β (TGF-β) protects against allergic encephalomyelitis. J Immunol 1993; 151:1116–1127.
55. Rott O, Cash E, Fleischer B. Phosphokiesterase inhibitor pentoxifylline, a selective suppressor of T helper type 1- but not type 2-associated lymphokine production, prevents induction of experimental autoimmune encephalomyelitis in Lewis rats. Eur J Immunol 1993;23:1745–1751.
56. Elliot M, Maini R, Feldmann M, et al. Treatment of rheumatoid arthritis with chimeric monoclonal antibodies to TNF alpha. Arthritis Rheum 1993;36:1681–1690.
57. Dwyer JM. Manipulating the immune system with immune globulin. N Engl J Med 1992;326:107–116.
58. Noseworthy JH, O'Brien PC, van Engelen BG, Rodriguez M. Intravenous immunoglobulin therapy in MS: progress from remyelination in the Theiler's virus model to a randomized double blind placebo controlled clinical trial. J Neurol Neurosurg Psychiatry 1994;57:11–14
59. Sicotte NL, Liva SM, Klutch R, et al. Treatment of multiple sclerosis with the pregnancy hormone estriol. Ann Neurol 2002;52:421–428.
60. Neuhaus O, Strasser-Fuchs S, Fazekas F,et al. Statins as immunomodulators: comparison with interferon-beta 1b in MS. Neurology 2002;59:990–997.
61. Zamvil SS, Steinman L. Cholesterol-lowering statins possess anti-inflammatory activity that might be useful for treatment of MS. Neurology 2002;59:970–971.
62. Cupps T, Edgar L, Fauci AS. Suppression of human B lymphocyte function by cyclophosphamide. J Immunol 1985;128:2453–2457.
63. Goodin DS, Arnason BG, Coyle PK, Frohman EM. The use of mitoxantrone (Novantrone) for the treatment of multiple sclerosis: Report of the Therapeutics and Technology Assessment Subcommittee of the American Academy of Neurology. Neurology 2003;61:1332.
64. Scheinman R, Cogswell P, Lofquist AK, Baldwin AS Jr. Role of transcriptional activation of IKB alpha in mediation of immunosuppression by glucocorticoids. Science 1995;270:283–286.
65. Kupersmith MJ, Kaufman D, Paty DW, et al. Megadose corticosteroids in multiple sclerosis. Neurology 1994;44:1–4.
66. Daynes R, Araneo B. Contrasting effects of glucocoricoids on the capacity of T cells to produce the growth factors interleukin 2 and interleukin 4. Eur J Immunol 1989;19: 2319–2325.
67. Beck RW, Cleary PA, Anderson MM, et al. A randomized, controlled trial of corticosteroids in the treatment of acute optic neuritis. N Engl J Med 1992;326:581–588.
68. Beck RW, Cleary PA. Optic neuritis treatment trial: one-year follow-up results. Arch Ophthalmol 1993;111:773–775.
69. Zivadinov R, Rudick RA, De Masi R, et al. Effects of IVmethylprednisolone on brain atrophy in relapsing-remittingMS. Neurology 2001;57:1239–1247.

70. Beck RW, Cleary PA, Trobe JD, et al. The effect of corticosteroids for acute optic neuritis on the subsequent development of multiple sclerosis. N Engl J Med 1993;239:1764–1769.

71. Cook SD, Devereux C, Troiano R, et al. Total lymphoid irradiation in multiple sclerosis. In: Rudick RA, Goodkin DE, eds., Treatment of multiple sclerosis: trial design, results, and future perspectives. Springer-Verlag, New York,1992, pp. 267–280.

72. Ahrens N, Salama A, Haas J. Mycophenolate-mofetil in the treatment of refractory multiple sclerosis. J Neurol 2001;248:713–714.

73. The Multiple Sclerosis Study Group. Efficacy and toxicity of cyclosporine in chronic progressive multiple sclerosis: a randomized, double-blinded, placebo-controlled clinical trial. Ann Neurol 1990;27:591–605.

74. Rudge P, Koetsier JC, Mertin J, et al. Randomized double blind controlled trial of cyclosporin in multiple sclerosis. J Neurol Neurosurg Psychiatry 1989;52:559–565.

75. Hughes RA. Treatment of multiple sclerosis with azathioprine. In Goodkin DE, Rudick RA, eds., Treatment of multiple sclerosis: trial design, results, and future perspectives. Springer-Verlag , New York,1992, pp.157–172.

76. Yudkin PL, Ellison GW, Ghezzi A, et al. Overview of azathioprine treatment in multiple sclerosis. Lancet1991;338:1051–1055.

77. Goodkin D, Rudick R, VanderBrug MS. Low-dose (7.5mg) oral methotrexate reduces the rate of progression in chronic progressive multiple sclerosis. 1995;Ann Neurol 37:30–40.

78. Sipe JD, Romine J, Koziol JA, McMillan R, Zyroff J, Beutler E. Cladribine in the treatment of chronic progressive multiple sclerosis. Lancet 1994;344:9–13.

79. Rice GP, Filippi M, Comi G. Cladribine and progressive MS: clinical andMRI outcomes of a multicenter controlledtrial. CladribineMRI Study Group. Neurology 2000;54:1145–1155.

80. Filippi M, Rovaris M, Iannucci G, Mennea S, Sormani MP, Comi G. Whole brain volume changes in patients with progressiveMStreated with cladribine. Neurology 2000;55:1714–1718.

81. Achiron A, Pras E, Gilad R, et al. Open controlled therapeutic trial of intravenous immune globulin in relapsing-remitting multiple sclerosis. Arch Neurol 19992;49:1233–1236.

82. Fazekas F, Deisenhammer F, Strasser-Fuchs S, Nahler G, Mamoli B. Randomised placebo-controlled trial of monthly intravenous immunoglobulin therapy in relapsing-remitting multiple sclerosis. Austrian Immunoglobulin in Multiple Sclerosis Study Group. Lancet 1997;349:589–593.

83. Noseworthy JH, O'Brien PC, Weinshenker BG, et al. IV immunoglobulin does not reverse established weakness in MS [In Process Citation]. Neurology 2000;55:1135–1143.

84. Weinshenker BG, O'Brien PC, Petterson TM, et al. A randomized trial of plasma exchange in acute central nervous system inflammatory demyelinating disease. Ann Neurol 1999;46:878–886.

85. van Gelder M, Kinwel-Bohre EP, van Bekkum DW. Treatment of experimental allergic encephalomyelitis in rats with total body irradiation and syngeneic BMT. Bone Marrow Trans 1993;11:233–241.

86. Burt RK, Burns W, Ruvolo P, et al. Syngeneic bone marrow transplantation eliminates V beta 8.2 T lymphocytes from the spinal cord of Lewis rats with experimental allergic encephalomyelitis. J Neurosci Res 1995;41:526–531.

87. Nash RA, Bowen JD, McSweeney PA, et al. High-dose immunosuppressive therapy and autologous peripheral blood stem cell transplantation for severe multiple sclerosis. Blood 2003;102:2364–2372.

88. Burt RK, Cohen BA, Russell E, et al. Hematopoietic stem cell transplantation for progressive multiple sclerosis: failure of a total body irradiation-based conditioning regimen to prevent disease progression in patients with high disability scores. Blood 2003;102:2373–2378.

89. Saiz A, BlancoY, Carreras E, et al. Clinical and MRI outcome after autologous hematopoietic stem cell transplant in MS. Neurology 2004;62:282–284.

90. Calabresi PA, Wilterdink JL, Rogg JM, Mills P, Webb A, Whartenby KA. An open-label trial of combination therapy with interferon beta-1a and oral methotrexate in MS. Neurology. 2002;58:314–317.

91. Lublin FD, Baiere M, Cutter G, et al. Results of the extension of a trial to assess the long term safety of combining interferon beta-1a and glatiramer acetate. Neurology 58 2002;58:A85.
92. Kalkers NF, Barkhof F, Bergers E, van Schijndel R, Polman CH. The effect of the neuroprotective agent riluzole onMRI parameters in primary progressive multiple sclerosis: a pilot study. Mult Scler 2002;8:532–533.
93. Paty DW. Magnetic resonance imaging in the assessment of disease activity in multiple sclerosis. Can J Neurol Sci 1988;15:266–272.
94. McFarland HF, Frank JA, Albert PS, et al. Using gadolinium-enhanced magnetic resonance imaging lesions to monitor disease activity in multiple sclerosis. Ann Neurol 1992;32: 758–766.
95. Khour SJ, Guttmann CR, Orav EJ, et al. Longitudinal MRI imaging in multiple sclerosis: correlation between disability and lesion burden. Neurology 1994;44:2120–2124.
96. Sharief MK, Hentges R. Association between tumor necrosis factor-α and disease progrssion in patients with mulitple sclerosis. NEngl J Med1991;325: 467–472.
97. Chofflon M, Juillard C, Julliard P, Gauthier G, Grau G. (1992). Tumor necrosis factor α production as a possible predictor of relapse in patients with multiple sclerosis. Eur Cytokine Net1992;3: 523–531.
98. Rossman HS. Neutralizing antibodies to multiple sclerosis treatments.J Manag Care Pharm. 2004;10:S12–S19.

Index